Indian Medicinal Plants

Vol. 1

(A-G)

Miss. Prakash Gupta

Originals

(an imprint of Low Price Publications)

Delhi-110052

Distributed by
D.K. Publishers Distributors (P) Ltd.
4834/24, Ansari Road, Darya Ganj,
New Delhi-110002
Phones: 23278584, 23278368, 23261465,
e-mail: dkpd@del3.vsnl.net.in
visit us at: www.dkpd.com

First Published 2003

ISBN 81-88629-04-9 (Set)
ISBN 81-88629-05-7 (Vol.1)

Published by
Originals
(an imprint of Low Price Publications)
A-6, Nimri Commercial Centre,
Near Ashok Vihar Phase-IV,
Delhi-110052
Phones: 27401672, 27452453
e-mail: lpp@nde.vsnl.net.in
visit us at: www.lppindia.com

Printed at
D K Fine Art Press P Ltd.
Delhi-110052

PRINTED IN INDIA

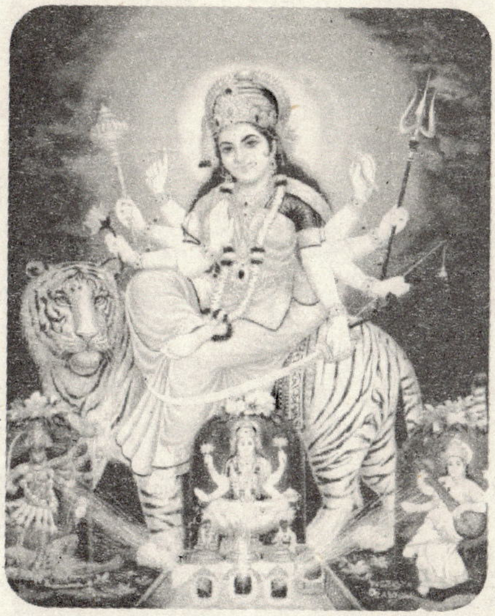

Dedicated to

Mata Vaishnoo Devi

Introduction

The history of Medicine proves that the 'Indian Medicinal Plants' used to exercise some magical influence upon people all over the world. And this knowledge was supposed to be more popular with hermits than educated people. At that time medicine prescribed by a hermit earned more favour and reputation than the one based on some test and experience. But as time elapsed and education spread everywhere, people started believing in allopathic medicine and surgery.

Until about fifty years ago, a sudden shift towards Indian medicinal herbs has been realized and since then the demand is increasing by leaps. The probable reason might be failure of English drugs in curing diseases completely. The cost of purchasing and the side effects of these medicines are few of the main causes due to which people have again shifted to Indian medicinal herbs which are much cheaper, more effective and do not have any side effects and these herbs do not suppress the disease but completely cure them. Easy availability of the herbs is another advantage. Due to the increasing popularity of Indian herbal medicine, foreigners are also attracted to the extent that they have started doing research and getting our plants patented. For example 'neem' (Margosa) is one of the examples.

To overcome this situation and give our people a more thorough understanding of our medicinal plants and to make teaching more effective, this subject was introduced in schools, colleges and universities where the students were systematically taught characters of the plants to identify them with medicinal uses to make them aware and save their natural wealth. In making this project successful the main hurdle was the recognition of the plant because howsoever perfect a student is in theory, he fails if he or she is unable to identify the plants. The author has made a humble effort to overcome this difficulty by collecting necessary systematic character availability of the different names, by which they are known and the medicinal uses in one book, along with respective photographs.

The literature on medicinal plants is so vast and scattered that there is scope of some more recent references and I shall gratefully welcome useful suggestions. I would close here by saying that nothing would ever be written if the author would wait to make her work so perfect that no improvement could be made.

Abbreviations

Abortif.	abortifacient
Absorb.	absorbent
Alk.	alkaloid
Alter.	alterative
Amenor.	amenorrhoea
Amorph.	amorphous
Antibil.	antibilious
Anthelm.	anthelmintic
Antid.	antidote
Antidysen.	antidysenteric
Antilith.	antilithic
Antimal.	antimalarial
Antiper.	antiperiodic
Antiphlegm.	antiphlegmatic
Antiphl.	antiphlogistic
Antipyr.	antipyretic
Antiscor.	antiscorbutic
Antisep.	antiseptic
Antisp.	antispasmodic
Antisyp.	antisyphillitic
Aper.	aperient
Aphrodis.	aphrodisiac
Arab.	Arabic
Arom.	aromatic
Astrin.	astringent
B.	Bengal
Bo.	Bombay State

Broncht.	bronchitis
Burm.	Burma
Carmin.	carminative
Catar.	catarrhal
Cath.	cathartic
Cholag.	cholagogue
Chr.	chronic
Constip.	constipation
Dec.	Deccan
Decoct.	decoction
Demulc.	demulcent
Deod.	deodorant
Diaphor.	diaphoretic
Diar.	diarrhoea
Digest.	digestive
Diur.	diuretic
Dysen.	dysentery
Dysmen.	dysmenorrhoea
Dyspep.	dyspepsia
Emmen	emmenagogue
Emol.	emollient
Essen. oil.	essential oil
Expect.	expectorant
Febge.	febrifuge

Galact.	galactagogue
Glucd.	glucoside
Gonor.	gonorrhoea
H.	Hindi
Haemat.	haematuria
Haemor.	haemorrhage
Ind. Baz.	Indian Bazaars
Indign.	indigestion
Inflam.	inflammation
Irrit.	irritant
Kan.	Kanarese
Kash.	Kashmir
Lactag.	lactagogue
Laxt.	laxative
Leucor.	leucorrhoea
M.	Madras State
Mal.	Malayalam
Mat. Med.	materia medica
Menor.	menorrhagia
Mucil.	mucilage
Nep.	Nepal
Nutri.	nutritious
P.	Punjab
Pers.	Persian
Phlegm.	phlegmatic
Purg.	purgative
Refrig.	refrigerant
Resolv.	resolvent
Restor.	restorative
Rheum.	rheumatic
Rubft.	rubefacient
S.	Sanskrit
Santh.	Santhal
Sialog.	sialogogue
Sing.	Singhalese
Stim.	stimulant
Stomch.	stomachic
Subst.	substitute
Syn.	synonym
Tam.	Tamil
Tel.	Telugu
Tox.	toxic
Var.	variety
Vern.	vernacular
Vet.	veterinary
Vesic.	vesicant

Contents

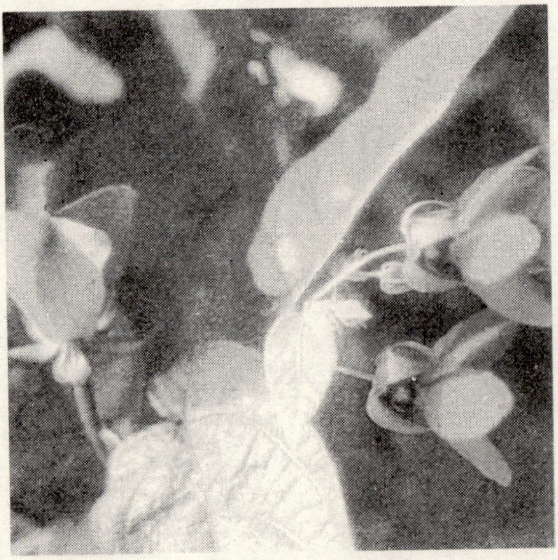

STERCULIACEAE

ABROMA AUGUSTA (LINN) WILLD

BENG.- OLATKOMAL., **MAR.**- OLAKATAMBOL., **ENG.**- DEVIS COTTON, GEVILS COTTON, COTTON ABROMA., **TAMIL**- SIVAPPUTLI., **SANS.** PISHASCARPASI., **GUJ.**- OLAT KAMBLE.

It is a small tree reported from hotter and drier region of India. Its branches contain hemp like fibers. Its flowers are deep red colour and their shape resembles !!!~~~~~the nail of a lion. The flower is turned inside.

It is cultivated throughout the hotter parts of India from Uttar Pradesh to Sikkim, Khasia Hills and Assam.

MEDICINAL USE : It roots, bark and leaves are mainly used. The decoction of its root is used for regularizing monthly cycle in women. Fresh and dry root bark is used as a uterine tonic and as an emenagogue. Fresh leaves, juice from root bark is useful in corrogative and neuralzic form of dysentry and diarrohea.

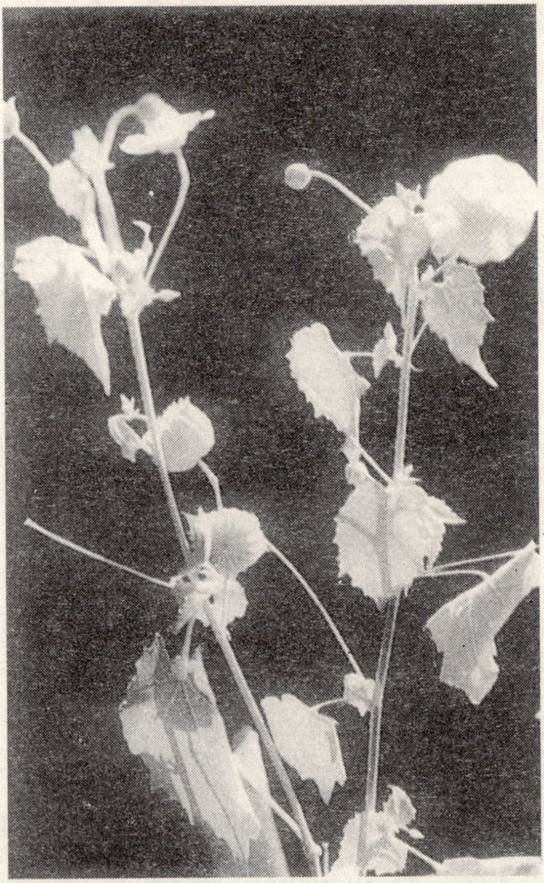

MALVACEAE

ABUTILON INDICUM (LINN) SWEET
SYN. A INDICUM. G.DON
COUNTRY MALLOW
SYN. SIDA INDICA LINN CENT.
LOCAL NAME : KANGHI; APHRA.

SANS.- ATIBALA, KANKATI., **HINDI.**- KANGHI., **BENG.**- POTARI., **TEL.**- TUTTURA BENDA., **TAM.**- PANIY ARATTUTTI., **KAN.**- TUTTI., **MAL.**- VELLURAM., **MAR. & BOM.**- KANGORI.

Annual or Perennial hairy under-shrub with golden yellow flowers, abundant throughout the hotter parts of India. Branches many, woody, stems on retting yield durable fiber. LEAVES : ovate to orbicular-cordate angular soft nearly entire or irregularly toothed covered on both surfaces with closely-felted white down with few or no hairs intermingled, Inflorescence:- axillary or terminal. Flower buds drooping. Flowers orange yellow on long pedicels; I"in diameter, opening in the evening. Bracteoles O stipules dettered peduncles longer than the petioles, jointed near the top Calyx:- Of 5 Valvate sepals, tubular below; sepals ovate acute. CAROLLA : of five petals, free above, connate below and adnate to the tube of the stamens. Staminal-tube divided at the apex into numerous filaments Carpels on ripening 15-20 longer than the Calyx glabrescent trumeate or shortly awned, awns spreading. Black at maturity, reniform, short - beaked. Styles as many as the carpels. Seeds black, tubercled, reiniform, upper ascending, lower decending. Flowers and fruits available during the major part of the year.

Generally distributed throughout tropical India (wanting in Malacca) Ceylon, Thwaites-Distribution Tropics.

MEDICINAL USE : The leaves are rich in mueilage and are used as a demulcent tonic. Heynelex. Burkill, I, II states that in sumatra a warm lotion is used for rheumatism. In, India an infusion of the roots is taken internally as a cooling medicine in levers. The seeds called balbij are such in mueilage and are laxative and demulcent.

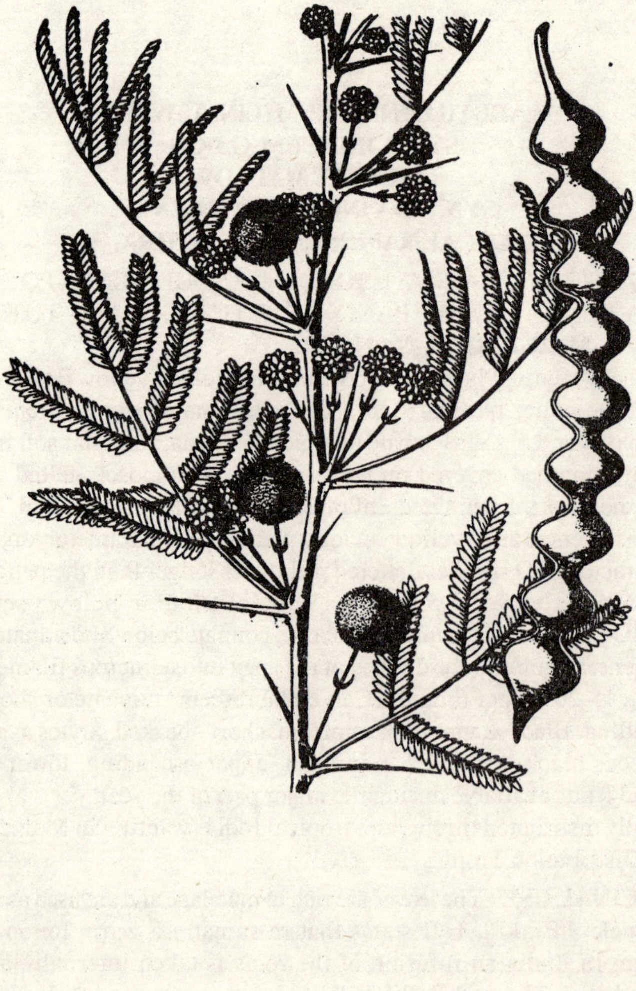

MIMOSACEAE

ACACIA ARABICA. (LAMK) WILLD.
(Syn. A. NILOTICA (L.) WILLD
EX DEL. SUBSP. INDICA (BENTH-) BRENAN
(Syn. MIMOSA ARABICA LAMK.)

ENG.- BABUL ACACIA., **HINDI**- BABUL, KIKAR., **LOCAL NAME**- DESI BABUL, BABUL, KIKAR., **SANS.**- BABUALA., **ARAB.**- UMMUGHILAN., **PUNJ.**- KIKAR., **GUJ.**- BAVAL., **TEL.**- NALLATUMMA., **TAM.**- KARUVELI., **KAN.**- JALI GOBLI; KARIJALI., **MAL.**- KARUVELAM., **BENG.**- BABLA, BABUL., **BOMB.**- BABHULA, KIKAR., **SANS.**- BABBULA+1, **GUJ.**- KALOAHAVAL., **KON.**- SHAMEERUKU., **MAR.**- BABHULA., **PUNJ. & KASH.**- SAK., **PERS**:- KHARE, MUGHILAN.

A. ARABICA is a moderate-sized spiny evergreen tree. Branches reddish brown, branching high above the ground with straight finely grey downy branchlets. Its bark is dark-brown or black, and longitudinally fissured. The spines are straight and sharp-pointed, and occur in pairs below the petioles. 3-7 cm. long, large, white ascending and pungent on the older branchlets. Leaves: Bipinnate, with minute leaflets; leaf rachises downy, with several glands; pinnae 6-12, ½ - 1½" long; leaflets 20-40, membranous, green, 1/8 - ¼"; glabrous or rather downy, Peduncles short, densely grey downy with the bracts above the middle, 4-6 nate, the subtending leaves of the upper nodes reduced or suppressed. The flowers are in yellow, fragrant in axillary, fascicled heads; ½" in diameter; Calyx 1/24"; campanulate; Corolla: twice the length of the calyx. Stamens, free; indefinite, much exserted; anthers minute; not gland-crested. Ovary stalked or sessile, many-ovuled; style filiorm, stigma minute capitate. Pod:- Straight-strap-shaped firm grey-downy with sutures deeply indented between each seed; rigidly-coriaceous, subindehiscent, densely persistently grey-downy, 8-12 seeded, 1¼ - ½ ft. by ½ - 5/8"; distinctly stalked.

It is reported from Punjab to Bihar, Western Peninsula and Ceylon. Distribution. Arabia, Egypt, Tropical Africa, Natal. The tree is indigenous to Sind, the Deccan & tropical Africa, and is naturalised in all parts of India locally it is planted along canal banks & in fields. It is a useful plant for afforeseting dried and arid areas. The flowering season is rainy season and fruiting season is cold and summer seasons.

MEDICINAL USE : Gum is useful is dirrohea; dysentry and in diabetes mellitus. Bark is astringent, demulcent and aphrodisise. Pods are expectorant. Extract of gum is styptic, tonic and astringent.

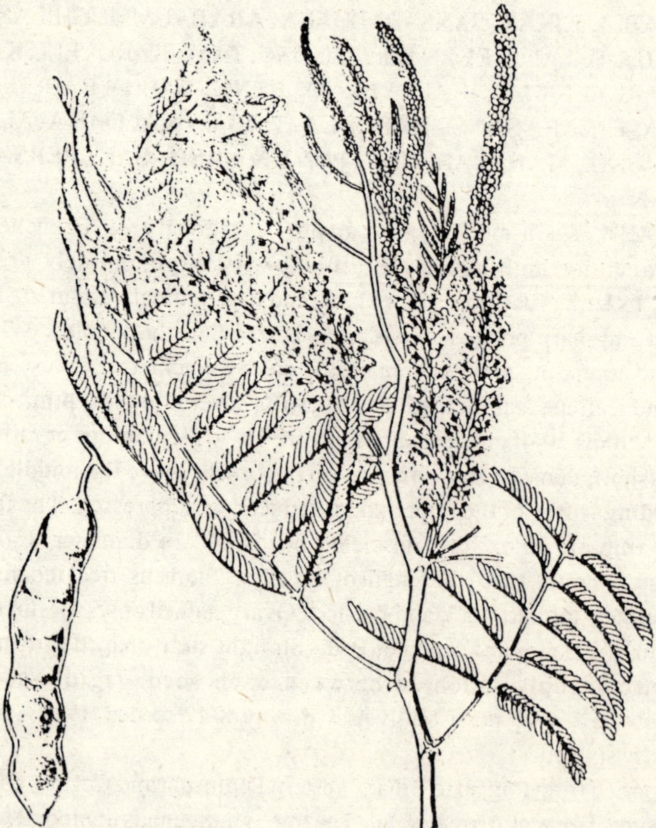

MIMOSACEAE

ACACIA CATECHU (LF) WILLD
(SYN. A. CATECHUOIDES BENTH;
(MIMOSA CATECHIOUIDES ROXB.)

ENG.- BLACK CUTCH, CATECHU., **BO**.- KHADERI., **B.**- KUTH., **HINDI**- KHAIR, KHADIRA., **S.**- KHADIRA., **TAM.**- KARANGALLI., **TEL.**- KHADIRAMU, SANDRA., **MAR.**-KHAIR., **KAN**.-KAGGALI, **BURMA**- SHA.

It is a small tree with grey white to black bark. The bark peels off in flakes and spines are present which are paired and hooked.Leaves bipinnate, pinnae more than 20 pairs and leaflets are numerous, flower buds are in cylindrical spikes, purple in colour but flowers are dark yellow and fragrant. Pods are strap shaped dark brown, dehiscent, torulose and long stalked. Calyx, corolla and leaf rachis are hairy. The seeds are black smooth elliptie and corm pressed Flowers and fruits are available from July to August.

It is reported from Punjab, N.W. Himalayas, Bihar, Ganjam, Madhya Bharat and all over India. Locally it is found in the hilly tracts of Delhi.

MEDICINAL USE : The bark is astringent and yields kaththa. Bark is also used for cough and diarrohea. Externally bark is applied to ulcers and boils and skin eruptions. Kaththa is used for cough, pan and throat irritations. It also enters into a number of compound preparations, few of the prescriptions are given by Birdwood and Birdwood G.T.1936-Practical Bazzar Medicines.

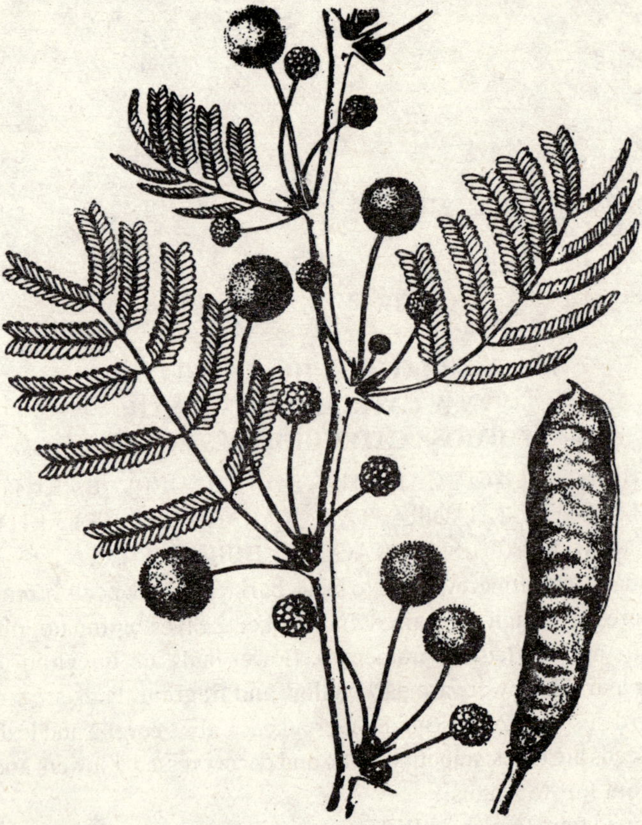

MIMOSACEAE

ACACIA FARNESTANA WILLD
(SYN. MIMOSA FARNESIANA L.)

SANS.- ARIMAEDAH., **HINDI**.- GAND - BABUL, DIWANA BABUL, VILAITI BABUL, VILAITI KIKAR., **ENG.**- SWEET ACACIA, CASSIE, CASSIA FLOWER., **BENG.**- GUYA - BADULA, GAYA BADULA., **BOM.**- DEOBABUL., **TAM.**- KASTURIVEL, PIKKARUVEL., **TEL.**- KASTURI TUMMA, KEMPUCUMMA., **GUJ**.- JABBAVAL., **KAN.**- KARI - JALI., **KON**.- KUSPI - JHAD., **MAL.**- KARIVEELUM., **MAR**.- GUIBADHUL., **LOCAL NAME**- VILAITIBABUL.

A shrub or low tree, with slender Zigzag branches, marked with grey dots, spines straight, often paired, 0.5 - 1.4 cm. long, stipular only, seldom over ¼ - ½ inch long on the branchlets. Leaves:- bipinnate, with minute leaflets; 20-40 leaflets, pinnae 8-16; leaf rachises downy, with a minute petiolar gland pinnae 1-1½ inch long; leflets green, subglabrous, rigidly corriaceous. Peduneles crowded in the nodes of full-grown leaves, shorter than the leaves with the ring of bracts at or near the apex. Flowers in globos heads or cylindrical spikes, hermaphrodiate or polygamous, usually pentamerus. Sepals or Calyx: Campanulate or funnel shaped, shortly toothed, very minute. Petals or corolla: exserted, united in the lower half; 1/24 inch; teeth short, obtuse. Stamens free, indefinite, much exserted; anthers minute, not gland crested. Pods 3.6 x 1.2 cm thick, cylindrical, hooked at the tip, pulpy inside, liqulate, or oblong, not jointed usually compressed and dry, dehiscent or indehiscent, rarely turgid or subcylindrical, sutures straight or wavy not thickened.

Its fruiting season is April to May.

It is reported from Himalayas to Ceylon and Penang, Cosmopolitan in the Tropics, but often planted. It is regarded as a native of West Indies, now occurring throughout India, Burma and Ceylon. It grows well in the plains of Punjab. Locally it is planted in gardens and road sides as a shade plant and for checking erosion of soil.

MEDICINAL USE : Bark is astringent, demulcent and aphrodisiac. Pods are expectorant. Extract of gum is styptie, tonic and astringent. Flowers are a source of cassie perfume.

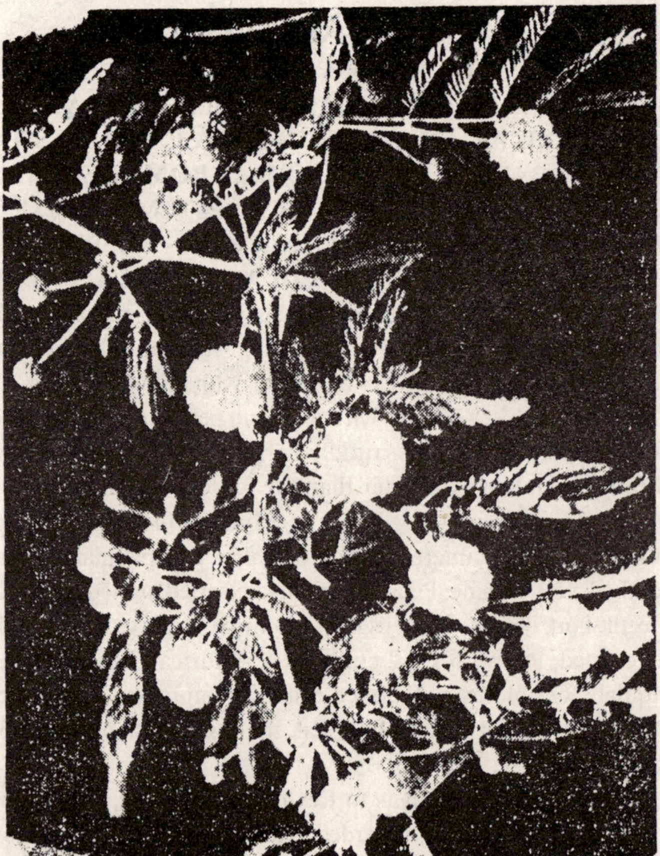

MIMOSACEAE

ACACIA LEUCOPHLOEA WILLD.
(SYN. MIMOSA LEUCOPHLOEA ROXB.)

HINDI- SAFED KIKAR, RONJ, ARINJ., **BENG.-** SAFED BABUL., **BOM. & MAR.**-HEWAR., **GUJ.**-HARIBAVAL., **TEL.-** TELLATUMA., **TAM.**-VELVAYALAM., **KAN.**-BILIJALI., **MAL.-** PATTACHARAYA MARAM., **BURM.-** TANAUNG., **SANS.-** SHVETA-BARBURA., **LOCAL NAME-** RONJ, JAND., **POPULAR NAME-** SHARABKI KIKAR.

A moderate-sized deciduous tree, ordinarily upto 3' in girth with an 8 - 10' bole. Bark yellowish-grey to white and light red inside. It is smooth and exfoliates in regular scales. It has strong, straight white spines nearly an inch in length. Leaves: bipinnate; pinnae 12 - 24, leaflets 30 - 60 pairs; leaf-rachises downy, with several glands; pinnae 1 - 1½" long; leaflets crowded, rigidly coriaceous, 1/8 - 1/6". Inflorescence is very bright and recognized from a distance. Flower heads small, pale yellow, sweet-scented, in large terminal, leafless, densely tomentose panicles. Panicles reaching a foot long and broad with long compound densely tomentose ascending branches the lower only from leafy nodes; heads yellow, not more them ¼" in diameter; peduneles with the bract medial, the upper very short. Calyx campanulate; corolla under 1/24". Stamens free, indefinite, much exserted; anthers minute, not gland-crested. Ovary stalked or sessile, many-ovuled; style filiforn, stigma minute capitate. Pod- 4 - 8" by ¼ - 1/3" sessile; narrowly ligulate falcate thin flat with straight sutres Subindehiscent, clothed with pale brown or grey persistent tomentum.

It is found in North West provinees to Ceylon and Burma. Distribution: Malay isles, Timor. The tree is very characteristic of dry regions. It is found in the plains of the Punjab and throughout the dry forest tracts of the peninsula. It is a characteristic tree of the hilly tracts of Delhi. Common on the ridge, the flowering season is Sept. - Oct. and fruiting season is November to February.

MEDICINAL USE : Bark is astringent; also used in preparation of spirits from Sugar and Palm Juice. Pods are considered poisonous and gum is used in indigenous medicine.

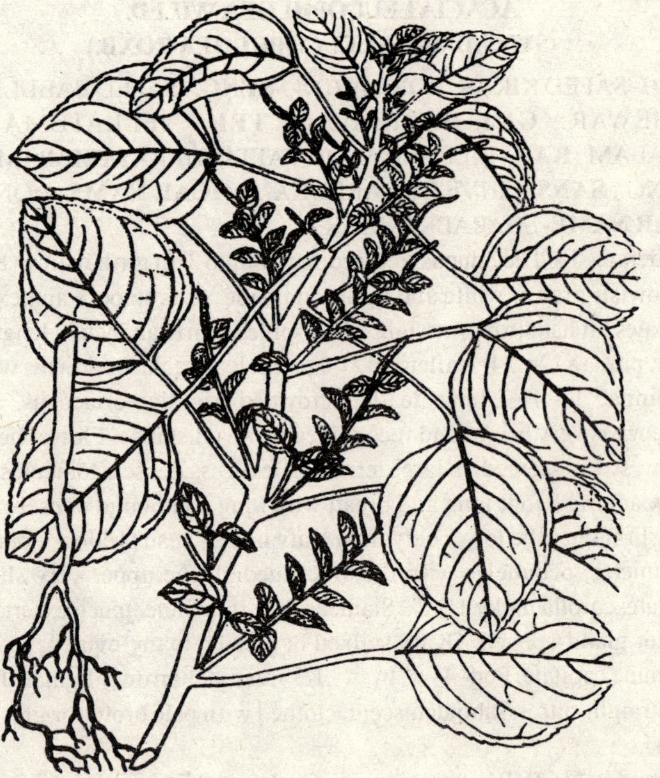

EUPHORBIACEAE

ACALYPHA INDICA LINN
SYN. A. INDICA
SYN. A. CILIATA.

BENG.- MUKTAJHURI., **ENG.**-INDIAN ACALYPHA., **GUJ.**-VANCHIKANTO, DADANO., **HINDI**- KUPPU., **KAN.**-KUPPIGIDA., **KON.**-KUNKMIPHAL., **MAL.**- KUPPAMANI., **MAR.**-KHOKI., **TAM.**- KUPPIVAEI., **TEL.**- KUPPICHETTU., **SANS.**- HARITA-MANJARI.

A small annual shrub 1-3' high occurring wild on the roadsides and waste places throughout the plains of India. Branches are many spreading or ascending. Leaves 1-2" herbaceous, pubescent, leaves long petioled ovate or rhombic - ovate crenate, serrate penninerved or 3-5 plenerved petiole slender, often longer than the blade. Spikes 1-3" slender, erect; bracts (¼-1/3") diameter cuneiform many nerved. Spikes all axillary androgynous elongate, males clustered towards the top; females solitary or paired each enclosed by a foliar 5 X 5 mm bract. Bracts many distant large broad 3-5 fid - truncate crenate much larger than the capsule. Females 1-2 is a peduncled solitary bract, monoecious, rarely diocious, apetalous; males very minute, ebraeteate; flower disk O. Calyx membranous, spilitting into four (4) valvate sepals. Stamens many, often 8 on a convex receptacle, filaments free; anther-cells divaricate, often twisted or flexuous. Pistaillode O Female Fl. Sepals 3-4, imbricate often minute ovary hispid 3 - celled; styles fifliform of ten very long and lacinate or fimbriate; ovules 1 in each cell- **Capsules:-** Quite concealed by the persistent bract, often only 1-seeded hispid. Seeds ovoid, acute, smooth.

It is Hotter parts of India from Bihar eastwards to Assam and Southwards to Singapore and Burma; and from the concan to Travancore. Ceylon, common in fields. Distribution westwards to Tropical africa, and eastwards to Timor and the Philippines. The flowering and fruiting season is September - June.

MEDICINAL USES : Plant emetic, expectorent used as a substitute for senega, useful in bronhities, pheumonia and asthma. Root - cathartic; leaves - laxative used in scabies.

Indian Medicinal Plants / 16

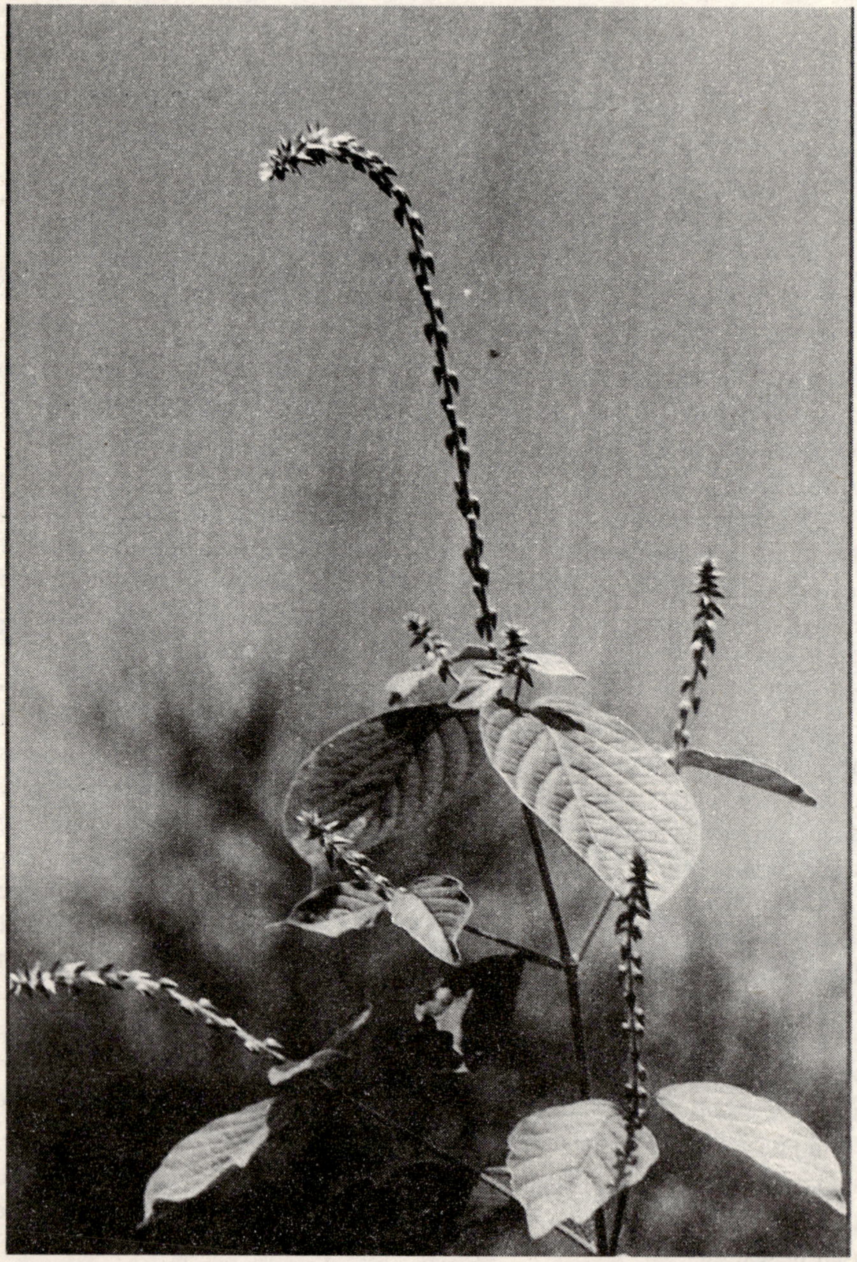

AMARANTHACEAE

ACHYRANTHES ASPERA LINN.
Var. PORPHYRISTACHYA HOOK. & SYN. A. PORPHYRISTACHYA WALL.

SANS.- APAMARGA., **ARAB.**- ATKUMAH., **PERS.**- KHARE-VAZHUN., **HIND.**-LATJIRA., **BENG.**- APANG., **MAR.**- AGADHA., **GUJ.**- AGHEDO., **TELGU**- UTTAREN., **TAM.**- NAYURIVI., **KAN.**- UTTARANE., **MAL.**- KATALATI., **LOCAL NAME**- PUTHKUNDA, LAPA, CHIRCHITTA, BALVALA CHIRCHITTA, MONGA.

It is popularly known as the Prickly chaff. Flower. It is a stiff erect herb, 1-3' high commonly found as a weed throughout India upto 3000'. Leaves large, ovate acute or accuminate, opposite, glaberous or nearly so. Flowers greenish white, deflexed in terminal spikes elongating in fruit. Spikes are slender or simple or panicled. Bracts and bracteoles peristent, ending in a spine. Sepals 4-5, subulate-lanceolate, gristate, shining, at length hardened and strongly ribbed. Stamens 2-5, filaments connate at the base with as many square staminodes, each of which is toothed or has a toothed scale at its back; anthers 2-celled. Ovary oblong, sub-compressed, style filiform, stigma capitellate, ovule-I, pendulous from a long basal funicle. Utricle oblong or ovoid, indehiscent top aerolate, or rounded. Seed inverse oblong, testa coriaceous; embryo annular. Twelve species, all of them are tropical or subtropical. It is also reported from China, Japan and Java for its medicinal properties. It is found throughout India upto 3000 ft. as a weed, up to Baluchistan.

MEDICINAL USE : It is considered as one of the important medicinal plant. It is astringent, diauretic, antiperiodic and purgative. It is used in renal dropsy. Piles, boils, skin eruptions colie pain, snake bite. It is also used in the treatment of bronchial affections and leprosy.

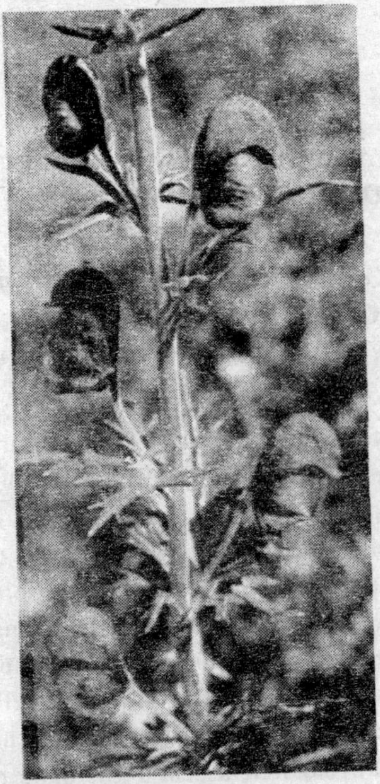

RANUNCULACEAE

ACONITUM FEROXWALL WALL
SYN. A. NAPELLUS (WALL) EX. SERY

HINDI- BISH., **SANS.**- VATSANG., **HINDI**-BACHNAG., **GUJ**.- BACHNAG., **M**.- BACHNAG., **ENG.**- ACONITE., **S.**- VISHA., **M & B.**- BISH., **BO.**- VACHNAG **M.**- VISHANARIE., **LATIN**- ACONITE FEROXWALL.

It is a herb grown in alpine Himalayas from sikkim to Garhwal and Assam.

MEDICINAL USE : It is lusterous root are used as antipyretic, diaphoretic and diuretic. The ointment is useful in treatment of rheumatism. skin diseases and neuralgia. It is also used in urinary troubles, diabeties, extensively used in, Leprosy, fever, cholra etc.

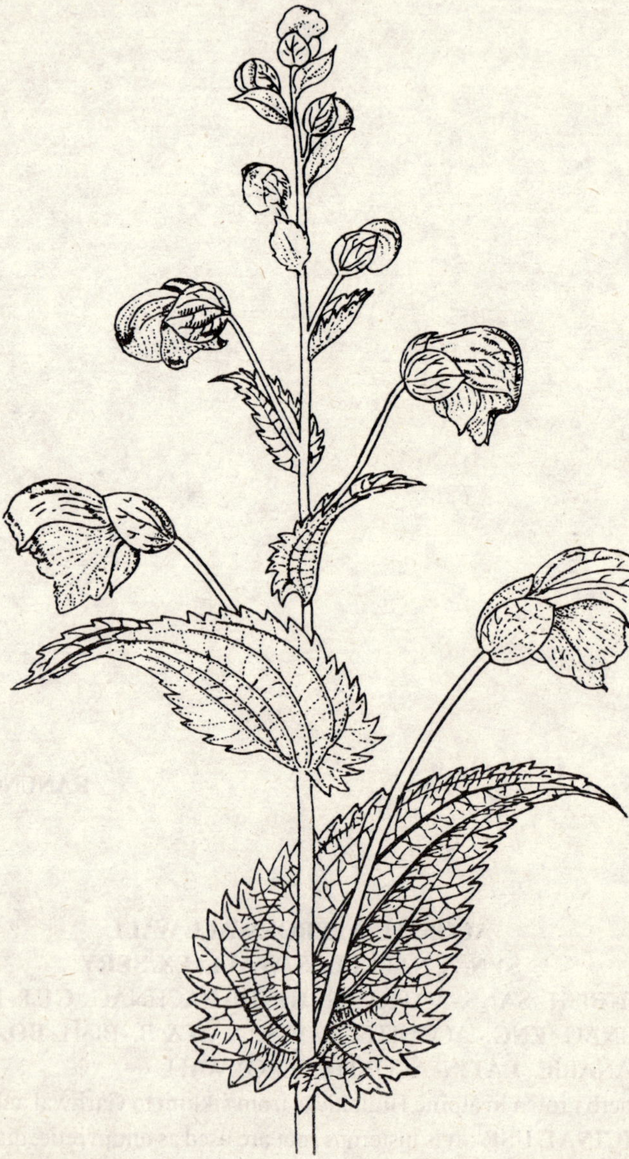

RANUNCULACEAE

ACONITUM FEROX WALL EXSER.
(SYN. A NAPEILUSAR. RIGIDUM HOOK. F. & THOMS)

SANS.- VISHA., **HINDI & BENG.**- BISH KATBISH, MITHAVISH, RISH., **BOMB.**- VACHNAG., **MAL.**- VASHANAVAL., **ENG.**- INDIAN ACONITE., **GUJ. & MAR.**- VUCHNAG., **HINDI**- MITHAZAHAR, BISH., **KAN. & KON.**- VATSANAABHI., **TAM.**- VISHANAVI, VISHNKNUIR VASHANARI., **TEL.**- VASANUBHI.

A Ferox proper is a rare and poisonous species found in the Northern Himalayas of Nepal and Kashmir.

They are perennial erect, rarely twining herb. Stem 3-6 ft; Puberulous, leafy, erect, simple below. Leaves: rounded or oval palmately 5- fid, raceme terminal dense flowered, helmet vaulted with a short sharp beak, testa plaited. Leaves 3-6", lobes cuneate ovate, incized; palmately 5 fid, racemed. Raceme 6-12", simple or sparingly branched below, tomentose, terminal dense flowered, helmet vaulted with a short sharp beak helmet about twice as long as high. Flowers: Irregular, pale dirty blue pedicles 1-2", thickened at the top; bracts pinnatifid; bracteoles linear. Sepals 5 petaloid, posterior helmet vaulted, the rest flat, 2 anterior narrower then the lateral. Petals 2-5/ 2- posterior clawed, limb hooded and enclosed in the helmet, 3 lower small or obsolete stamens many. follicles 5 erect, usually densely villous, glabrous in some garwhal specimens. Seeds many testa plaited.

Distributed temperate subalpine Himalya, from Sikkim to Garwhal, alt. 10-14,ooo ft. Recently it has been collected from Darjeeling and Assam.

MEDICINAL USE: Its tuberous roots are used as antipyretic, diaphoretic and diuretic. In small doses it has got stimualatory action on heart. In large doses it acts as poison, narcotic and as a powerful sedative (Chopra at al. 1956, Nadkarni, 1954). Aconiline ointment is useful in treatment of rheumatism, skin diseases and neuralgia.

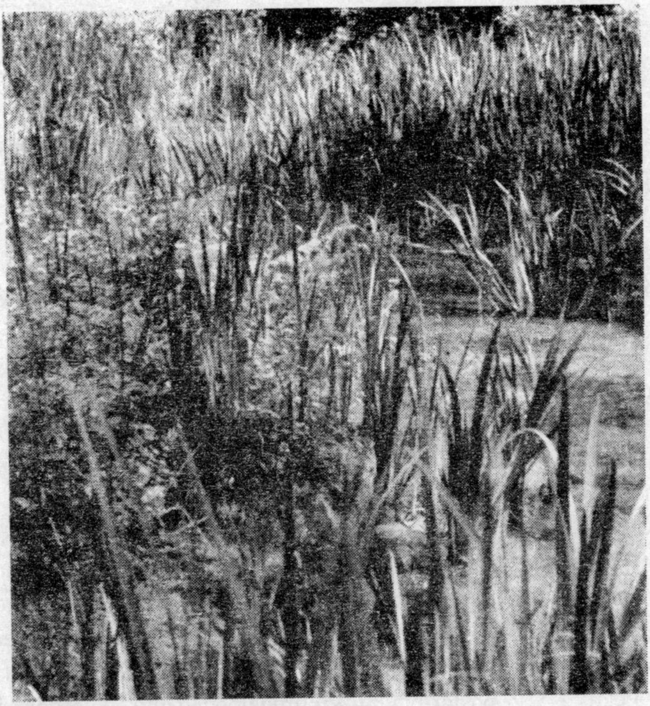

ARACEAE

ACORUS CALAMUS L.

HINDI- BACH, GHORABUCH, SAFED BACH., **ASSAMES-** THEMEPRII., **BENG.-** BACH., **GUJARATI-** GANDHLORAZ., **KANNADA-** BAJEGIDA., **MALYALAM-** VUSHAMPE., **MARATHI-** VEKHAND., **SANSKRIT-** BHUTANUSHINI., **TAMIL-** VASAMBU., **TELGU-** VASA., **ENG.-** SWEET FLAG.

It is a marshy and aromatic herb growing chiefly in marshy and moist habitats. It is much branched consisting of a rhizome leaves and flowers.

It is found throughout India and ceylon in marshy, wild or cultivated habitats in Himalayas and Sikkim upto 6000 ft. It is plentiful in the marshy tracts of Kashmir, Manipur and Nagaland Hills.

MEDICINAL USE : The aromatic rhizomes are used as carminative; stimulant for central nerous system, and as a tonic. It is useful in diarhoea and dysentry. It relieves flatulence and in the power form used as vermifuge. Alcoholic extract of the plant has sedative and analgesic effects and causes moderate depression in blood pressure.

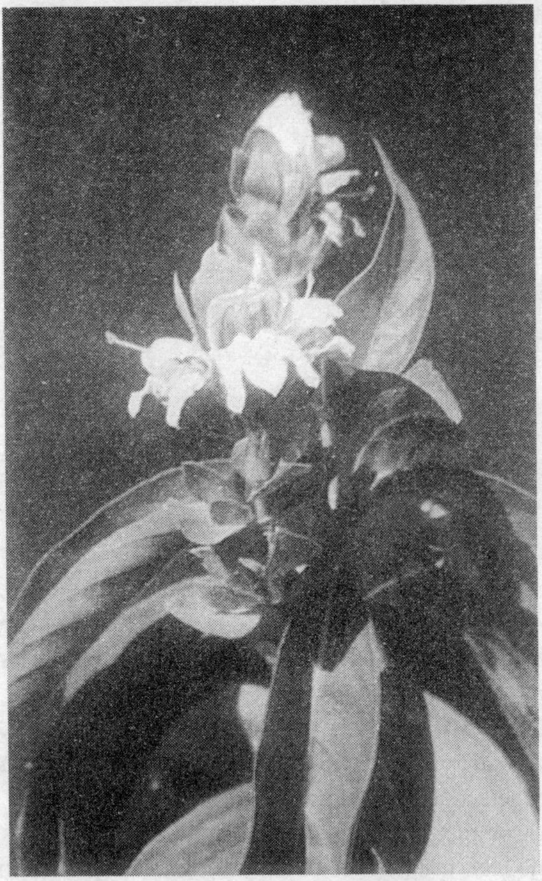

ACANTHACEAE

ADHATODA VASICA NEES

SANS.-VASAKA., **HINDI**-ADULASA., **BENG.**-BAKAS., **TAM.**- ADADODAI., **TELUGU**- ADASARAMU.

LOCAL NAME.- BANSA; ARUSA, PIABANSA BEKAD; BASUTI.

A diffused, branched evergreen dense shrub, reaching a height of 4-8 ft. Sometimes it becomes arborescent and reaches a height of 20 ft. Internodes short. Leaves upto 20 x 8 cm.; ovate or elliptic, lanceolate, entire minutely pubescent acuminate. Petiole 1" spikes dense, short 1-3", terminal often several together bracts 3/4" by 1/4", eliptic, subacute puberulous or glabrate; bracteoles 1/2 by 1/8" falcate-oblong. Flowers white, with pink or purple stripes, in dense, axillary, peduncled spikes at the ends of branches. Calyx 1/3 - 1/2", deeply 5- lobed, lobes equal lanceolate. Corolla tube 1/3 - 1/2" broad; lips white palate transversely rose-barred. Stamens glabrous anther cells acuminate at base, sometimes minutely white-tailed. Ovary and style base minutely hairy. Bracts conspicuous capsule 2.5 x .8 cm or more clavate, pubescent 4-seeded. Seeds 1/3" in diam; glabrous, tubercular suborbicular venucose or rugose. Flowering and fruiting period is from December to April.

It is reported from Punjab and Assam to Ceylon and Singapore, common, frequently cultivated. Malaya and S.E. Asia. Locally it is common and abundant, often gregarious on the ridge and adjacent hills. Where it occurs as co-dominant shrub with Capparis sepioria, Linn.

MEDICAL USE : Flowers, leaves and roots are antiseptic. Leaves have got insecticidal value and used in rheumatism. Roots are used in fever. Leaves and roots are used in cough, chronic bronchitis, asthma, phthisis.

COMMERCIAL USE : It is one of the Chief ingredient of Commercial Glycodine Terp Vasaka.

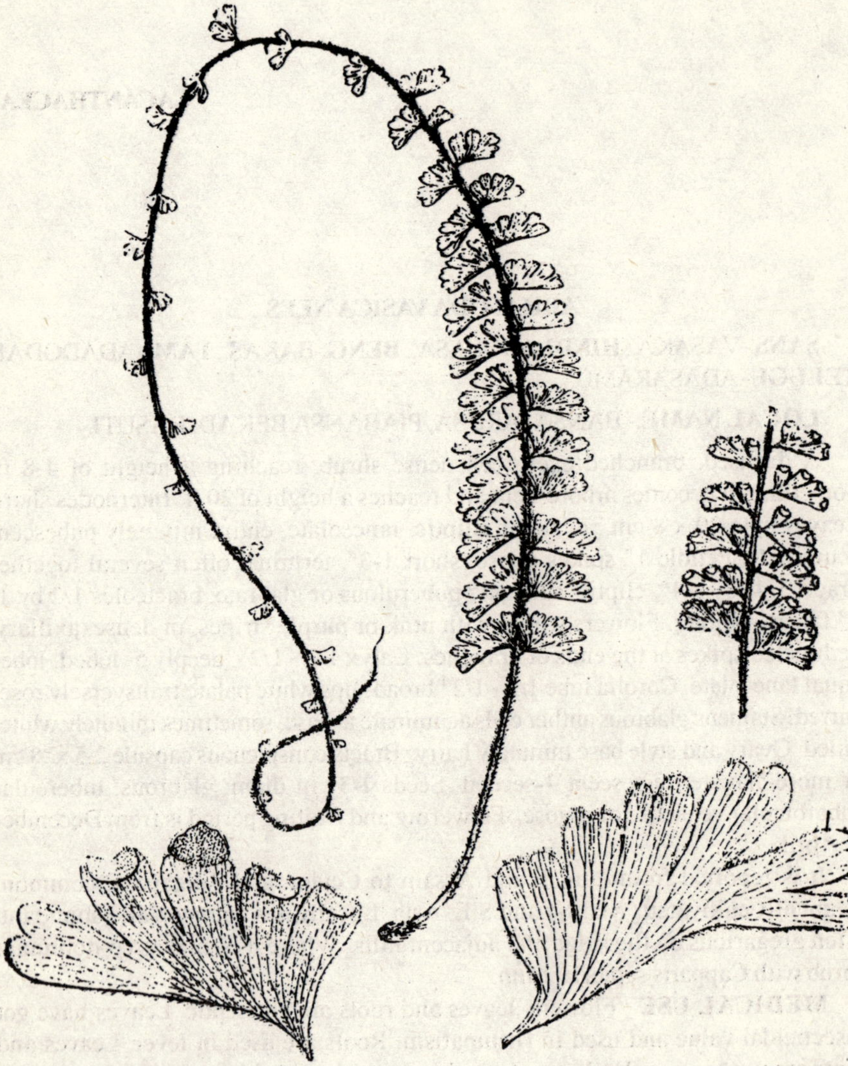

ADIANTACEAE

ADIANTUM CAUDATUM LINN.

SANS.-MAYUROSHIKHA., **P.- ADHSARITA**-KAJARI.

This plant is known as Fern commonly. The stipes are 2-4 inches long tufted, wiry of dark chestnut-brown colour, fronds 6-12 inches long, simply pinnate and elongated rooting at the extremity, pinnae 1/2-3/4 inches long 1/4 inch deep, dimidiate, sessile and lower line straight and horizontal, the upper rounded and cut deeply and repeatedly, the point blunt the lower ones slightly stalked, texture is corracious, the veins are prominent. The rachis; dorsal and ventral surfaces are hairy; sorl roundish to oblong on the edge of the lobes.

It is reported from all over India, in the plains and lower slopes of the hills.

MEDICINAL USE : Fronds are used for skin diseases, diabetes, cough and fever.

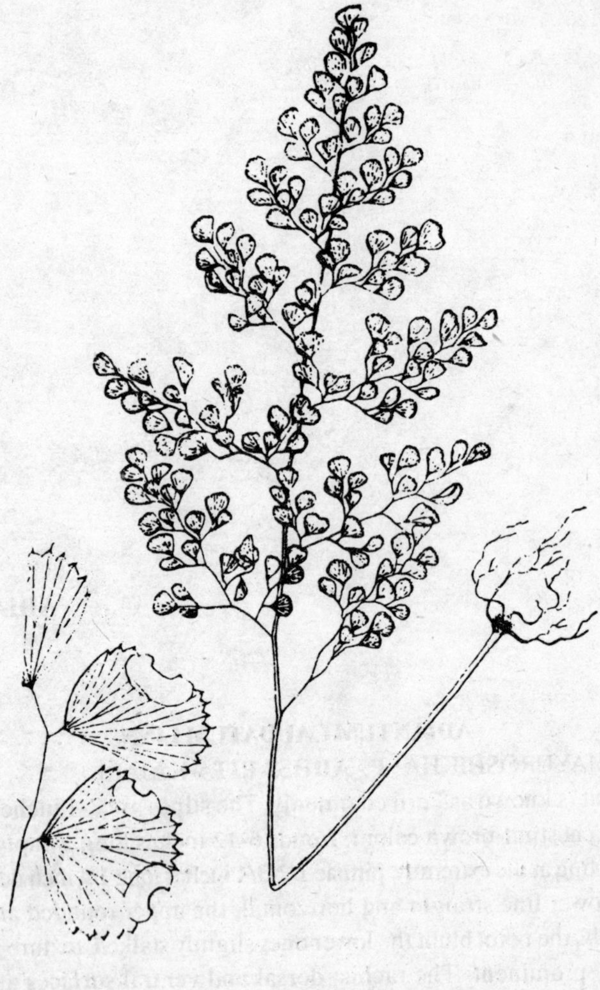

ADIANTACEAE

ADIANTUM VENSUTUM G. (DON.)

H.-HANSARAJ., **BO**.-MUBARAK., S.-HANSAPADI., **TAM**.-MAYIRSIKKI.

This plant is also known as fern. It is glossy, glabrous and ebencous coloured. The involucres are reniform to cordate submembranceous; stipes and rachis slender; Fronds are 3-4 pinnate, pinnules firm membranous, chartaceous, glabrous and slightly glaucous beneath, shortly petiolate, obovate-cuneate, rarely subrhomboid acuminate straited, the superior margin rounded but 2 or 3 lobed, finely dentate-serrate fertile lobes with 2, rarely 3 notches, each notch bearing a large sorus at the bottom.

It is reported from Himalayas from 3000 to 10,000 ft. very common in Simla.

MEDICINAL USE : Fronds act as tonic, resolve, expect. diuretic, eommen, astringent, emetic, in scorpion sting.

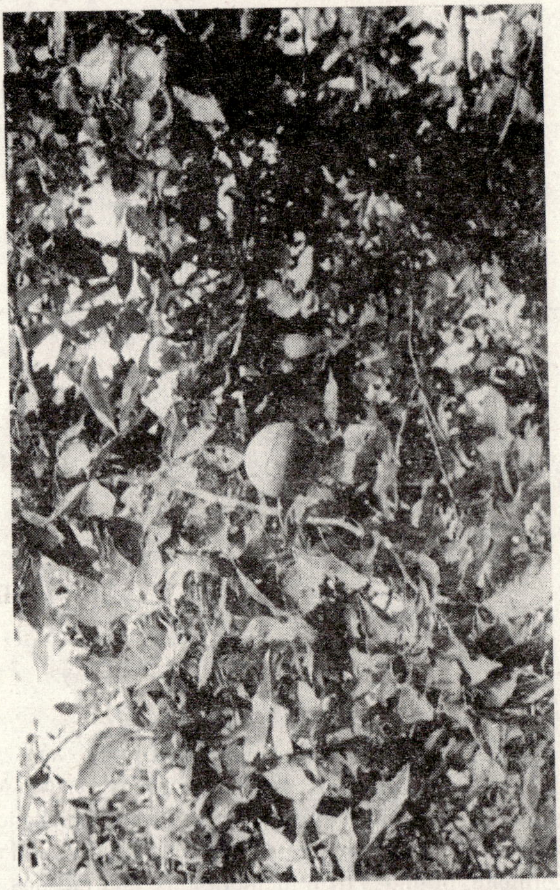

RUTACEAE

AEGLE MARMELOSE (L) CORREA

HINDI- BEL., **ASSAMESE** - BEL., **BENGALI**- BELA., **GUJARATI**- BILIVAPHAL., **KANNADA**- BILPATRA., **MALYALAM**- VILVAM., **MARATHI**- BALLAS., **SANSKRIT**- BILVA, SRIPHAL., **TAMIL**- VILVAM., **TELGU** - BILVAMU.

It is a tall, leaf shedding and very significant medicinal plant. Its leaves are tripartite and odourless. The whole tree is spiny, and spines are straight and pointed. Every-year old leaves are shed off from Jan. to March and then new leaves emerge. From May to July while aromatic flowers bloom and globular round fruits are formed. The size of the fruit varies from 2 - 8 inches in diameter. Fruits ripe up to December. The fruits are round, thick and very hard olive coloured when unripe and golden yellow when ripe. The pulp of the unripe fruit is white and pungent while ripe fruits contain orange coloured pulp with white seeds. The seeds are oblong and surrounded by a mucilatinous material.

It is found wild in the sub Himalayan tract, Central and south India. It is often planted all over India.

MEDICINAL USE : The fruit is used for chronic diarrohoea and dysentry. The ripe fruit is very good for removing constipation. It is also used for making cold drink in summer which is aromatic cooling and laxative. The root bark is used in intermittent fevers. The decoction of leaves is good for reducing blood pressure. The presence of whole tree in the garden is very good for eliminating harmful insects. Aegelin derived from the plant has been tried in the treatment of bronchial spasm (Das Gupta, and Chakravarti, 1958).

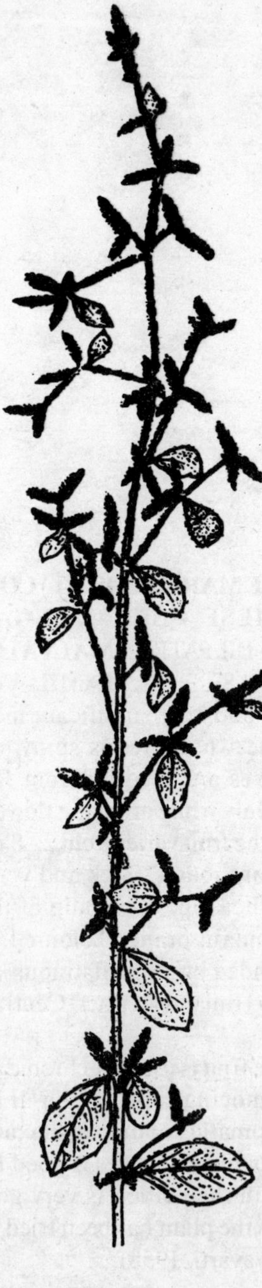

AMARANTHACEAE

AERVA LANATA (LINN) JUSS.

S.- ASTMABAYDA., **H.- & B**.- CHAYA., **P.-** BUIKALLAN., **TAM.-** SIRUPHULAI., **TEL.-** PINDICUMDA., **LOCAL NAME-** GEDHA KICHAI.

A sub erect, prostrate herb, stems and branches are woolly tomentose leaves alternate, white woolly beneath, obovate or elliptic - rounded, spikes 1.5 x 0.5 cm. clustered in the axils. Flowers greenish - white, bisexual. Anothers yellow seeds black, shining. It is abundant after rains.

Commonly found in open lands especially in shady spots in garden hedges and fields. It is found throughout the plains of India ascending to 3,000 ft. in the hills.

MEDICINAL USE : Plant anthelm, diur. Root - Demule, diur in the treatment of headache (apothekerzig, Berl, 1895, 346). It is also used in the treatment of wounds.

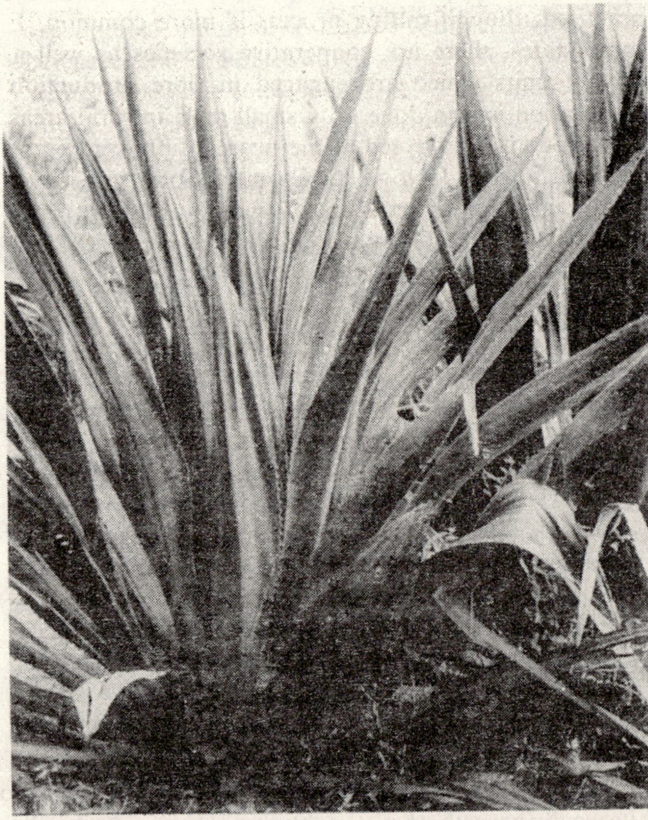

AMARYLLIDACEAE

AGAVE SISALANA PERR EX. ENGELM.
(SYN. A. RIGIDA MILL VAR. SISALANA (SISAL)

ENG.- SISAL, AGAVE.

Sisal is a xerophytic short-lived, monocarpic perennial with a short thick stem or bole and a dense rosette of leaves. A long stout flowering shoot or pole is produced after 5 to 12 years and after the production of flowers and bulbils the plant dies. Root: fibrous; arising adventitiously from the base of leaf scars at the bottom of the bole; 2-4 mm. in diameter, extend 1.5-3 cm. and upto 5 mm. in plants with free range, in the top 30-40 cm. of the soil. The stem is short and thick reaching a height of about 100 cm. with a diameter of 20 cm. It bears an apical meristem and a close rosette of about 100 leaves. Leaves : are produced in an ascending spiral with a phyllataxy of 5/34, which may be clockwise or anticlockwise in direction. Mature leaves are sessile, rigid, linear-laneolate; about 120 cm. long but may attain a maximum length of 2 meters, widest in middle where 10-15 cm. wide, dark bluish green in colour, concave above convex below; leaf bases thick, fleshy, bulbous; closely interlocking; lamina gradually broadening in the middle and narrowing towards terminal sharp, lignified, dark brown spine, 1-1.5 cm. long, shallowly grooved, leaf margin spineless in CVS; cuticle well developed & Waxy. Inflorescence : This emerges from the centre of the plant and bears 50-60 purple brown bracts; each bract is 10-15 cm. long, tipped with a sharp spine. Flowering : branches are produced from lower buds of panicle. Perianth pale green, superior, regular or irregular, tube long short or 0, limb 6. lobed; Stamens : 6, attached to base of tube and exserted about 6 cm. above perianth; filaments thin, yellow, anthers versatile, 2-lobed speckled; pollen yellow, dusty. Strong smelling, ovary interior, 3-locular; ovules numrous in two rows in each loculus; anatropous. Style : awl shaped; stigma; simple or cleft; 3-lobed. Fruit : Usually capsular, loculicidal; rarely fleshy and bursting irregularly. Seeds : few or many, they are flat, papery black rounded-triangular enclosing the small embryo.

It is reported from all over India and has naturalized in the sub-Himalayan tract and the outer Himalayas and many other parts of India. SISAL has now been widely introduced throughtout the tropics and is used locally in many countries, but the only other countries outside East Africa with substantial production are Brazil, where Sisal was introduced at the end of the nineteeth century, Haiti; Angola, Mozambique and the Malagasy Republic. Java was formerly an important producer; South Africa requirements are grown in Natal.

MEDICINAL USE : The leaf plup is used for the isolation of hecogenin which serves as raw material for manufacturer of Cortesone and sex harmones.

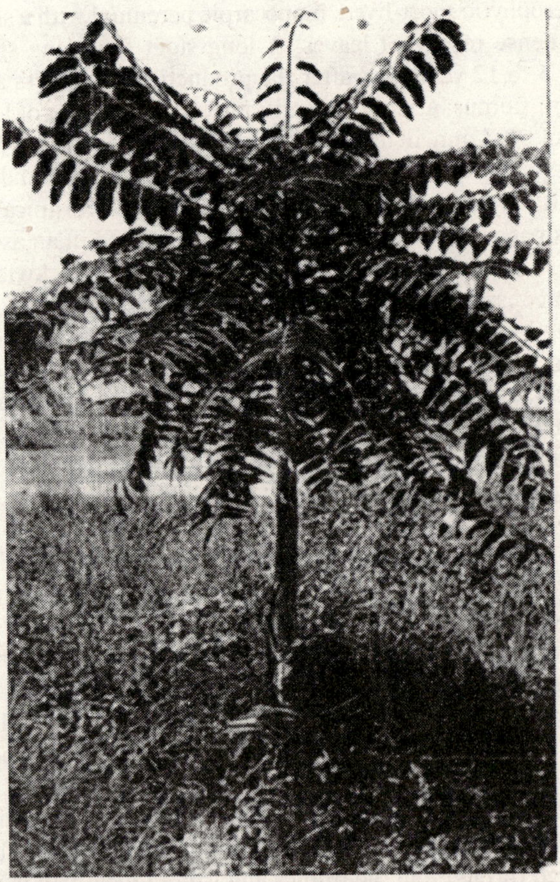

SIMAROUBACEAE

AILANTHUS EXCELSA ROXB.

HINDI - ARUA, MAHARUKH., **ENGLISH** - TREE OF HEAVEN., **MARATHI**-MAHARUKHA., **LOCAL NAME** - ULLOO, URU., **SANS.**-MAHANIMBA., **TAM**-PERUPPI., **TEL.**-PEDDAMANU., **MAL.**-MATTIPONGILYAR.

It is a large beautiful avenue tree, wood is soft and white. Leaves are large pinnate and in the autumn conspicuous with terminal clusters of young reddish winged fruits, known as Samara. Flowers greenish 5-8 cm. across in erect branched clusters 10-20 cm. Leaves 45-60 cm with 13-25 large oval lanceolate leaflets, each with 2-4 coarse glandular teeth near the base. Leaflets 7-12 cm long. Fruits in hanging clusters, each with a single central nut and propeller-like wing 3-4 cm twisted at the top. A freely occurring tree. The flowering season is January-March and fruiting season is May-July.

It thrives well and has been planted along several roads of New Delhi. It is reported from Bihar, Chota Nagpur, Madhya Pradesh, forests of Ganjam, Vizagapatnam and Deccan.

MEDICINAL USE : Arom. used for dyspeptic complaints. tonic, febge, expect. antisep. given in chronic bronchit and asthama. Used as cure in diar. and dysen. Bark and leaves - tonic used especially indebility after child birth. The leaves are boiled and their extract is used for washing wounds and skin eruptions.

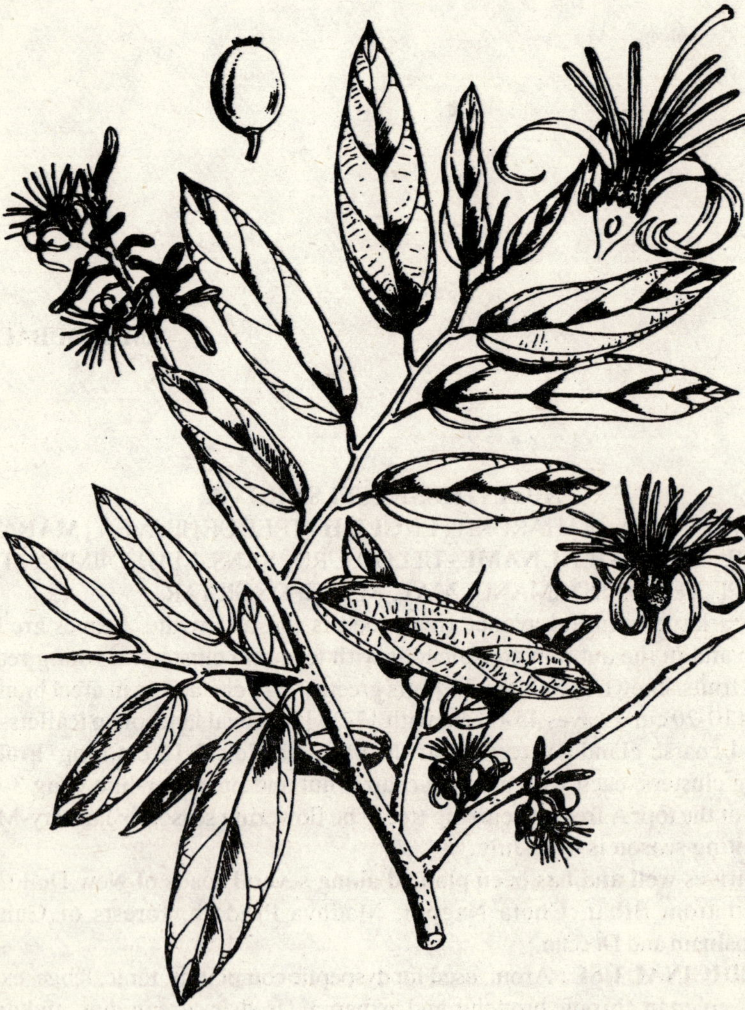

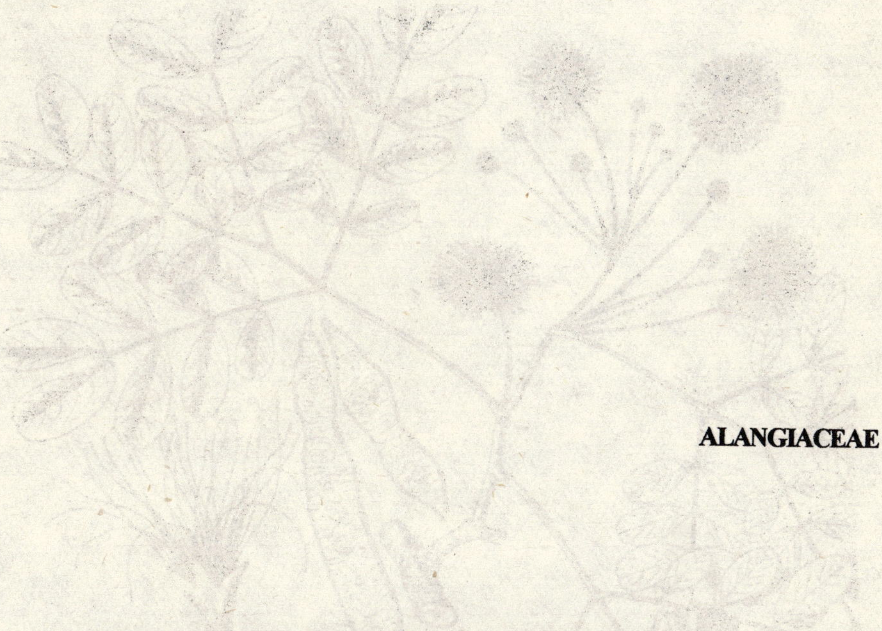

ALANGIACEAE

ALANGIUM LAMARCKII THWAITES
(SYN. SALVII FOLIUM (LINN. F.) WRANG

BENG.- AKAR - KANTA., **MAL.**- ANKOLAM., **MAR.**- ANKOLI., **TAM.**- ALANGII., **TEL.**- ANKOLAMU., **ENG.**- SAGE-LEAVED ALANGIUM., **GUJ.**- OUKLA., **HINDI**- AKOLA., **KAN.**- ANKOLEMARA.

The plant is spiny and 25 - 40 ft. in height. Its leaves are 3 - 6" long and 2 - 4" broad like kaner leaves. The flowers are yellow and white or red and white. The fruits are very tasty and of mouve colour.

It is reported throughout the drier parts of India grows vigrously in the forests of South India.

The leaves and seeds are the chief sources of medicine. They are used in piles, as blood purifier for removing poisonous effect from blood. The fruits are cooling; tasty and destroying cough; tonic; and allergy killer. The powder of leaves is used to remove fever and reduce cold and thrust. It is very useful in removing all types of skin infection. Leaves are also used in poultice in rheumatic pain.

The bark is said to lower blood pressure.

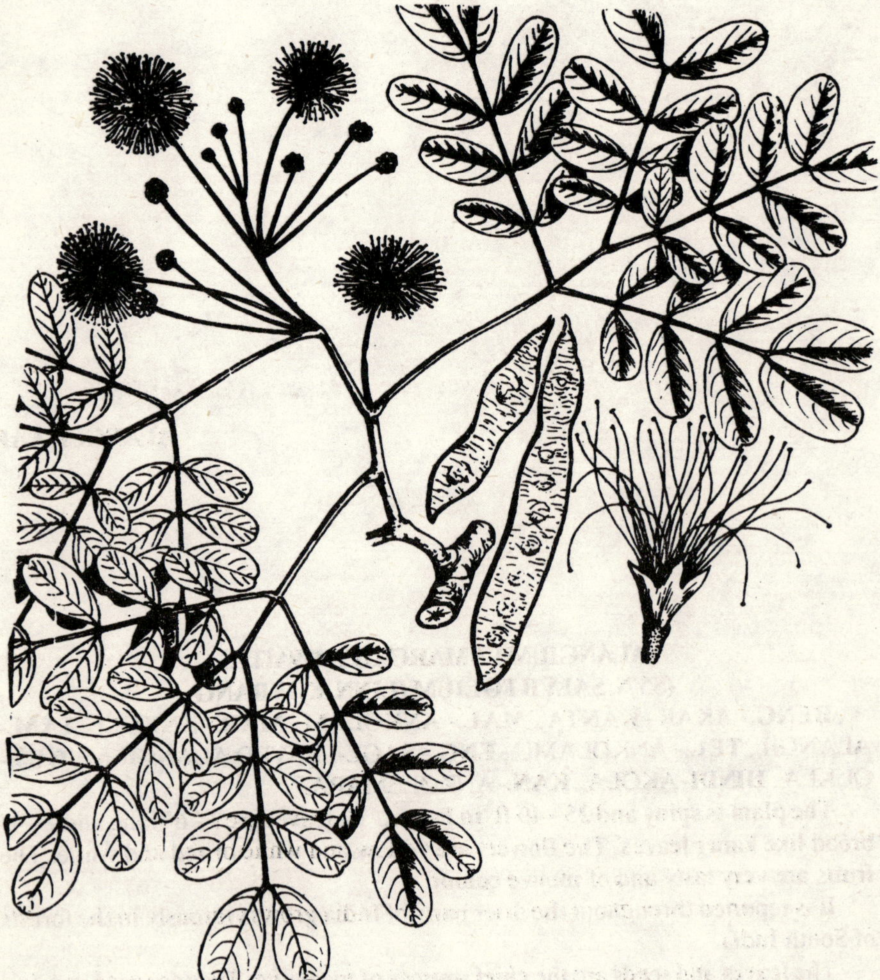

MIMOSACEAE

ALBIZZIA LEBBECK (LINN) BENTH
SYN. HIMOSA LEBBECK L ACACIA LEBBECK WILLD

BENG., & HINDI, BOM. - SIRIS., **SANS.** - SHIRISHA., **KAN.** - BAGEY., **TAM.** - VAGHEY, VAGAI., **MAR.** - MOTHA SIRIS., **TEL.** - DIRASSANA., **ENG.** - KOKKO, LEBBECK - TREE. **LOCAL NAME** - SIRAS.

It is a deciduous tal l tree without prickles. Trunk is grey. Leaves: glabrous or downy - rachises and a large gland near the base of the main petiole; bipinnate, pinnae- 4-8 with or without a gland between the lowest; leaflets 8-18, oblong ¼ - 1/3" broad sheet - stalked, rigidly sub-coriaceous, oblique, 1-1½ " long, glabrous or finely grey - downy. Heads not panicled many - flowered, short - peduneled, 3-4 together from the crowded upper nodes on downy ercto-patent peduncles. Flowers in the Indian species in globose heads, sessile or pedicellate, usually pentamerous and all hermaphordite. Calyx 1/6", downy, companulate or pedicellate funnel- shaped, distinctly toothed.

Corolla: Funnel- shaped, petals firmly united below the middle; greenish yellow, twice the Calyx, the teeth short lanceolate. Stamens: Indefinite (monadelphous at the base, filaments several times the length of the Corolla; anthers minute, not gland crested Ovary: Sessile or shortly stalked; style filiform, stigma capitate minute, Pod: Large, thin, flat, strap-shaped, straight indehiscent or sub-indehiscent, continuous within, the sutures not thickend firm, yellow-brown, ½-1 ft, by 3/4 - 1½", 6-10 seeded.

The flowering period is April-July and fruiting period is September. Distribution species 25-30, spread through the Tropics of the old World. AIOPHANTHA is naturalised on the Nilghiris. In India a common road side tree suitable for avenue planting, wind breaks and shelter belts. The largest supplies of Kokko came from the Andamens. In lesser amounts it is found in Bengal, Assam, Tamil Nadu, M.P. Punjab and U.P.

MEDICINAL USE : Bark is used as a remedy for bronchitis. leprosy, paralysis, gum inflammation and helminthie infections. Whole plant is used in snakebite and scorpion-sting. Root-bark in powder form is used to strengthen the gums. Leaves are useful in night blindness.

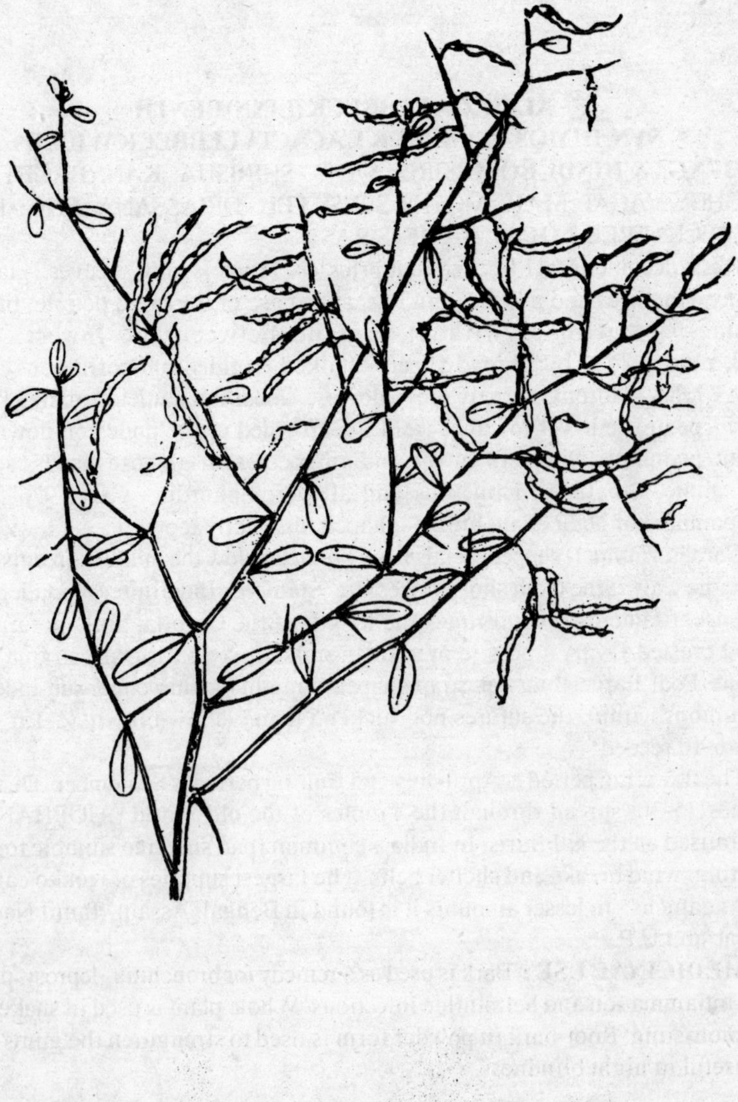

PAPILLIONACEAE

ALHAGI-PSEUDALHAGI BIEB DESW
Syn. A MACRORUM BAKER
Syn. A. CAMELORUM FISCH
Syn. HEDYSARUM PSEUDAL ALHAGI BIEB
AND ALHAGI CAMELORUM FISCH

Popularly known as Camel thorn, Persian Manna Plant.

PERS.- KHAREBUZ., **HINDI**.-JAWASA., **MAR. & GUJ**.- JAWASO., **BENG.**- DULA LABASH., **SANS.**- DURLABHA., **TEL.**- TELLAGINIYA., **LOCAL NAME** - JAWASA AUD BHARBHARRA.

A low spreading spiny shrub 2-3' high. The shrub is armed with copious subpatent hard pungent spines 1/2-1" long. Leaves: Simple, droping from the base of the spines or branches, oblong, obstuse, rigidly coriaceous, glabrous. Flowers 1-6 from a spine, axillary on short pedicles. Calyx: Glabrous, 1/12-1/8", Campanulate, teeth 5, distinct, minute. Corolla: reddish, 3 times the calyx; exserted; standard broad, keel obtuse. Stamens: Diadelphous; anthers uniform. Ovary linear, sessile, 6-8 ovulate, style filiform, incurved; stigma minute, capitate. Pod: Linear; 1" long or less, falcate or straight, sub-continuous or moniliform; joints oblong, small turgid, smooth.

Species 1 spread from Songaria to Greece and Nubia. It is found in drier parts of Gujarat, Sind, the Punjab, the United provinces, Rajputana & Baluchistan.

MEDICINAL PROPERTIES : Plant is used as laxative, diuretie and expectorant; and oil from the leaves is used for curing rheumatism; and flowers are used for piles.

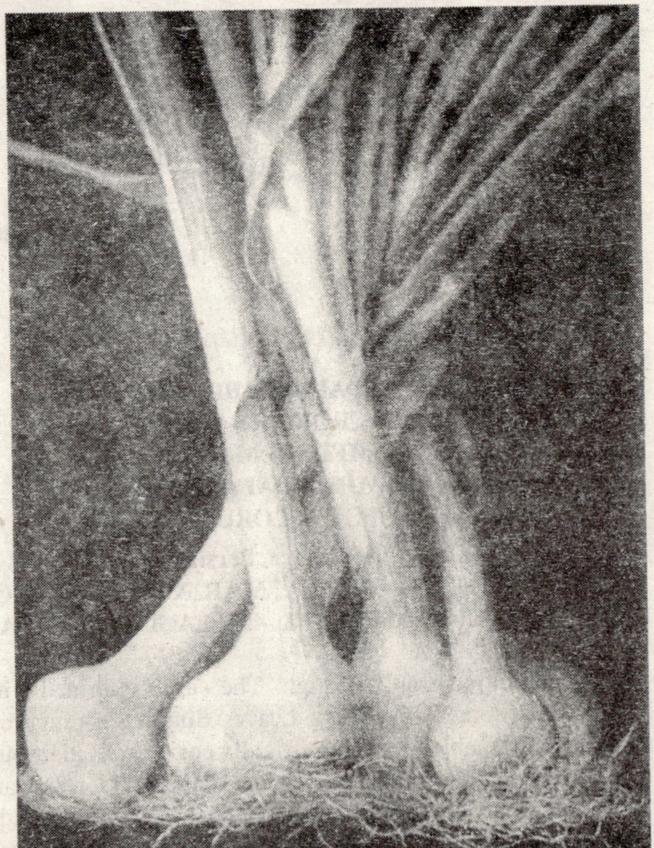

ALLIACEAE

(LILIACEAE)

ALLIUM CEPA LINN

HINDI.- PIYAJ., **ENG.**- ONION., **GUJ.**- DUNGARI-KANDO., **MAL.**- EERULLI, CHUVANNAULLI., **MAR.**- KANDA., **TAM.**- IRULLI, VENGAYAM., **TEL.**- NIRULLI, YERAGADDA., **SANS.**- PALANDU., **BOM.**- KANDA., **ARAB.**- BASL., **PERS.**- PIYAZ., **BENG.**- PYANJ., **KAN.**- NIRULLI, IRULLI.

The plant is a bulbous, biennial herb, bearing linear hollow, flesh cylindrical leaves and umbels of small white flowers. Bulbs 6.8 x 4.6 cm. ovoid. Primary root produced by the seedling, after which all other roots are adventitious arising from the short stem. New adventitious roots are produced as the plant top enlarges and older root may die as the plant ages. Stem: very short flattened stem is produced at base of the plant which increases in diameter as growth continues to form an inverted cone. The new leaves are produced by the apical meristem; Leaves: radical, hollow; bifarous, distichous, glaucous are produced in succession from the broadening stem apex. Bulbs: large, the outer leaves are thin and dry, the inner leaves are fleshy. As the bulb matures, the leaf sheathes weaken above the bulb and fallover. On reaching the bulb into full maturity an inflorescence is formed by the elongation of the internode to produce the scape which is hollow and nearly 30-100cm. long. It is swollen below the middle. Flowers many, white, in dense umbels with both flowers and bulbils subtended by 2 or 3 reflexed. Pedicel slender; perianth 6 in bracts, 2 whorls, greenish white in colour, reflexed, free ovate, accuminate; 5mm with prominent nerve. Stamens: 6 in 2 whorls, alternating with and longer than perianth segments; anthers bilocular, introrse; filaments of inner whorl of stamens expanded at base often with a single tooth on either side; ovary superior, 3-locular, with nectary at base of each septa and 2-anatropous ovules per loculus; style simple, filiforn, shorter than stamens at anthesis. Fruit globular capsule, splitting loculicidally down each loculus. Seeds: few compressed, testa black.

It is extensively cultivated all over India; It is both a field crop and garden crop. The flowering period is November to December of the year.

MEDICINAL USE : The Onion is said to possess stimulant diuretie and expectorant properties and is considered useful in flatulence and dysentery. Freshly expressed onion juice has moderate baetericidal properties (Fuller and Higging. Ghem, Abstr; 1941, 35, 2627 & 2552.)

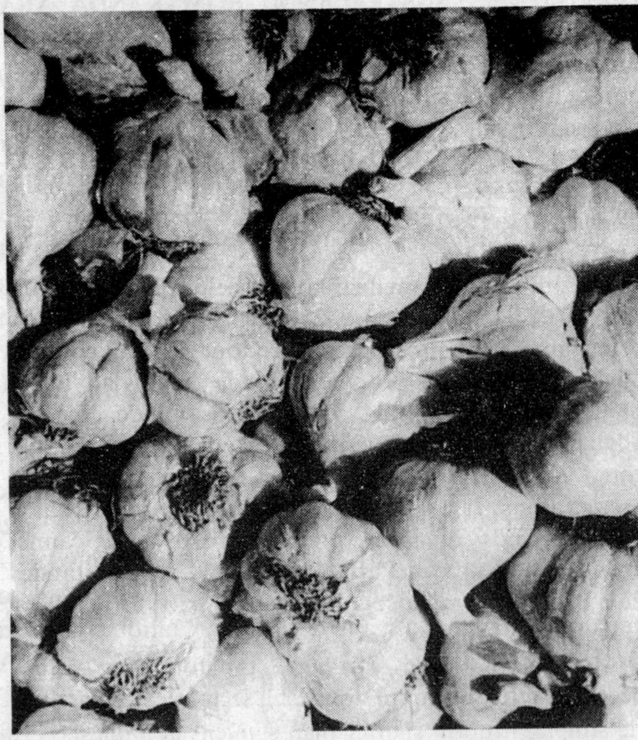

ALLIACEAE
(LILIACEAE)

ALLIUM SATIVUM LINN

BENG.-RASUM, LASAN., **ENG.**-GARLIC., **GUJ.-& MAR.- & HINDI**.-LASAN., **KAN**.- BELLULI., **MAR.- & TEL.**- VELLU; TELLAGUDDA., **TAMIL**-VELLAIPUNDU., **SAN**.-LASAN, ARISHTHA., **ARB.**-SAUM., **PERS**.-SIR., **BOMB**-LASAN.

It is a hard perennial foetid scapigerous herb. The root is reduced to a disc bearing the root hairs on its lower side. The stem is modified into a form of bulb.

It consists of several smaller bulbs called ' cloves' or 'bulblets' and is surrounded by a thin white or pinkish membrane. Leaves : Usually narrow, often fistular and flat, scape slender, spathes long beaked. Flowers often displaced by bulbils pinkish, in lax umbels and a long terete scape exceding the leaves: Capitate or umbelled, all at first. enclosed in 1-3 memberanous spathes, stellate or accuminate; sepals 6 free-laneolate or acuminate. Stamens : hypogynous or inserted on the perianth; filaments free or connate below, inner filaments 2 - toothed; anthers excerted, oblong Ovary 3 - gonous, 3 - celled; style exserted filiform, stigma minute, cells few-ovuled. Capsule small, loculicidal. Seeds few, compressed, testa black.

It is cultivated in the cold region and is reported from all over India. It is a native of central Asia.

MEDICINAL USE : 1. Garlic is strongly antiseptic and antibacterial properties and is widely used for infections diseases and intestinal disorders. Taken internally it kills bacteria and worms while externally garlic juice kills skin infection used as rubifacient in skin diseases, as are drops in earache and in colie and flatulence. It also cures reheumatism, clears chest and improves lungs It has got a negative and germicidal effect and helps curing typhoid and paratyphoid. Bulbs are used in cough fever and relieves of pain in rheumatism.

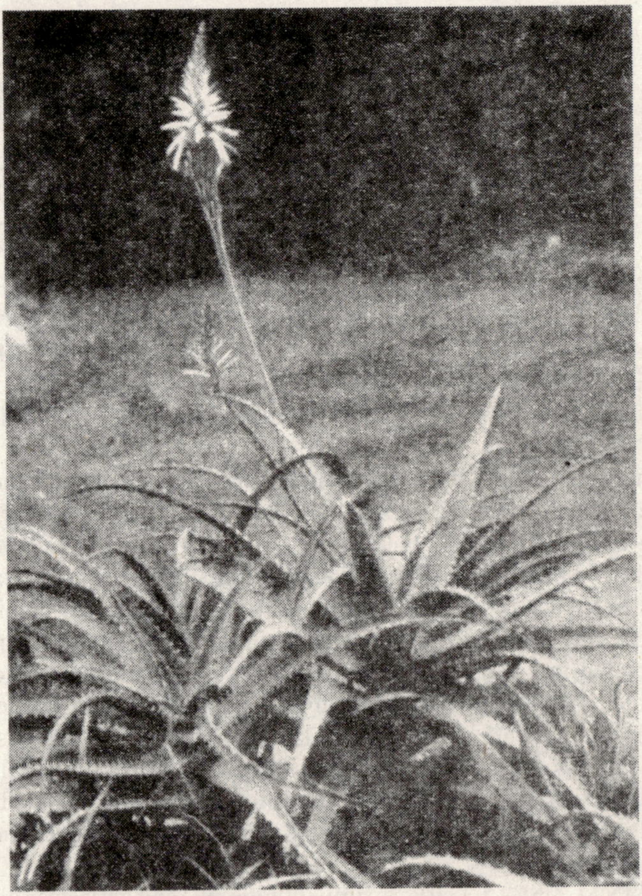

LILIACEAE

ALOE BARBADENSIS MILL

SYN. A PERFOLIATA L; A. VERA WEBBAND BERTH

SAN. & BENG.-GHARITA KUMARI., **HINDI**-GHIKANVAR., **TAMIL**-CHIRA KATLAI, KALTALAI., **TELUGU**-CHINNA-KALEBANDA., **MAL.**-KUMARI., **ENG.**- INDIAN ALOE., **GUJ.**-KANVAR., **KAN.**-KUMARI., **KASH.**-MUSABAR., **MAR.**-PIVALABOEL., **PUNJ.**-ELWA.

It is known as a caulescent and stoloniferrous plant, the leaf rosettes arising from the ground upto 60 cm. high; leaves are numerous thick glaucous, erect green lanceolate and long pointed, thorn edged on both sides. Flowers vermillioin coloured in simple errcet racemes, the lower flowers falling off as the receme elongates, stamens equalling the perianth. Flowers are available in March and April.

It is planted in Indian gardens. Many species are found in a semi-wild state in all parts from the westward valleys of the Himalayas upto Cape Comarin.

MEDICINAL USE : The plant is stomachic, tonic in small doses and in larges doses it acts as purgative and used in piles and rectal fissures. Dried leaf powder is given in constipation and fresh juice is cooling and used in fever. Root is given in colic.

This species form an active ingredient of ABANA, Herbolex (Himalaya Drug Co.).

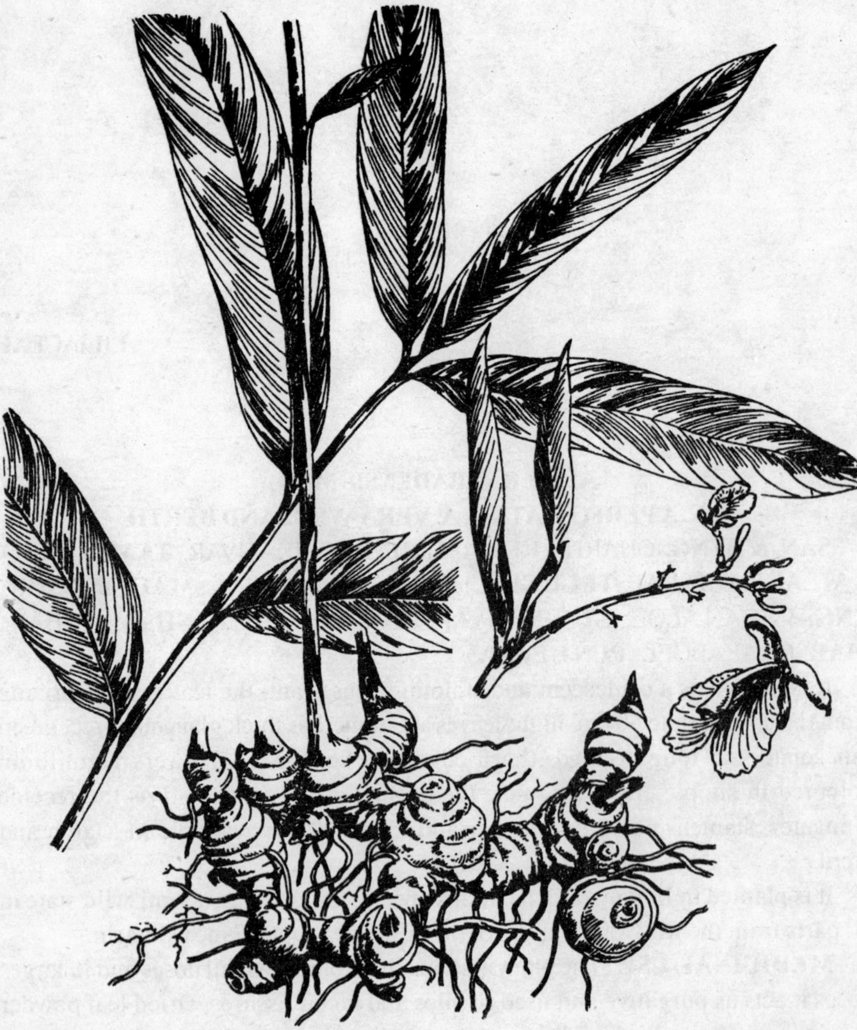

SATAMINACEAE

ALPINIA GALONGA WILLD
(SYN. A. CALEARATEI)

GUJ.- KULANJAN., **FA.**- KHIRDARM., **ENG.**- EKKHARGIN GREATER., **BENG.**- SUGANDA - VACHA., **MAL.**- CHITTA - RATTA., **ENG.**- JAWA GALANGAL., **MAR.**- KOSHT - KUTINJAN., **HINDI**- SPHED -PANAKI - JHAD., **TAM.**- PERIARETAI., **KAN.**- DHUMARASHMI., **TEL.**- PEDDA - DHUMPA., **BO.**- BARIPANKIZAR., **LATIN**- ALPINIA GALANGA.

It is a robust herb native to Indonesia and Malaysia now mostly cultivated in North India and E. Himalaya.

It is reported from the eastern Himalayas and South - West India.

MEDICINAL USE : The plant is useful for throat, mouth, cough and stomach diseases. Rhizomes used in Rheumatic fever and, specially in bronchial catarrh. affections, oil extracted is useful in respiratory troubles, specially for children.

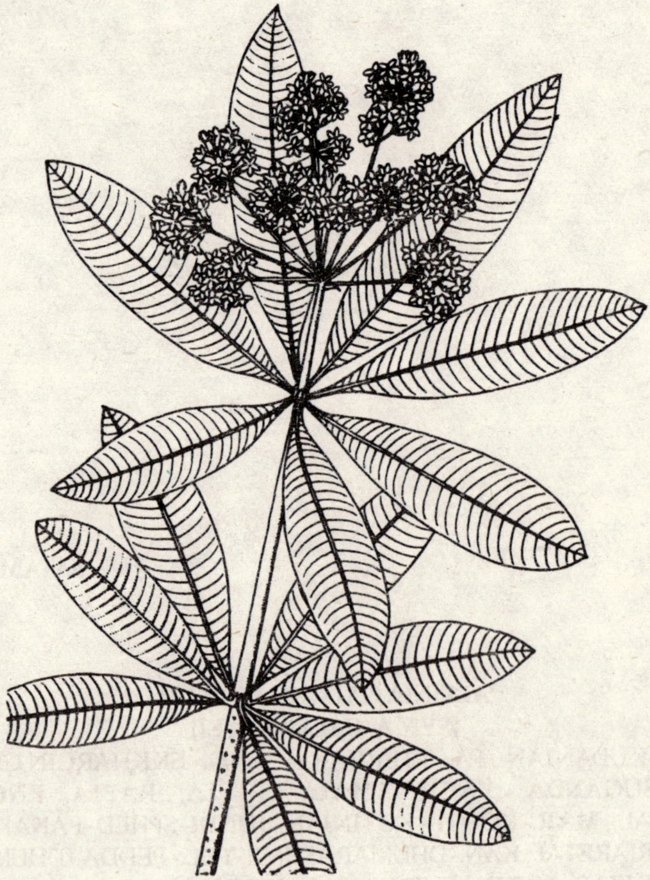

APOCYNACEAE

ALSTONIA SCHOLARIS (LINN) R. B. R.
Syn. ECHITES SCHOLARIS L.

BEN.- CHHATIN, CHATTIM., **ENG**.- DITA BARK, DEVIL'S TREE., **HINDI** DATYUNI, CHATIAN., **KAN**.- HALE, MADDALE., **KON**.- SANTHNI, ROOKU., **MAL**.- DAIVAPAL, PALA., **MAR**.- SATVEEN., **TAM**.- EZWILAYPATAY, PALA, ACLILAMPLAI., **TEL**.- PALAGARUDA, EDAKULAPALA., **TRADE**.- CHATIYAN OR SHAITANWOOD., **SANS**.- SAPTAPARNA.

An evergreen large tree with a straight, often fluted and buttressed stem, 40' ft. high at times 80 - 90 ft. (Brandis) and upto 8" in girth. The bark is grey white; the trunk is tall and the branches are whorled. The bark is yellow from inside and exudes a bitter milky juice.

Leaves: 4 - 7; 10 - 20 x 4.5 - 5.5 in a whorl obovate or elliptic - oblong white beneath, base acute, tip obtuse rounded or obtusely accuminate. Coriaceous, whitish beneath where 30 - 60 pairs horizontal veins joining an intra marginal one. Petiole stout ¼ - ½" cymes - peduncled or sessile, capitate, umbellately branched peduncle 1-3". rarely O, very stout; branches numerous flowers pubescent sub-capitate corymbose cymes, greenish white (Benthem and Hookers greenish yellow (Delhi Flora). Calyx: Short, 5 - lobed or partite. Corolla: 1/3 - ½" in diameter, throat villous annulate or with reflexed bars, lobes rounded over lapping to the right or left. Stamens Near the top of the tube, included anthers sub-acute. Disc: annular; zero (0); carpels 2; distinct; hirsute; style filiform, top ovoid or oblong stigma minute or 2 - many to infinate serriate in each carpel. Follicles 2, linear slender; 1-2ft. Pendulous in clusters only 1/8 in diameter, terete.

Seeds: 1/3" long slender toothed; ovule flattened, peltately attached, often cilliate, albumen scanty; cotyledons oblong, flat radicle superior - The flowering. Dec - March; and fruits - May-July. It is found throughout the moist regions of India, particularly in the W. Coast forests.

MEDICINAL USE : Bark bitter - tonic, after, febge, in Malaria, useful in diarr and dysen, in snake-bite and deafness. The fresh bark juice + milk is used for leprosy and dyspepsia.- Leaves extract with fresh ginger is given after confinement; also used for beri-beri in Malaysia and against congestion of liver. The leaves boiled in oil is given for dropsy poultice of the leaves is used for ulcers. The milky juice is applied to ulcers sores/tumours and in rhumatic pain and is used for curing tooth ache. It is reported to be an antidote for Antiarias - poisoning mixed with oil, it is reported to cure ear ache, boiled with coconut oil it is used in itches.

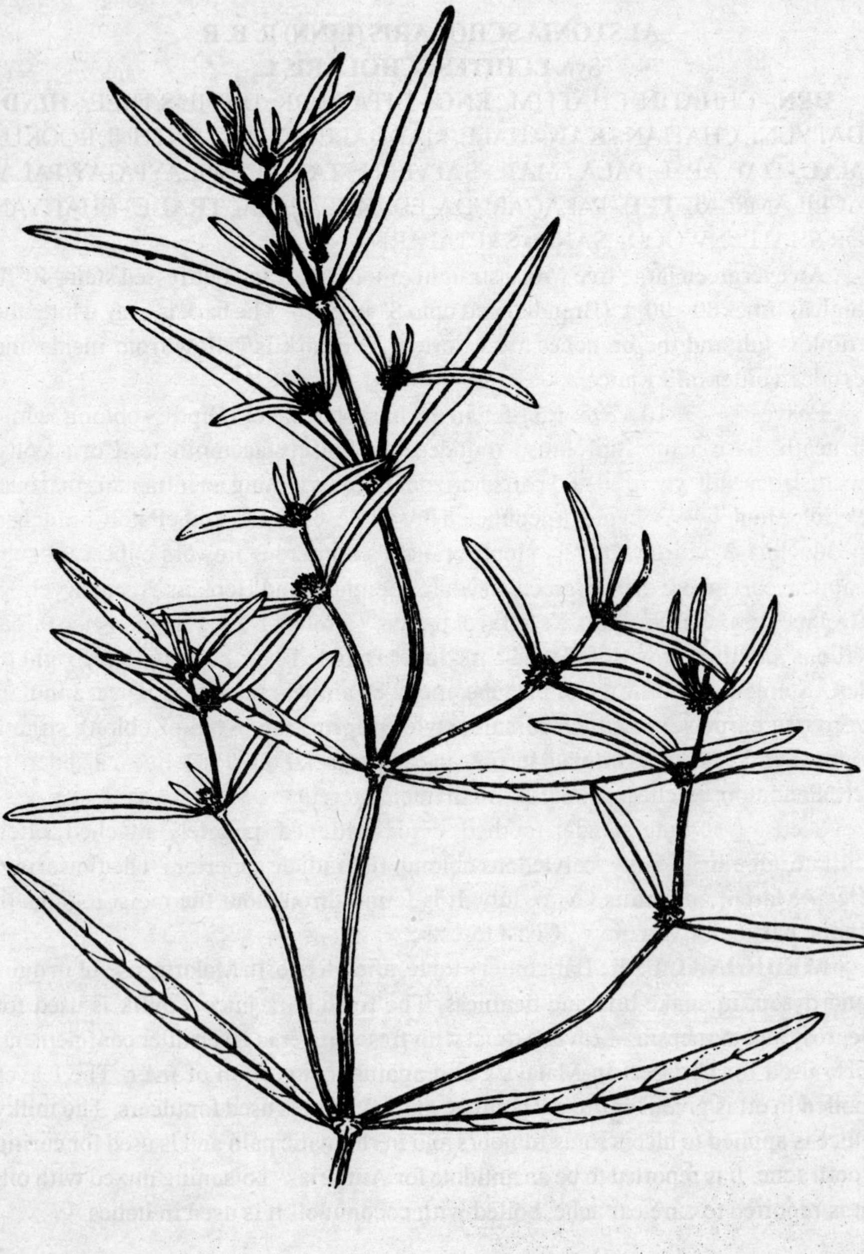

AMARANTHACEAE

ALTERNANTHERA SESSILLES (LINN) R. BR.
(SYN. A. REPENS J.F. GMEL; GOMPHRENA SESSILLES LINN.

BO.- KANCHARI., **M.**- PONNANGANNI., **TAM.- & MAL.**- PONNAUGANNI-KECRAY., **TEL.**- PONNAGANTA - KURA.

A polymrophic, glabrous, prostrate spreading herb, often rooting at the nodes. Branches many often arising two equal and opposite in position alongwith the main branch, often light pinkish, grey, leaves glabrous, elliptic, linear - oblong or oblanceolate tapering towards the base. Flowers white, shining in small axillary sessile, chaffy heads. Perianth segments not spine tipped; stamens - 3; utricle broadly obcordate or orbicular. Seeds sub-oroicular. Flowers and fruits - rainy seasons.

A weed in cultivated fields and waste lands. Also common in damp places slongwith the borders of ponds and tanks or grows as an aquatic in shallow water. It is a highly variable herb, depending on habitat conditions.

It is a weed found throughout the warmer parts of India.

MEDICINAL USE : Plant -galact, cholag, febge, Stem and leaves used in snake bite.

Young shoot are nutritous and contain protein iron and megnesium (H1 th. Bull. No. 23, 1941, 30.)

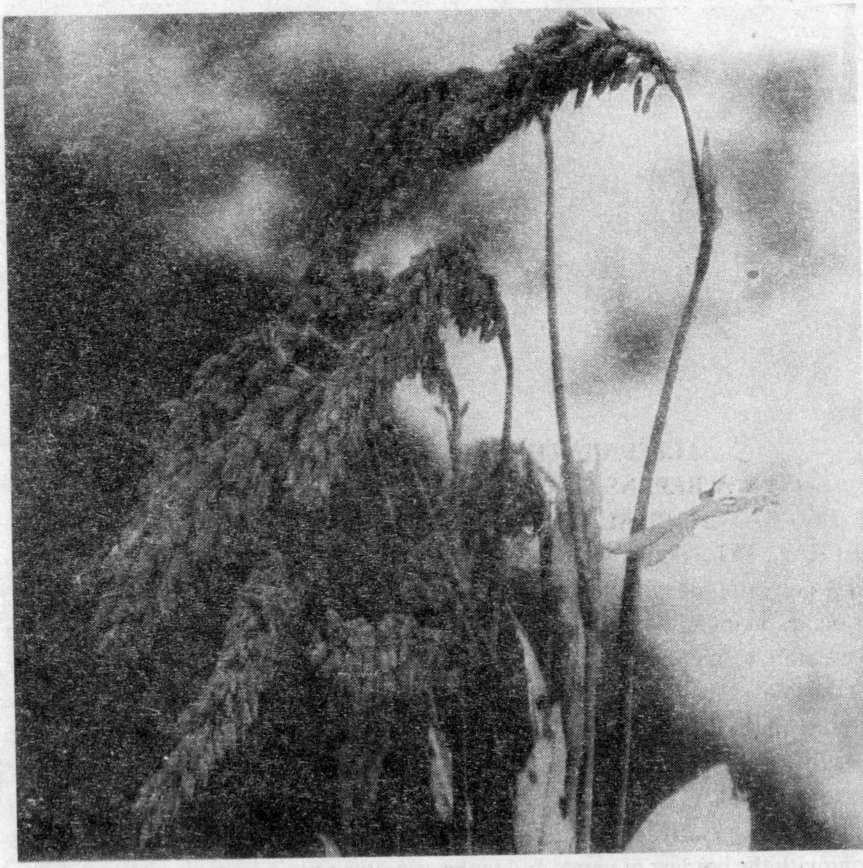

AMARANTHACEAE

AMARANTHUS CAUDATUS LINN
(SYN. A. PANICULATUS (LINN) THELL.

HIMALAYAN NAME- KEDARI CHAU., **GUJARATI**- CHUKO., **BENG.**- ANANTHMOOL and CHUKO NATYA., **BO.**- KAHOLABHOJI., **H.**- CHAULAI, RAMADANA, CHURAMARSA., **KASH**- BUSTANOFROZ., **TAM.**- SRIRUKERA, PAUGI KIRAI., **SANS.**- RAJAGIRI., **ENG.**- AMRANTH (GRAIN), VELVET FLOWER., **TELGU**-KAYI-KERA.

The plant is an annual herb tall and robust with profuse branches. The stem is errect and grooved. The leaf is entire elliptical to oblong and blunt. The stalk is long and leaf is prominently nerved. The base of the leaf is cuneate.

The flowers are small, 1 - 2 mm. long bright red or yellow arranged in long pendulous clusters forming a cobra panicle, the central spike is the longest. The flower has got a papery perianth, oblong five pointed bracts owl shaped larger.

It is cultivated throughout India, chiefly in mountains upto 2400 meters in the Himalayas from May to August.

MEDICINAL USE : The leaves are rich in oxalic acid. Plants used for purifying blood. It is used in piles, and it is also used in strangury also given in scrofula and applied to scrofulous sores.

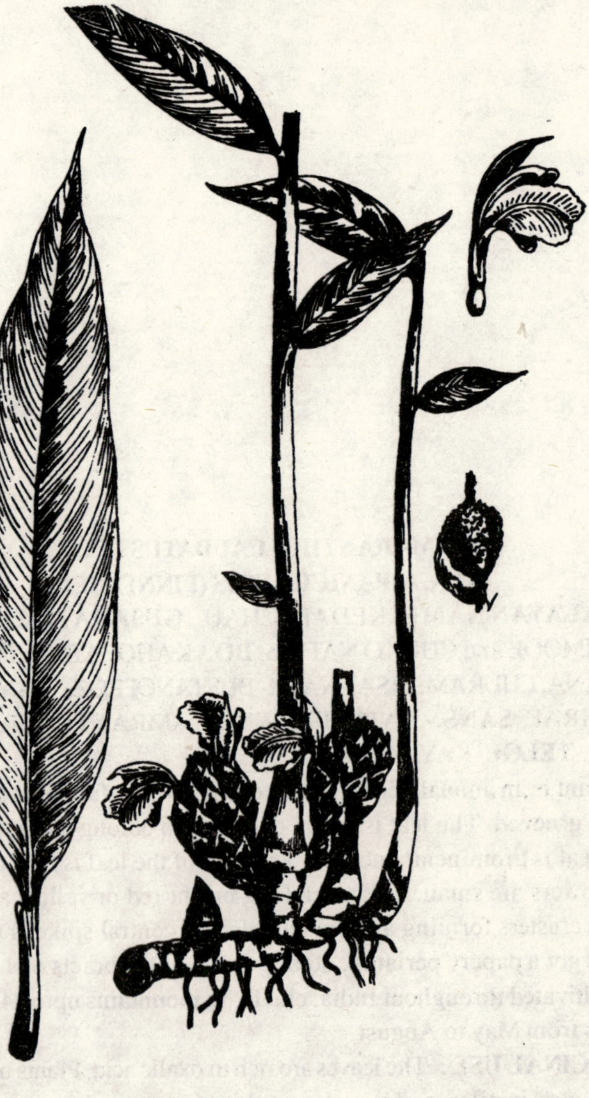

ZINGIBERACEAE

AMOMUM SUBULATUM ROXB.
(SYN. A. AROMATICUM ROXB).

S.- BRIHADAELA., **H & B**- BARA- ELACHI., **TAM**- PERIYAYELAM., **TELGU**- PEDDAYCLAKI., **ENG**.- BENGAL CARDAMOM.

It is a perennial herb like palnt with distinct leaf and flower - stems, arising from short rhizomes. Fruit is dark brown red globose capsule containing several cells held together by a sugary syrup. Each cell contains numerous seeds. Each fruit contains 60 - 100 seeds. The seeds are aromatic.

It is cultivated in swamy places along the sides of mountain streams in Nepal, Bengal, Sikkim and Assam and Tamil Nadu.

MEDICINAL USE : Seeds, stomach, useful in Neuralgia used in gonorrhea as aphrodis, antatid to seorpion sting and snake bite.

Oil from seeds is aromatic, stimulant, stomach, applied to eyelids to allay inflammation. The oil is also used for mouth gargle and tooth ache.

ELETTARIA CARDAMOMUM forms an important ingredient of Abana, Bonnisan and Geriforte. These three being HImalayan Drug Medicines.

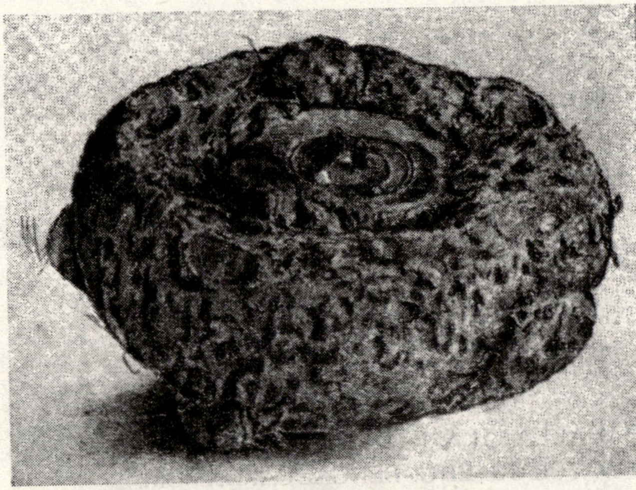

ARACEAE

AMORPHOPHALLUS COMPANULATUS (ROXB) B1.
(SYN. ARUM COMPANULATUS (ROXB)

S.- ARSAGHNA., **BOM.-** JUNGLI SURAN., **B.- OL; H.** ZAMIKAND., **TAM.-** KARNAIKILANGU., **TEL.-** KANDA., **MAL.-** CHENA., **SANS.-** ANSHODDAN, SURAN., **ENG.-** TELUGU POTATO, ELEPHANTFOOT YAM., **BENG.-** OL., **MARATHI.-** SURAN., **GUJ.-** SURAN., **LATIN.-** AMORPHOPHALLUS COMPANULATUS.

It is of two types 1) which is sown, (2) which grows on its own. It is a perennial stemless herb, native to tropical Asia and it is now cultivated throughout India for its large calms.

MEDICINAL USES : In fresh condition, it is much used in acute rheumatism. Tuber helps in increasing apetite, used in piles; colon and dysentry. It also help in reducing gas problems and obesity.

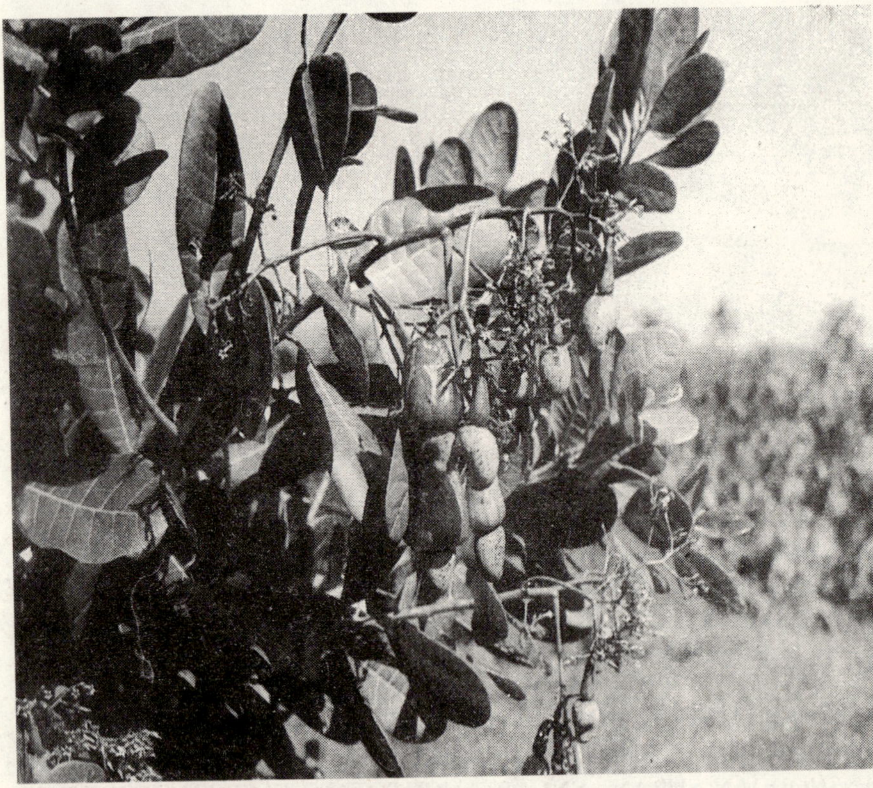

ANACARDIACEAE

ANACARDIUM OCCIDENTALE LINN.

H. & BO.- KAJU., **B**.- HAJLIBADAM., **MAL.**-KASHUMAVU., **S.**-KAJUTAKA., **TAM**.-MUNDIRI., **TEL.**-MOKKAMAMIDI., **ENG**.-CASHEWNUT., **HINDI, KON., MAR. & GUJ.**-KAJU., **K.**-GERUMARA.

It is a small evergreen tree. Leaves are pinnate, flowers small, regular in clusters. Sepals 5 fused, petals 5 (five) free, stamens 5-10; between the stamens and ovary, there is a fleshy disc. Ovary superior and five carpels fuse with 1-3 style. Fruit usually a drupe with a single seed. Fruit is special, the pedicel is enlarged & swollen into a pulpy structure known as cashew apple and the seed forms the cashew nut.

It is found cultivated in the coastal districts of India, especially in the western Ghats, Ratan Giri & N. Knaera district in Bombay, Goa, S. Konera L; Malabar districts in Madras, Cochin, and Travancore.

MEDICINAL USE : Bark is rough alternative and astringent. Tar or aerial oil from the bark applied in leprosy, corns, ulcers-counter irritant, rupifacient, vesicant. Root is pergative Kernel is nutritious, demule. and fruit. is antidiarrhoeal.

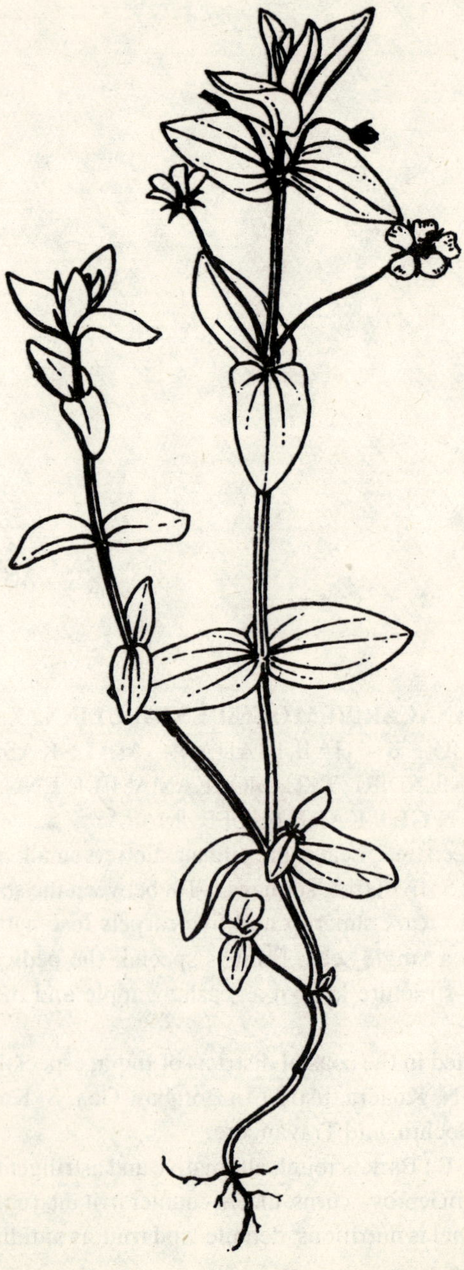

PRIMULACEAE

ANAGALLIS ARVENSIS LINN.

HINDI.- JONKH-MARI., **GUJRAT.**- ANAGALLIDE, MORGELLINA., **PUNJAB.**- DHABBAR.

It is a small annual, erect or procumbent herb found all over India with small red and blue flowers. It is glabrous, gland-dotted; branched from the base, branches four-angled, ascending. Leaves 1/2 - 1 1/2", rarely whorled, sessile ovate cordate or lanceolate acute dotted. Peduncles 1-2", erect in flower, decurved in fruit. Sepals narrow, lanceolate, accuminate, almost equalling the blue and red corollas. Corolla 1/3 - 1/2" diameter closing in dull weather, segments often ciliate. Capsule size of a small pea. Seeds 3-gonous. Both the blue and red flowered varieties are found in Western India; the blue being the common one eastward.

It is reported from Bengal, North-Western India, and the Himalaya from Nepal Westward ascending to 50,000 ft. Central India, the Nilgri Hills and Ceylon (whether introduced.)

MEDICINAL USE : Plant as a whole is used in gout, cerebral infections, hydrophobia, leprosy, dropsy epilepsy, mania, as fish poison, in snake bite.

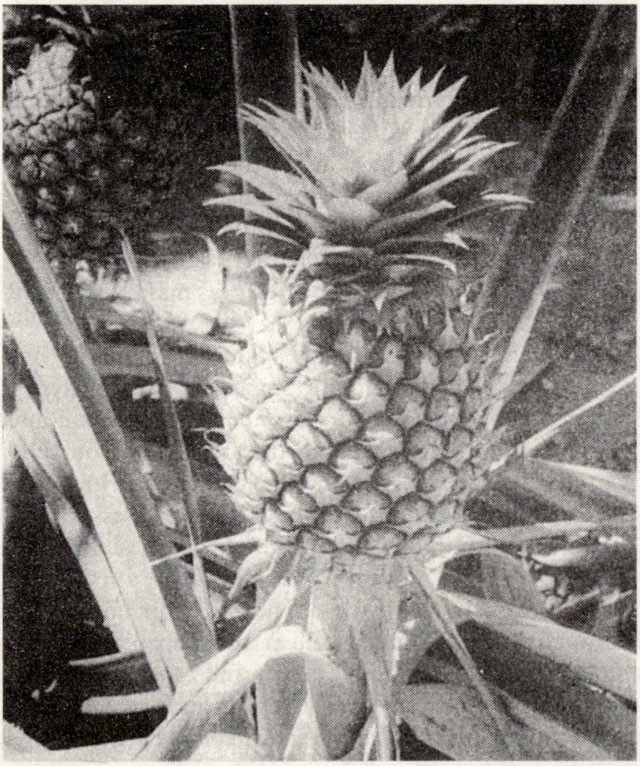

BROMELLIACEAE

ANANAS COMOSUS (L.) MERR.
(SYN. A. SATIVUS SCHULT. F.)
BROMELIA COMOSA L)

BEN.-ANARAS., **MAL.**- ANNANAS., **ENG.**- PINEAPPLE., **TAM.**- PARANGITHALAI., **GUJ.**, **HINDI & MAR.**- ANANAS., **TEL.**- ANANASH., **KAN.**- ANASU.

It is a biennial herb consisting of root stem leaves and fruit. In general when fruit is ripe the whole plant is uprooted and after removing the fruit the rest of the plant is thrown off. Since the time it is known as the plant contains an enzyme bromelin, the whole plant has become very important medically. Now the efforts are made to raise two or three crops in a year. Not only the enzyme is extracted out of the plant but the whole plant is used in making a powder which is of extreme importance in medicine as follows.

Pineappele are triennials with a very short main axis and a rosette of leaves, often the stem elongating slightly and carries spiral of closely packed leaves. The leaves are long, flashy, fibrous and shield like, reaching a length of 1 mtr. and 5 - 8 cm. wide, inflorence is densely purple, sessile flowers are subdivided by a painted bract.

It is a multiple fruit i.e. is a fusion product of the main axis of the inflorence and small berry like fruits produced from each flower, arranged spirally. The fruit contains a digestive enzyme the bromelain.

It is cultivated in Tamil Nadu, Coastal Andhra Pradesh, Assam, Kerala, Karnataka, West Bengal, Tripura and Orissa.

MEDICINAL USE : The bromaline power is capable of removing blood clots from veins and artries and thus save people from death. Besides this in the healthy condition also the bromelin powder helps in maintaining a regular blood circulation and eliminates formation and distribution of blood clots.

A scientist named Towsing states that bromelin is very useful in Tonsilites, neck swellings and swelling in any part of the body.

It is also found extermely useful in skin grafting where it dries the skin and wound very quickly. It is considered as one of the chief medicine for Diphtheria and throat irritation.

A paste of the fruit when applied to sores and boils helps in quick recovery while the juice of the fruit is a very good tonic for the body and heart and reduces thirst in summer. It kills worms and helps in extracting stones from kidney and gall bladder, reduces kidney and urinary troubles. It purifies blood and helps in maintaining skin in good condition.

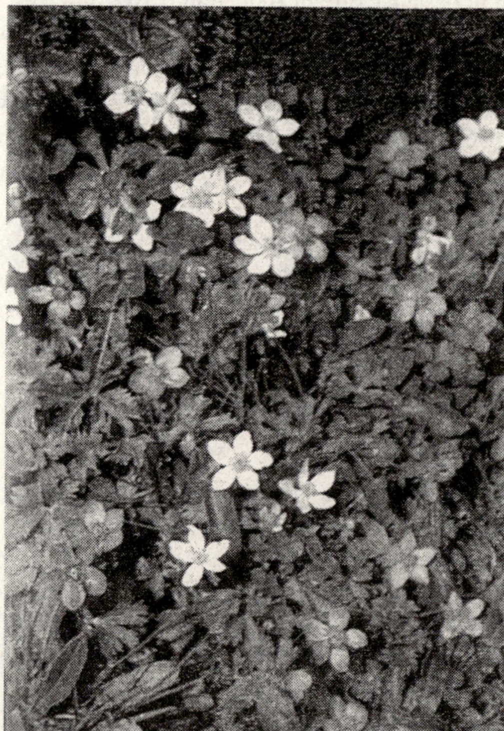

RANUN CULACEAE

ANEMONE OBTUSILOBA D. DON
P. & KUMAON.-RATTANJOG, RATANJOTA.

It is a small plant 5-8 cm., with flowers which are white within and bluish outside and which becomes dull red when old; and with in involuere of lobed leaves below the 1-3 stalked flowers. Flowers 2-3 cm. across; stalks hairy; Basal leaves long stalked; blade lobed, roots tuberous ovoid. Achenes embeded in dense woolly hairs.

It is distributed to temperate and alpine Himalayas, from Kashmir to Sikkim, 7,500 to 15,000 ft.

MEDICINAL USE : Roots mixed with milk given internally for contusions and used externally as a blistering agent.

Seeds produce vomiting and purging.

All dried plants have got similar properties to anemonin.

It's one species known ANEMENE PATENS is actively used in rheumatic medicine by Himalaya drug Co.

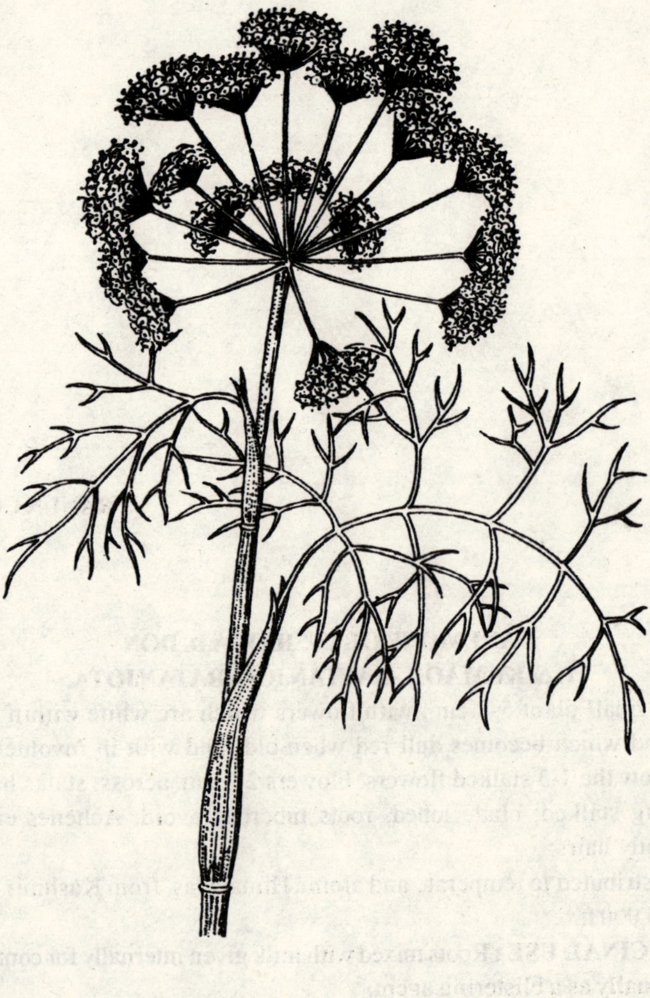

UMBELLIFERAE

ANETHUM GRAVEOLENS LINN
(Syn. PEUCEDANUM GRAVEOLENS (LINN) BENTH.

BENGAL- SOOLPHA., **ENG.-** DILL, DILL SEED., **GUJRATI.-** SURVA-NUBI., **HINDI-** SOWA., **KAN.-** SABBASIGE., **KASH.-** SOI., **MAL.-** CHATUKUPPA., **MARATHI-** SHEPU., **PUNJ.-** SOYA., **TAM.-** SATAKUPPAY., **TEL.-** SHATAKUPIVITTULU.

A. SOWA, the Indian species is sometimes regarded as a variety of A. GRAVEOLENS.

It is a winter crop and is cultivated all over India. The plant is a herb, glabrous perennial and branched as high as 1-3"; the flowers are yellow and the leaves are pinnately divided. Leaves-finely dissected; fennel-like; 2-3 pinnate; ultimate segments of the leaves ½ - 2"; linear-oblong or ovate, entire or remotely sparingly toothed; Pedicels many bracts and bractioles O. Flowers polygamous, yellow. Calyx teeth obsolete or small. Petals yellow obovate, emarginate or 2-fid; styles small dorsal and intermediate ridges distinct, slender; vittae large solitary in each furrow, 2 on the commissure ovary glabrous. The fruits are as broad and narrowly winged being 4 x 2 mm. plano-convex 2 - 3 times as broad as thick. Either mericarp or cremocarp. Seed much dorsally compressed, inner face plane. It is found throughout tropical and subtropical India; often cultivated.

It is Cultivated in south Europe and W. Asia. Flowering and fruiting season is from Jan to March.

MEDICINAL USE : The fruits are used as carminative stomachic and stimulant. The seeds yield dill oil and dill water. Dill water is an excellant remedy for children flatulence and digestion problems. Dill oil is used in pharmacutical Industry.

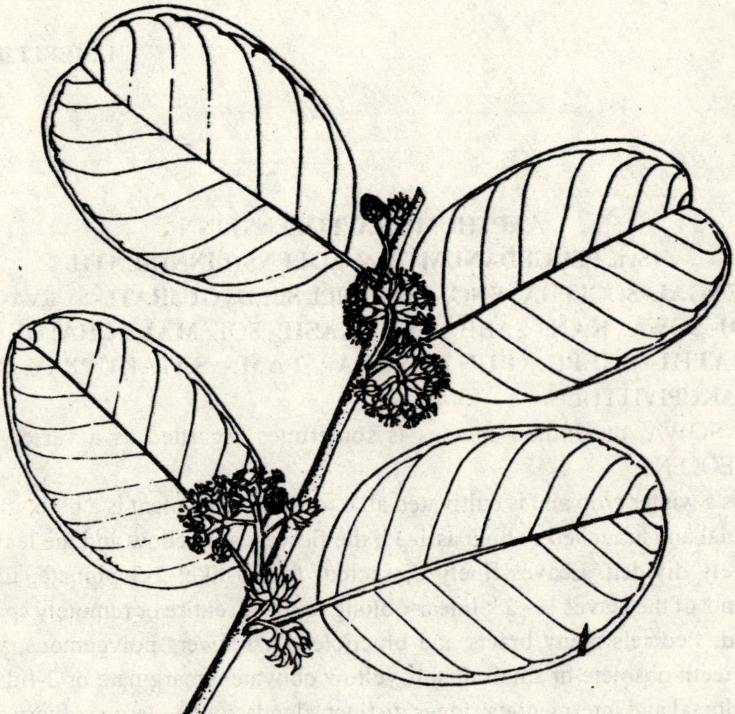

COMBRETACEAE

ANOGEISSUS LATIFOLIA WALL

ENG.- GHATIGUM., **JAM.**- VELLAYNAGAMARAM., **B.**- DHOOYA., **HINDI**- BAKLA, DHEWA, DHAWRA., **LOCAL NAME** : DHOY, SIRAS., **BO.**- DHAVADA., **S.**- SHAVA., **TEL.**- CHIRIMANU., **MAL.**- MARUKINEHIRAM.

A shrub or small tree branching from base. Young parts are purplish. stems ash coloured or grey white. Leaves variable, ovate to elliptie, apiailate. Flower buds vermilian coloured. Flowers - greenish - yellow in axillary and terminal globose heads. Calyx tube shorter than the fruits, and terminal, globose heads branches pendulous turning dull red in fruits. Fruits nearly orbicular, 2 winged, 4 x 4.5 mm. Flowers and fruits August - September.

Occurs commonly near Delhi ridge and Faridabad. Common in dry decidous forests throughout India except E. Bengal and Assam. Found in the Sub Himalayan tract from Ravi to Nepal Bihar, Chota Nagpur, Madhya Bharat and Southwards to Ceylon. Ascends to 4000 ft. in the Himalayan and the South Indian hills.

MEDICINAL USE : Bark - bitter, astringent, plant in scorpion sting and snake bite. The plant tannin, yields gum which is a good substitute for gum arabic; gum is chiefly built up of pentoses and galactose (Weber, I) 824.

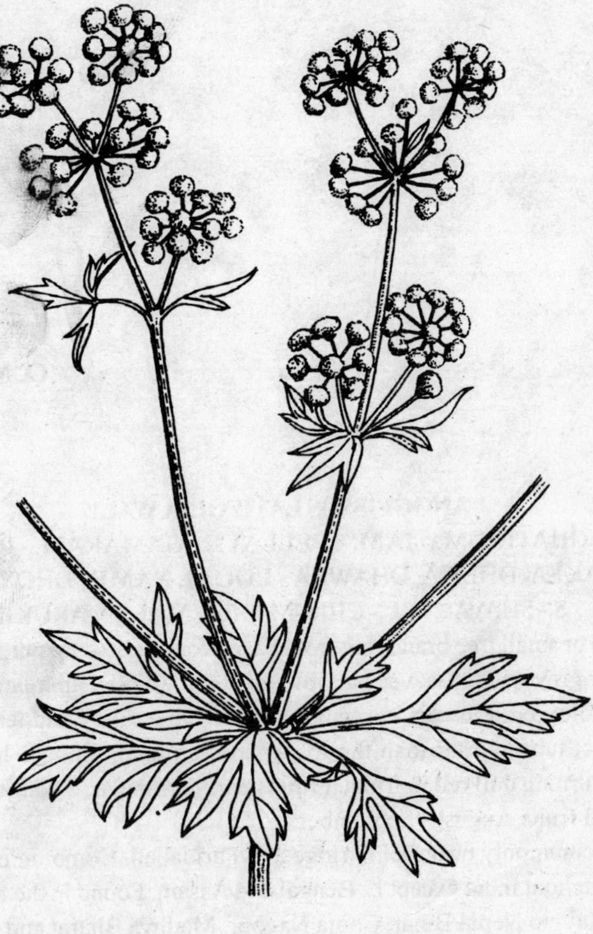

APIACEAE

APIUM GRAVEOLENS L.

BENG.-RANDHUNI., **HINDI**-AJMUD, SOWA, SOYA, BORAJMUD, KARAFS., **GUJ.**- BODIAJAMODA., **MARATHI**-AJMODA., **PUNJ.**-BHULJHATA., **SANS.**-AJMODER, BRAHMAKOSHI., **BENG.**-SALMAMUSHAL, SYNO-HASTIKAVARI, HAYAGANADHA, MAYURA, MURKATI, VASTAMODA., **ENG.**- CELERY, INDIAN DILL.

It is a glabrous branched, perennial herb. Leaves finely dissected. Leaves radical, pinnate, deeply lobed segments, toothed at the apex, pedicellate, umbel inflorence. Seeds are ridged.(funnel like) flowers yellow, fruits are winged.

It is found all over India.

MEDICINAL USE : It prevents rheumatism and gout. The root is considered to be altrative diurertic and given in anasarca & colie, Seeds are stimulant and cardio-tonic. They are used in bronchitis asthma and to some extent in liver + spleen diseases. (Nadkarni 1954).

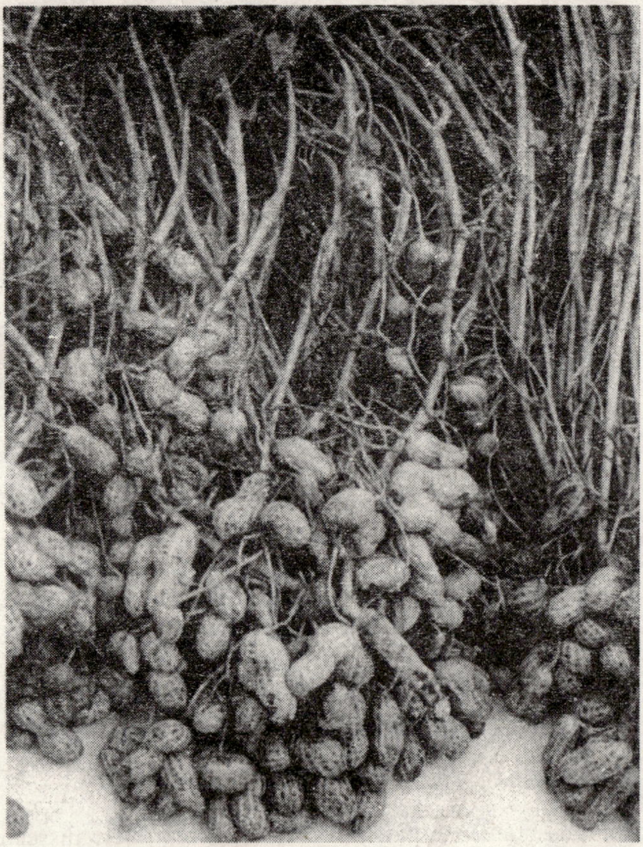

PAPILIONACEAE

ARACHIS HYPOGEA LINN.

BENG.- CHINEEBADAM., **ENG.**-EARTHNUT,GROUNDNUT, PEANUT., **GUJ.**- BHOISING., **HINDI**- MUNGPHALI., **KON.**- BHI-MUG., **MAL. & KAN.**- NELAKADALE., **MAR.**- BHUICHANA., **SANS.**- BUCHANAKA., **TAM.**- VERKADALAI, NILAKADALAY., **TELUGU**.- VEERUSA NAGALU.

A. HYPOGAEA is one of the most important oil-seed crops of the warmer regions of the World.

It is a small diffused herb which grows errect (height 1-2'), or trails on the grounds and bears small yellow flowers. The leaves are hairy and compound. Each leaf is having two pairs of opposite leaflets. The flowers are 5 to 7 cms. long, yellow and sessile and develop singly or in clusters of two to four. The calyx consists of 5 fused sepals in the form of a tube, often mistaken for a pedicel. The corolla is a papilionaceous and the staminal column (consisting of ten monadelphous stamens) are adnate at the base and attached on the margin of the calyx tube. The ovary is monocarpellary and is surrounded by a long filiform style. The development of the seed after fertilization is underground and the pods are produced in the form of bunches. The pod is about 1-2" long cylindrical reticulate and indehiscent, each containing seeds, Each seed is covered by a coloured papery covering or skin i.e. the seed coat. The seed coat ranges from white to pink, purple, shades of brown or red, and consists of two white fleshy cotyledons rich in oil and protein. Brazil is considered as the home of the groundnut, but now it is cultivated in all tropical and subtropical countries. The major countries producing this crop are India, China, the U.S.A. and West Africa. It is also cultivated in Burma, the East Indies, Nigeria and in Southern Europe.

The plant is reported to have been introduced into India in the 16th century. Its cultivation extended at a phenomenal rate since 1900, and today India is the largest producer of groundnuts accounting for more than 35% of World Production.

MEDICINAL USE : The fruit and oil are astringent to the bowels. The oil is aperient, emolient and used as subsitute for Oilve Oil.

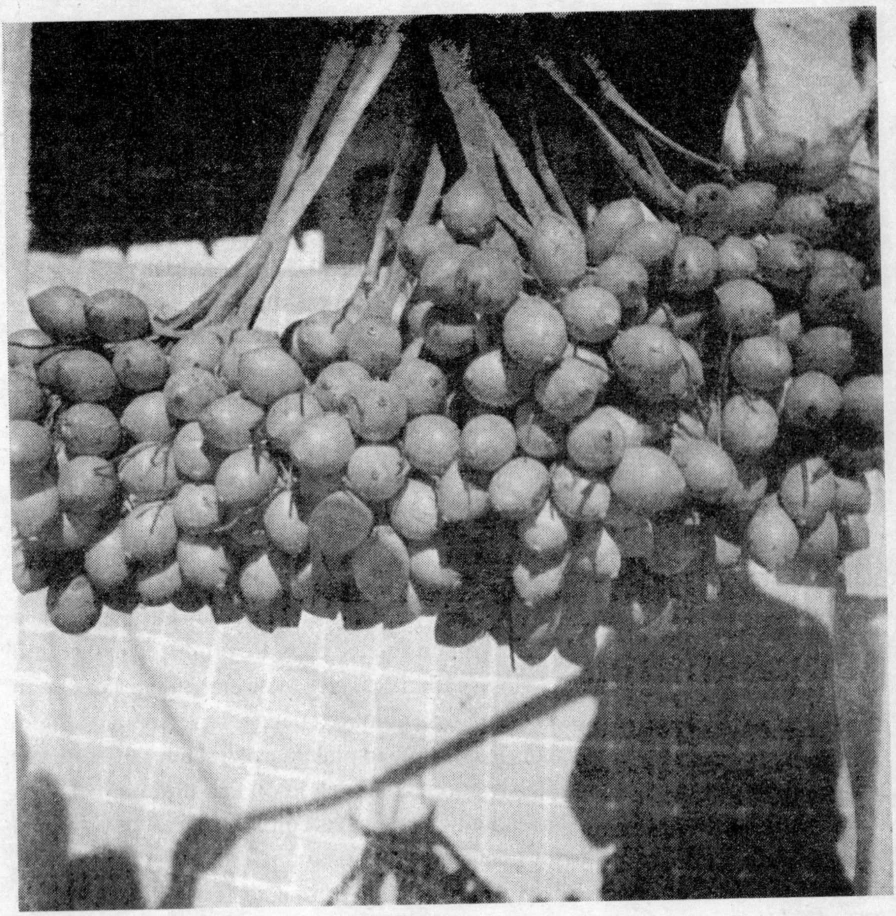

PALMACEAE

ARECA CATECHU LINN
(ARECA NUT, SYN. A. CATHECUL)
BETEL NUT (PALM)

SANS.-POOGIPHALAM., **ARAB.**-FOJAL., **PERS.- HINDI.**-SUPARI., **TELGU**-VAKKA, KAZHANGU., **TAM.**- PAKKU, PAAKKUMARAM., **KAN.**-ADIKE., **MAL.**- ADAKKA., **BEN. GUJ. & MAR.**- SUPARI., **ENG.**-ARECANUT, BETALNUT PALM., **BOM.**-SOPARI.

This is a erect palm tree with a tall slender, smooth and whitish stem. Stem: erect, annulate, trunk solitary, 40-100 ft. Leaves: Pinnate; 4-6 ft; leaflets numerous, 1-2 ft; upper confluent, quite glabrous. The lower portion of the petiole is expended into a broad tough, sheath like growth. The inflorenscence is a spadix encased into spathe and comprises much branched rachis which bears male and female flowers. Spadices intrefoliar, branched spathe glabrous, compressed. Rachis start compressed, branched with filiform tips bearing more or less distichous minute male flowers. solitary at the bases and axils of the branches; I. Female flower much larger, few at the base of the branches; perianth acrescent; sepals and petals, Orbicular, imbricate the petals with acute valvate tips, Ovary 1-celled, Stigma 3, Sessile, Ovule basal, erect male flowers many, minute, sepals small; petals obliguely lanceolate, valvate, stamens 3 or 6 anthers, basifixed, connate, erect.

Fruit 1½-2", smooth, orange or scarlet betalnut; ovoid or oblong, stigmas terminal seed with a truncate base, embryo basilar-

There are about 24 species belonging to tropical Asia and Australia cultivated in the hot damp regions of Asia and the Malayan Islends. It is now grown along the coasts or Karnataka, Kerala, Tamil Nadu, West Bengal, Assam and Maharashtra. It is also grown in Ceylon and Burma and it has been extended to Medagaskar and East Africa.

MEDICINAL USES: Nuts are chiefly used in Veterinary practice as a vermifuge for tapeworm and for the preparation of dentrifices. Powdered nut is useful in checking diarrhoea and also in urinary diseases. It is also used in snake-bite.

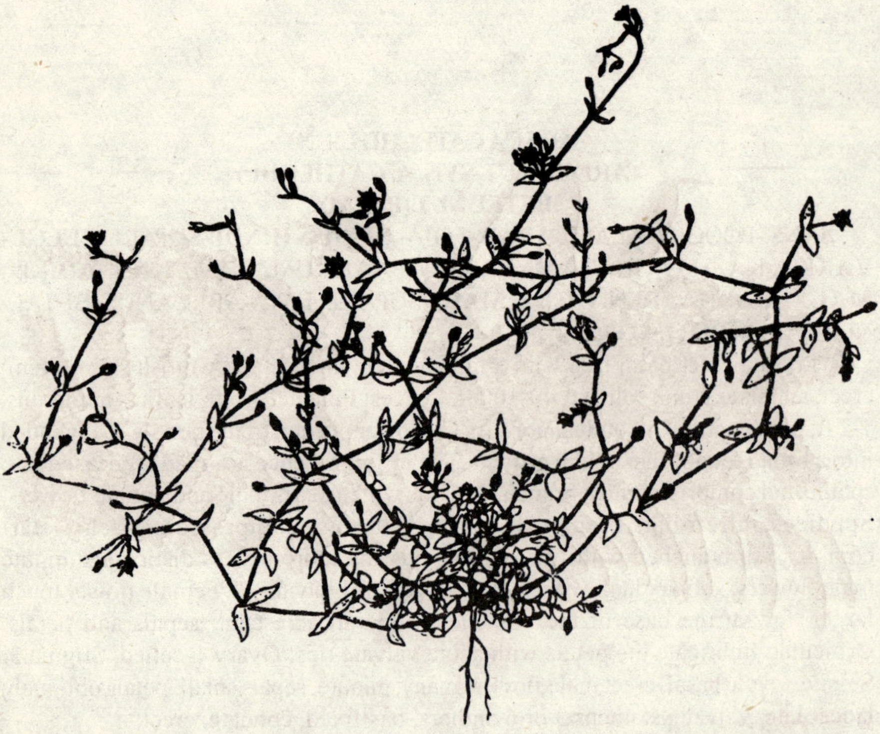

CARYOPHYLLACEAE

ARENARIA SERPYLLIFOLIA LINN

It is a small, decumbent or suberect, much branched tufted annual. Branches glandular throughout. Leaves ovate or elliptic ovate. Flowers white in many flowered cymes. Stamens 5-6 anthers pinkish or whitish. Style 3. Capsules ovoid, seeds black, tubercles.

Flowers and fruits from February to March.

Found as weed in moist places at the end of the winter season, subtropical and temperate Himalayas from Nepal to Kashmir, Rohilkhand and the Punjab and West Tibet.

MEDICINAL USE : It is used in china for bladder, diseases, considered valuable for calculus troubles and acute and chronic cystitis.

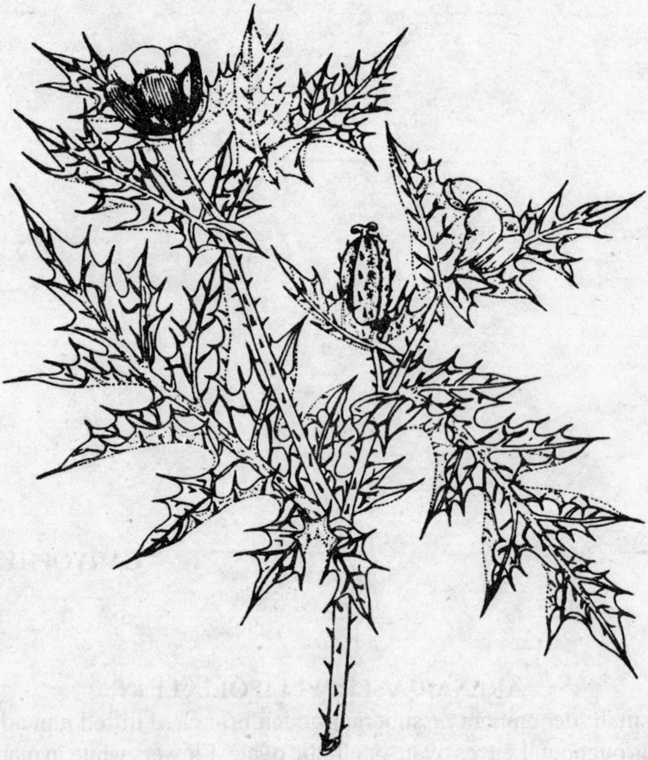

PAPAVERACEAE

ARGEMONE MEXICANA LINN

SANS.- SRIGALA-KANTAKA., **MAL**.-PONNUMMATTAM., **H&B**.-SHIOLKANTA., **P.**-SIAKANTA., **TAMIL**- BRAMADANDU., **TELGU**-BRAHMADANDI., **LOCAL NAME**- UNT- KATERA, KATELI KANDIA., **BEN**.-SHIEL-KANTA., **ENG.**- TELLOW THISTLE, PRICKLY POPPY., **GUJ.**- DARUDI., **HINDI**-PITADHATORA., **KAN.**- ARASINA, UNAMATTA., **MAR.**-KANTA-DHOTRA., **PUNJABI**-KANDIARI.

It is distinguished by its prickly stems & leaves and yellow-poppy like flowers. It is a short herb. Stem and branches are woody. Leaves are clasping sinuate, pinnatifid, prickly and glaucous. Flowers yellow with red stigma. Capsules are erect, prickly dehising by valves. Seeds black. The flowers and fruits are found in october to April.

It is naturalized world wide in warm countries. In India it is found up to 5000 ft. in waste lands and along road sides.

MEDICINAL USE : The root is used in chronic skin diseases. Seeds are laxative; euretic; expectorant demulcent, yellow juice of plant used for dropsy, jaundice and cutaneous infections. Its oil is purgative used for nervous affections. seeds are entid to snake poison.

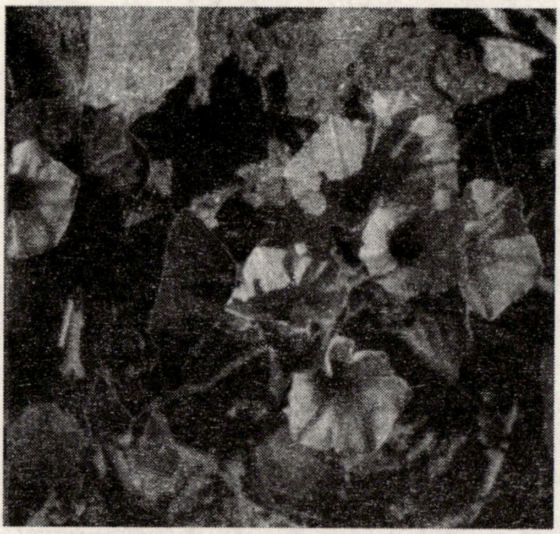

CONVOLVULACEAE

ARGYREIA SPECIOSA SWEET
SYN. A NERVOSA (BRUM F.) BOJ. ALSO)
(LETTOSOMIA NERVOSA ROXB.)
THE ELEPHANT CREPPER

SANS.-SAMUDRA PALAKA., **HINDI.**-SAMANDAR-KA-PAT., **BENG.**-BICHTARAK., **MAR.**-SAMUDRA SOKA., **S. INDIA.**- SAMUNDRA PALA., **LOCAL NAME.**-GHABEL, BANSA.

It is a large extensively climbing herb. Stems stout, white tomentose. Leaves 3-12" in diameter, glabrous above even before unfolding, ovate-cordate acute glabrous above persistently white tomentose beneath; petiole long. Peduncles long and stout usually 3-6", white tomentose; Bracts large, foliar, outer bracts 1 and 1/2". Bracts ovate-lanceolate acute thin soft woolly and decidous. Flowers rosy-purple in sub capitate cymes. Sepals ultimately 2/3" diameter, ovate, coriaceous woolly. Corolla 2-3" tubular, woolly funnel-shapped, rosy. Fruit brown yellow stout nearly dry; 3/4" in diameter, globose apiculate.

It is found throughout India (except in the dry. Western regions) upto and elevation of 1,000. It is found from Assam to Belgium and Mysore; frequent in Bengal plain. Distribution Java; also from China, Mauritius, cultivated.

MEDICINAL USE : The root is regarded as alterative and tonic, and is useful in rheumatism and diseases of the nervous system. The under surface of the leaf is densely pubescent, and is an irritant. It is used to promote maturation of boils, and as a rubifacient in skin diseases.

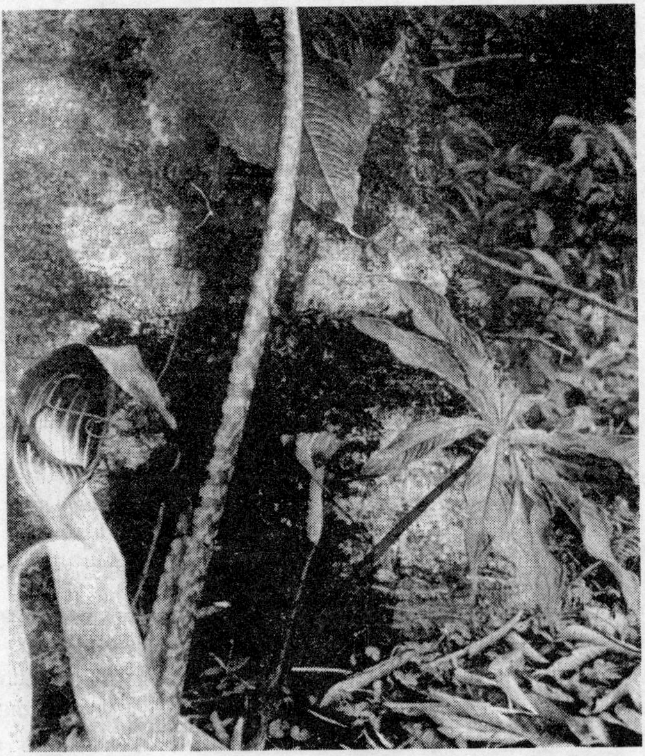

ARACEAE

ARISAEMA CURVATUM KUNTH
Syn. A TORTUOSUM SCHOTT
Syn. A. JACQUEMONTIL RLUME-RUMPH
Pun.-DON, NEP.- BIRBANKA

BENG: BIRMON., **HINDI & PUNJABI-** GURIN, KIRI KI KURI, SAMP KI KHUMB., **KAN.-** AWU-MARI-GIDDA., **MAR.-** SAPKANDA, SAPKENELA., **TAM.-** KATTU-SENAI, MUNDARI-HURING CHAKKED, SANTAL - BIRMANI, TUUYA-JONDRA

A curvatous herb, tubers spheroidal attaining 5"in diameter. Leaves 2-3, leaflets 5-18 semile or petrolulate ovate or linear-laneeolate sub-candately-acuminate, tube of green spathe about as long as the large incumbed broadly cymbiform acuminate limb, appendage narrowed from the base to the tip erect then porrect and again erect. Petiole 1-3 ft. green or with the sheaths mottled with pumple. 1 leaflets 8-18", pale green or purplish, lobe sub-cylindrical, gaping, gradually dilating into the limb. Spadix uni or bisexual, appendge like a rat's tail, quite smooth very common and varying greatly in shape, the numbers and proportions and breath of the leaflets, colour of the spathe, and monoccious or dioceious flowers.

They are rendered from temperate and sub-tropical Himalayas, alt, Brooft; from Simla and Bhutan. The Khasia Hills, Mannipure, the Western Ghats, from the Konkan to Malabar; at 3000-7000 ft.

MEDICINAL USE: Roots are employed to kill worms which infest cattle. Plant is poisonous and seeds are given with salt for colic in sheep. Root is also antheromintic (Chopraetal; 1956 Nadkarni 1954).

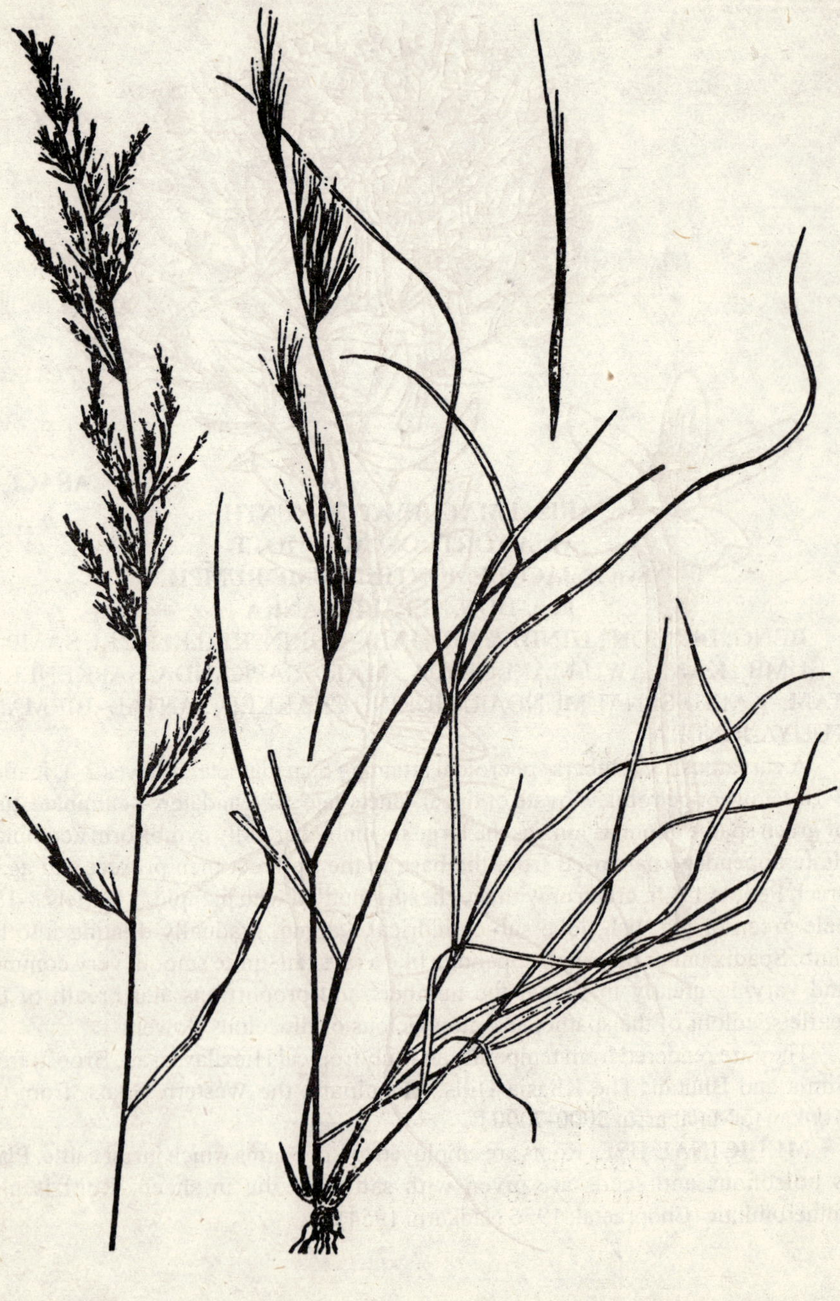

GRAMINEAE

ARISTIDA ADSCENSCIONIS LINN.
(Syn. A. DEPRESSA RETZ
Locally known as LAMP :

It is a genus of slender, annual or perennial grasses, comprising about 160 temperate and sub-tropical species. About 12 species are known to occur in India. These are low grasses with little foliage and are characterised by narrow, awned spikelet.

It is annual or perennial, panicle contracted, branches short or elongate and naked below, spikelets ¼-1/3" acute, glume I accuminate not awned, II obtuse or emarginate and mueronate not awned articulate at the base. Stem 6"-3, tufted, usually almost filiforn, rarely as thick as a crowsquill, smooth. Leaves very narrow, smooth or scaberulous 30 X 0.2 cm. Panicle 3-12"; subsimple or compound, rachis and capillary branches nearly smooth; branches very short with green or purplish, glume. I, 1/3-¼"; acute; II ¼-1/3"; tip truncate mueronate, III 1/5-¾"; smooth or scabrid; middle branch of awn 1/3-2/3"; rarely". Caryopsis as long as the glume. The flowering and fruiting season is from July to October. It is found throughout the plains and low Hills of India, Burma and Ceylon, ascending to 8,000 ft. in Kashmir.-Distribution. Most warm countries.

Locally it is common and abundant on the ridge in dry, gravelly soils and depressions and also in cultivated fields and near canal banks, forming dense tufts in local patches.

MEDICINAL USE : In Madagascar an Ointment consisting of Land and the ashes of the flowers is used topically for itch and ring worm.

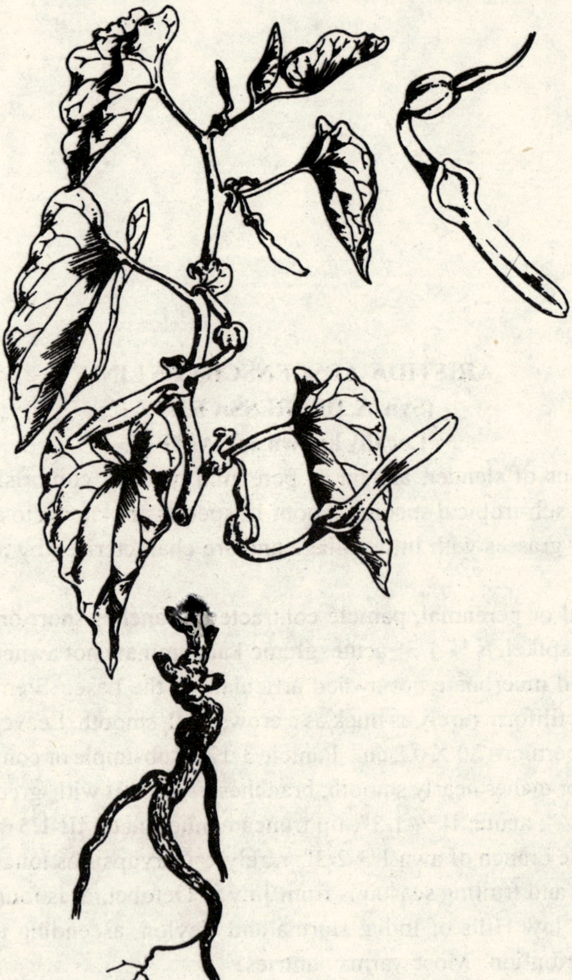

ARISTOLOCHIACEAE

ARISTOLOCHIA BRACTEATA RETZ.
(THE BRACTEATED BIRTHWIRT)

SANS.- DHUMRA - PATRA., **HINDI.**- KIRAMAR., **GUJ.**- KIDAMARI, GUDHATEE., **MAR.**- KIDEMAR, GANDHANI., **TAM.**- ADUTHINAPALAI., **MAL.**- ATU-TINLAP., **TEL.**- GADIDHA - GADAPPA., **KAN.**- ADUMUTTADA-GIDA, SANNAJALI - HULLU., **URIYA.**- PANIRI., **ENG.**- WORM - KILLER., **BOMBAY**.- KIDAMARI., **LOCAL NAME**- KIRAMAR.

It is slender, prostrate perennial herb Leaves entire or lobed. (4-6 X 3.5 - 4.5 cm.; glaucous, reiniform or broad ovate, deep cordate, basal lobes rounded, Petiole with a dilated base 1-1 ½" and with often the stipule like leaf of an undeveloped bud in the axil. Stem often twining, decumbent slender branches 12-18", angled and straight Perianth coloured tube inflated at the base, then contracted, hairy within; limb dilated, obliguely 1-2 lipped. Flowers 50x5 mm. dark purple, solitary, tubular with trumpet-shaped mouth with revolute edges, villous, with purple hairs. Anthers 6 rarely 5, or more style very short, 3-6 lobed. Capsule pyriform, oblong-ellipsoid, ribbed, 2-5 x 1.5 cm. It is septicidely 6-valved or splitting through the placentas. Seeds various, often covered with the remains of the placenta 7 triangular, cordate.

It is found in the upper Gangetic Plain, Bengal, the Western Peninsula, and in the North-West upto Bundelkhand. It grows abundantly on the black soil of the deccan and Gujarat and keeps on bloming for the most part of the year. It is also reported from Ceylon, Arabia and Tropical Africa.

MEDICINAL USE : The whole plant is used as purgative and anthelmintic. A decoction of root was found efficacious in expelling round worms.

The juice of leaves is applied to foul and neglected uleers to kill the worms and maggots. Bruised leaf powder mixed with castor oil is applied in cases of obsinate eczema.

It is also given in syphilis, gonorhoea and skin diseases (Nadkarni, 1954).

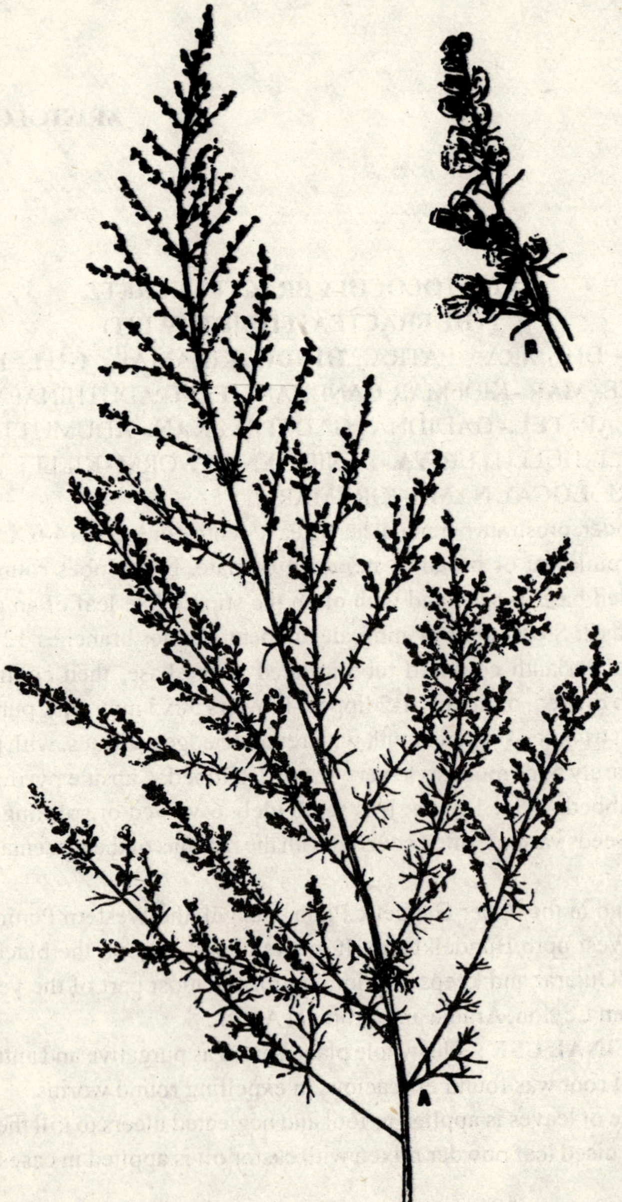
B
A

COMPOSITAE
ASTERACEAE

ARTEMISIA VULGARIS LINN.
(Syn. A. VULGARIS AUCT, NON L.)
(Syn. A. NILAGIRICA CLARKE) PAMP,

SANS.-NAGADAMANI, **HINDI.**-NAGADOUNA, **BENG.**- NAGADONA, **TAM.**-MASHIBATTIRI, MACHIPATRI, **TEL.**- MACHIPATRI, **PUNJ.**-TERKHA, **ENG.**-INDIAN WORM WOOD FLEA BANE.

Artemesia is a bitter aromatic herb or low shrub, often with much divided leaves and inconspicucous flowers borne on numerous small heads, often forming thickets 6-8 ft. high, with branches as thick as the thumb, hoary pubescent or tomentose, stems leafy paniculately branched. Leaves: Large ovate lobed laciniate or cut into filiform segments or 1 - 2 - pinnatipartite white-tomentose beneath rarely hoary or green on both surfaces, lobes acute, ir regularly serrate or lobulate lower petioled, upper sessile or petioled with stipule-like basal lobes, upper most linear-lanceolate entire; nearly 7" long and broad: heads 1/8 - 1/6" long ovoid or subglobose clustered or senate subsecured in short or long suberrect or horizontal panicled racemes, heterogamous or homogamous disciform; outer fl. female, 1-serrate, fertile, very slender 2-3 toothed; disk fl. heremaphrodite, fertile or sterile, limb 5-fid. Involucre ovoid, subglobose or hemispheric; bracts woolly or glabrate, outer small herbaceous, inner almost wholly scarrious; receptacle flat or raised, naked or hirsute. Anther-bases obtuse, entire. Style-arms of hermaphrodite, with truncate usually penicillate tips, often connate in the sterile flower. Achenes very minute, ellipsoid oblong or subovoid, faintly striate; pappus O.

It is reported throughout the mountainous districts of India, at an elevation of 5-12000 ft. in the Western Himalaya, and 5-8000 ft. in Sikkim, the Khasia, Ava and Martaban Mts. Mt. Aboo, in Marwar. The Western Ghats, from the concan, Southwards to Ceylon, Distribution Temperate Europe and Asia, Siam, Java.

MEDICINAL USE : Roots are used as tonic and antispasmodic, and herb as anthelmintie, antispasmodic and stomachic. An infusion of leaves and flowering tops, given in nervous, spasmochi infections, and in asthma.

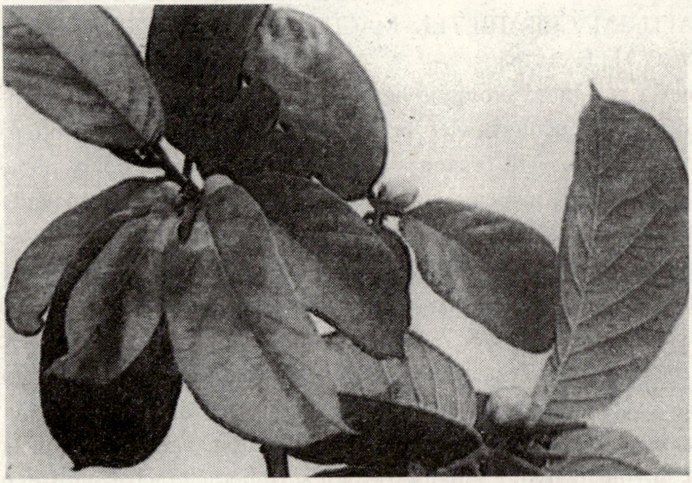

MORACEAE

ARTOCARPUS LAKOOCHA ROXB

LOCAL NAME- BARHAL., **SANS.**- LAKUCHA., **HINDI.**- DAHUA, BARHAL., **BENG.**-DAHUA, DEPHAL, **BOMB.**- LAHU., **TEL.**- KAMMAREGU, LAKUCHAMU., **TAM.**- ILAGUSAM., **MARATHI.**- WOTOMBA., **ENG.**- MONKEYJACK, LAKOOCH., **KAN.**-VATEHAULI., **BURM.** MYANKDOK., **TRADE.**- LAKUCH.

A deciduous tree with a clear straight or bent stem, generally 20 - 30 ft high and upto 8' in girth with a spreading crown branchlets softly tomentose or villous. Bark fissured, dull black. Leaves thinly coriaceous very large 20 - 25 x 10 - 15 cms; alternate, entire or denticulate, or pinnately lobed, penninerved nerves 8 - 12 pairs. Oblong elliptic or subobovate cuspidate softly pubescent reticulate beneath base usually rounded, stipules small, caducous, ½ inch, lanceolate; pubescent. Petiole: ½ - 1"; pubescent at length glabrous. Flowers: monoecious, densely crowded on globose or oblong unisexual solitary axillary (rarely terminal) receptacles, often mixed with bracts. Male flower: receptacles orange yellow; flowers monandrous ½ - 1" in diameter, oblong or globose, pubescent; bracteoles clavate, puberulous; Perianth 2 - 4 lobed or-partite; lobes obtuse, cancave, valvate or slightly imbricate. Stamen 1, erect, Pistillode O. Female flower: Perianths tubular, connate and comfluent below with the receptacle, mouth minute. Ovary - straight: style central or lateral, stigma entire, rarely 2 - 3 fid. Ovule pendulous. Fruit clusters lobulate, nearly smooth yellow, velvety when ripe. Large fleshy oblong cylindrical globose or sublobed receptacle, clothed with the greatly enlarged fleshy perianthus and carpels (anthocarps) which have hardened spinous or truncate or pyramidae or plain tips. Achenes deeply sunk in the fleshy mass. Seeds exalbuminous; embryo straight or incurved, cotyledons fleshy equal or unequal, radical very short, superior. Flowering and fruiting season is April to June, every year.

It is reported from Tropical Himalaya, ascending to 4000 ft; from Kumaon eastwards to Burma, and South wards to Travancore and Malacca. It is met within Bihar, Orissa and the Central Provinces. In the West Coast it is found from Konkan Southwards to Malabar and Travancore. Locally it is commonly cultivated in the Sabzimandi and Sarai Rohilla fruit orchards for its edible fruits, used either raw, ripe, cooked or as pickle.

MEDICINAL USE : Ripe fruit is demulcent, nutritive and laxative, while unripe fruit is astringent. Seeds are purgative. Bark in powder form applied to sores to draw out purulent matter in infusion applied to small pimples and cracked skin. The picee of Cotton soaked in its latex when kept inside tooth cavity is a good source of remedy from pain.

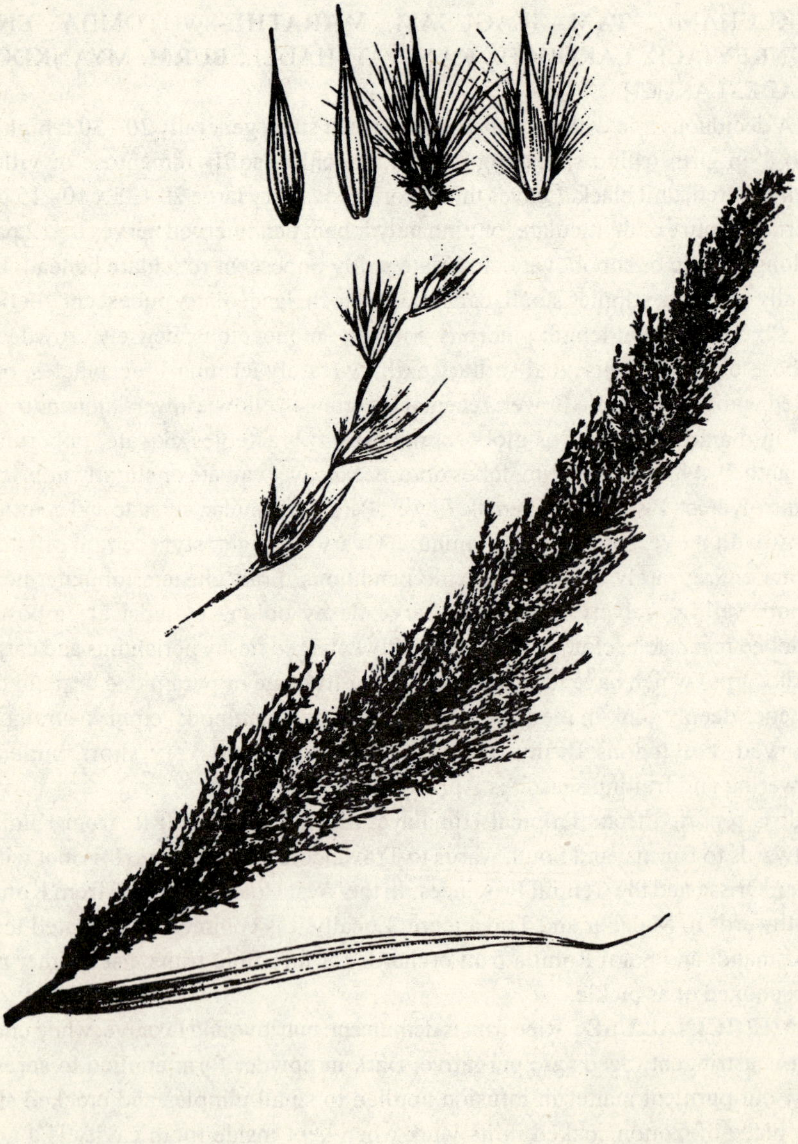

GRAMINEAE

ARUNDO DONAX LINN

H- BARANAL., **B.**- GAHANAL., **P.**- BANSI., **SANS.**- KADILAKA., **TAM.**- KORUKKAI., **TEL.**- ADAUI-KEEKASA-GADDI., **ASSAM**-GABANALI., **GARWAL**- NALDURA., **U.P.**- NAL, NARKUL., **LOCAL NAME**- NARHAL, NARSAL.

A tall, perenenial grass with stout erect culms 3 - 6 m. high stems hollow, many - noded, green, glabrous and smooth. Leaves linear lanceolate, tapering to a fine point 30 - 60 x 2.5 cm. inflorescence a large erect terminal plumose panicle, 30 - 60 x 10 cm. Branches scabrous erect or dropping. Spikelets 8 - 10 x 2 mm. light brown, usually 2 flowered. Involucral glumes glabrous, floral ones long hairy on the beek in the lower half. Flowers and fruits - September to February.

It is cultivated often as hedges in gardens. It is also reported from lower Himalayas from Kashmir to Nepal upto 1200 ft. from Punjab to Sylhet and the Naga hills upto 1600 - 2000 m. Coorg and Nilgiris hills.

MEDICINAL USE : A decoction of rhizome is used as an emollient and diuretic. It is also used as a stimulant for menstrual discharge and to diminish the secretion of milk.

It contains an alkaloid donoxine and donaxarine which shows a rise in blood pressure and contracts isolated intestine and uterus in domesticated pets.

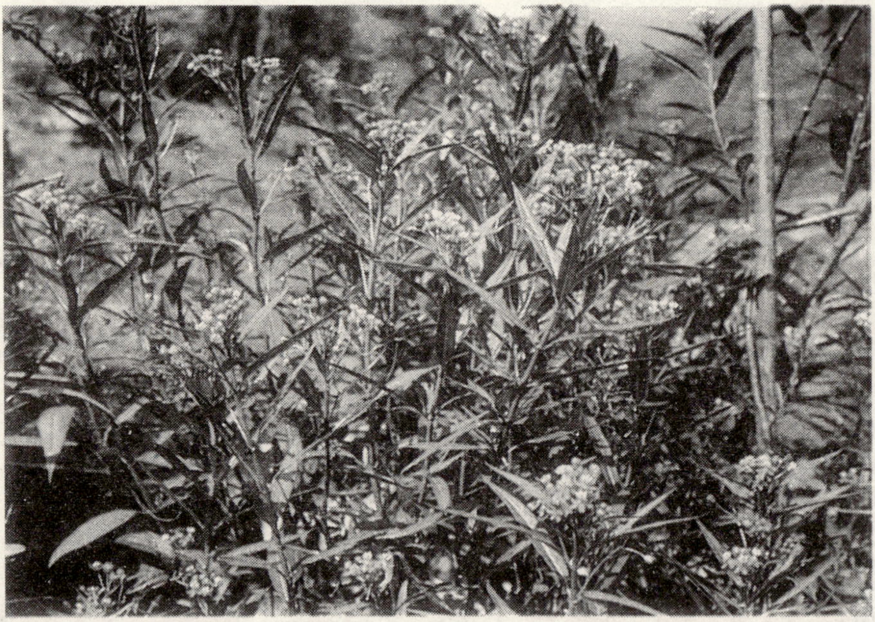

ASCLEPIADACEAE

ASCLEPIAS CURASSAVICA LINN.

MARATHI.- KURKI HH., **BO & P.**- KAKATUNDI.

It is a perennial herb, leaves ovate to chordate thin and acute having long leaf stalks twinning plant. Flowers white tinged with pink in long stalked branched rounded clusters. Each flower is 18-12 mm across with 5 narrow lanceolate spreading lobes & a much shorter deeply 5 lobed cup-shaped corona; calyx lobes lanceolate, hairy. It is grown in gardens naturally occuring in south India & Bengal.

MEDICINAL USE : Root is purgative, remedy for piles and gonorrhoea, also used as an emetic and in the treatment of warts and caneerous growths. Juice of the leaves is anthelmintic, sudorific, used for arresting haemorages and gonorrea. Plant is used in phthisis and is poisonous.

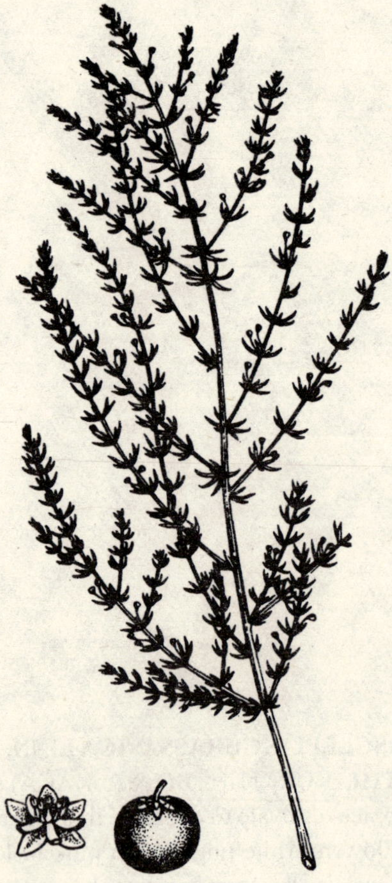

LILIACEAE

ASPARAGUS ADSCENDENS ROXB.

HINDI, MARATHI & GUJ.- SAFED or SAFETA MUSLI, SATAVAR., **MAL.**- SHEDEVELI., **TAM.- TAUNIRVITTAN**- KIZHANGU., **TELUGU**- TSALLOGADDA., **LATIN**- ASPARAGUS ADSCENDENS., **SANS.**- SAFED MUSLI, GARHWAL JHIRMA., **BENG.**- TAL MULI., **M.**- PANDRI MUSLI., **GUJ.**- UJALI MUSLI.

It is a small herb nearly 1 ft. tall. The leaves are 8 - 10 "long and broad." The roots are double and jointed.

It grows in Punjab, Raiwala forests near Hardwar and Mussoorie hills.

MEDICINAL USE : It is helpful in checking leucorrea and increasing milk production during lactation.

Root is used as demulchant and also in diarrohea and dysentry.

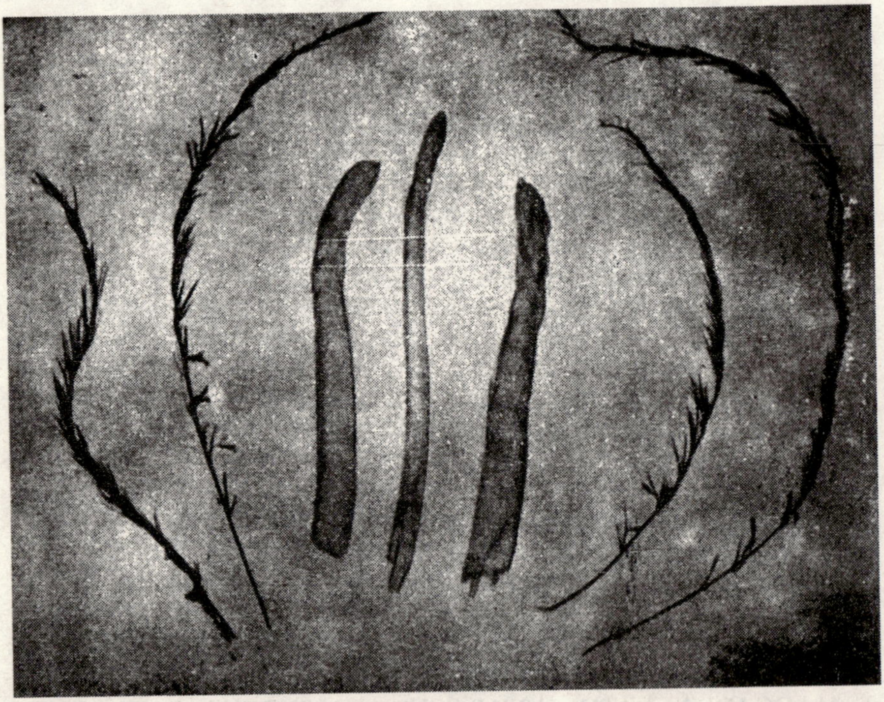

LILLIACEAE

ASPARAGUS OFFICINALIS LINN

H- HALYUN., **B-** HIKUA., **ARAB & PERSIAN-** HALGUN.

It is a herbaceous dioceious perenial hardy strongly erect, much branched. It is distinguished by the absence of leaves, in their place are clusters of needle - like cladodes (stem performing the function of leaves) and the leaves are reduced to scales or spines. Stem tall, glabrous and slightly glaucous; the shoots bearing prominent scale - like leaves. Cladodes thread like, one to several in the axil, flowers 1-4 axillary tiny, companulate, yellowish, green dioceous fruit a berry small red and on maturing rounded 3 cells, seed 1-9 per berry; fleshy. Woody rhizome black in colour rounded underground, developed with fleshy cord like roots, fibrous, extending over a large area.

Its principal producer are Germany, U.S.A., Spain, France and Taiwan. It is also cultivated in India for more than last 50 years.

MEDICINAL USE : The plant is demul, diure, laxt, cardiac sedative, tonic aphrodis, roots are more diur. than shoots in infusion used against jaundice and conjestive torpor of the liver.

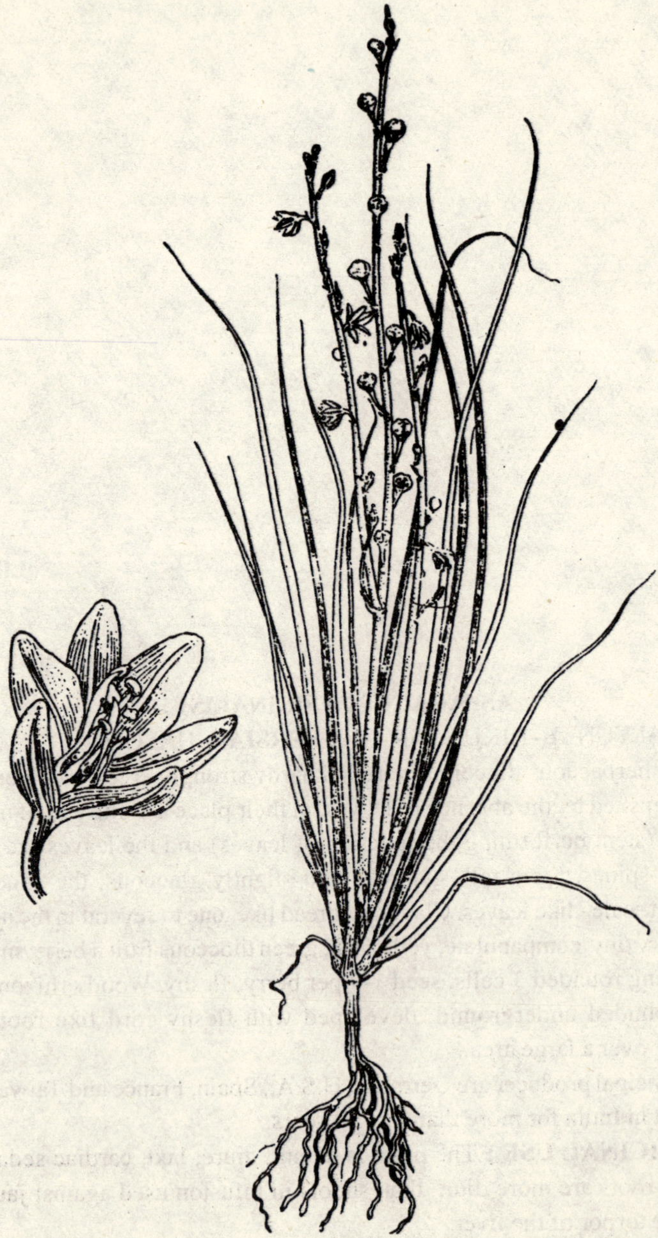

LILIACEAE

ASPHODELUS TAENIOFOLIUS CAV

HINDI- BOKAT, PYAJH., **PUNJAB-** BINGNAK-BIJ, BOKAT, PIAZI., **GUJ.-** DUNGRUN., **ARAB & PERS.**-ASHRASH., **LOCAL NAME-** PIAZI.

It is an errect, glabrous annual, Stemless herb variable insize. It is with short rhizomes. The leaves are radincal, teretc hollow 15-30 cm. linear, accuminate scapes several, simple or branched in tghe upper part, 45-90 cml flowers white with a central red brown streak, in lax racemes. Bracts broad obate. Perianth lohes oblong. Capsules globose loculicidel, valves deeply wrinkled, seeds black trigonous. The flowering and fruting season is Jan. to June.

It is common winter weed of Cultivation in mosit locatities. Also found in moist, waste and unused ground, It is distributed through out Indo-Gangetic plain, from Bengal to Punjab.

MEDICINAL USE : Seed yield an oil which may be of therapeutic value in preventing aterosclerosis due to its high linoleic acid content. The seeds are diuretic. They are applied externally to ulcers and inflamed parts. (Ind. J. Pharm. 1964,26,80)

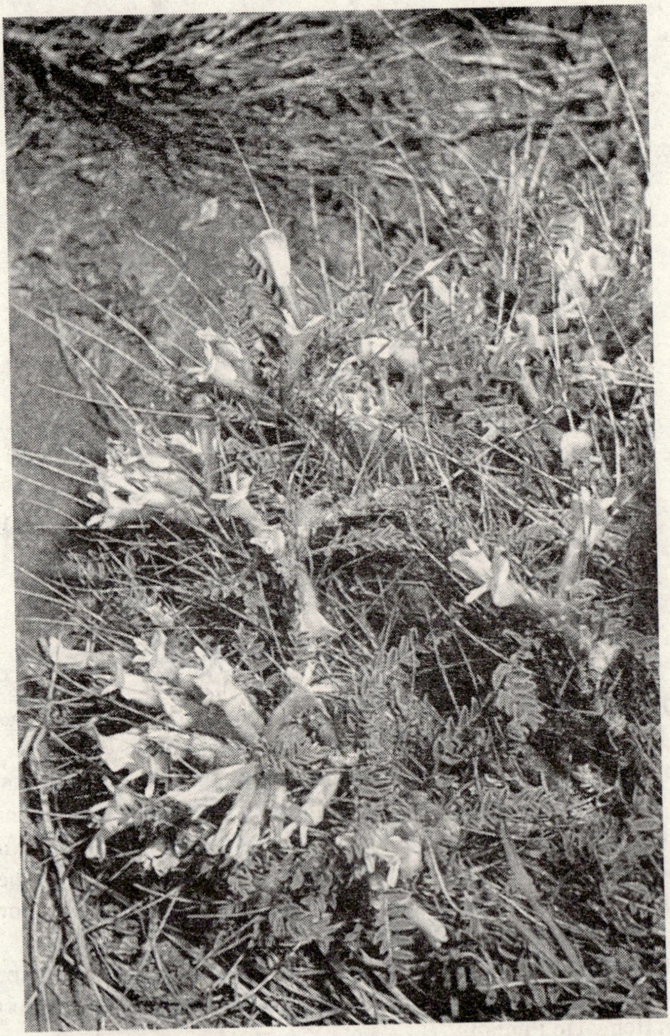

PAPILIONACEAE

ASTRAGALUS CANDOLLEENUS LINN

It is a large shrub, spinous, the spines commonly formed by the stiffening of the petiole or midrib of the leaves when the blade falls off. It is distinguished from related genera by the tubular Calyx with 5 short teeth or lobes, by the blunt-tipped keel and by the pod which is often longitudinally divided into two chambers. Stems woody, not more than a few inches long, beset below the tufts of leaves with the copious ascending woody rachises of the old leaves with the laneeolate membranous stipules still persisting.

Leaflets 17-25 leaf-rachises indurated persisting long after the leaflets. Leaves 3-4' long; leaflets oblong, obtuse, glaucous 1/4 - 1/2' long more or less silky; petioles 1-2' finely downy. Heads subsessile, dense, many flowered; pedicles 1/8 -1/6'; densely silky; bracets linear; calyx 1/2'; densely silky, teeth linear; a third as long as the tube. Corolla an inch long; wings shorter than the standard, Keel than the wings, Pod 3/4-1' long, curved, short, stalked, firm, tugrid, bilocular, 12-16 seeded.

It is reported from West Himalayas, temperate and alpine region, about 8-13,000 ft. West Tibet, Kunawar, Kashmir, Gurwhal, Kumaon. (Benthem and Hooker). It is considered a large genus of herbs or undershrubs comparising about 1600 spaces distributed in the mountainous regions, from Asia Minor through Kardistan to Iraq, Persia and North Western India.

MEDICINAL USE: A few of these species especially A. GUMMIFER labill of the source of the commercially important gum tragacanth. The best grades are used in Pharmacy, In Pharmacy it is used as a demulcent of emulsifier, and as an adhesive agent for pills and tablets, and for the suspension of insoluble powders. The best grades come from Sinyrana and other parts of the Persion gulf, and are known.as Persian or Syrian tragacanth. (Wealth of India Vol. I. Page No. 133-134).

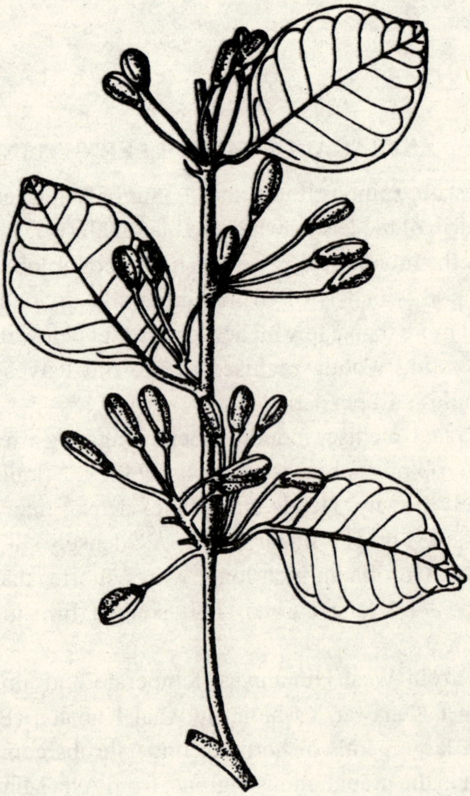

RUTACEAE

ATALANTIA MONOPHYLLA (ROXB.) DC CORREA (Syn. LIMONIA MONOPHYLLA ROXB.) (Syn. A Malabarica (Rafin).

ENG.- WILD-LIME., **GUJ.**- DODI-NIMBU., **KAN.**- KAADU-LIMBE, KADU-NIMBE., **MAL.**- MALENARAKAM, KATTUNARENGA., **MAR.**- MAKADLIMBU, THE WILD LIME., **SANS.**- ATAVI-JAMBEERA, **TAM.**- KATTUELUMICCAMPAZHAM., **TEL.**- ADAVI-NIMMA.

A large woody glabrous shrub or small tree and usually strong axillary single spine. Leaflet 1-3", ovate-oblong or elliptic, obtuse, notched or 2-lobbed at the tip, coriaceous, bright green, quite entire petiole very short, often pubescent, stipular scales subulate. Flowers 1/3- 1/2". diameter; always fascicled in the leaf axils pubescent; pedicels 1/4 - 1/2"; minutely bracteolate; buds subglobose or pyriform. Calyx rupturing irregularly. Petals obovate-oblong, obtuse. Filaments 8, rarely 5-7, connate into an irregularly cleft tube, which is anthoriferous at the top, anthers broadly ovoid ovary sessile on small. disk, 3-5 celled. Berry as large as a nutmeg, globose, like a lime. Usually 4-celled; cells 1-seeded. Roxburgh describes the flowers as shortly racemose and calyx as 4-5 parted.

It is reported from Silhet, at the foot of the Khasia Mountains, throughout the Western Peninsula, from the Concau and coromandel South Wards; Ceylon not uncommon towards the North of the Island. In India it is very popular in South, Assam and Ceylon extending to the Andamens and Burma.

MEDICINAL USE : Root is regarded as antiseptic and stimulant and leaves are used in snakebite. The berries are used in fever also yield an oil which is used in chronic rheumatism and paralysis.

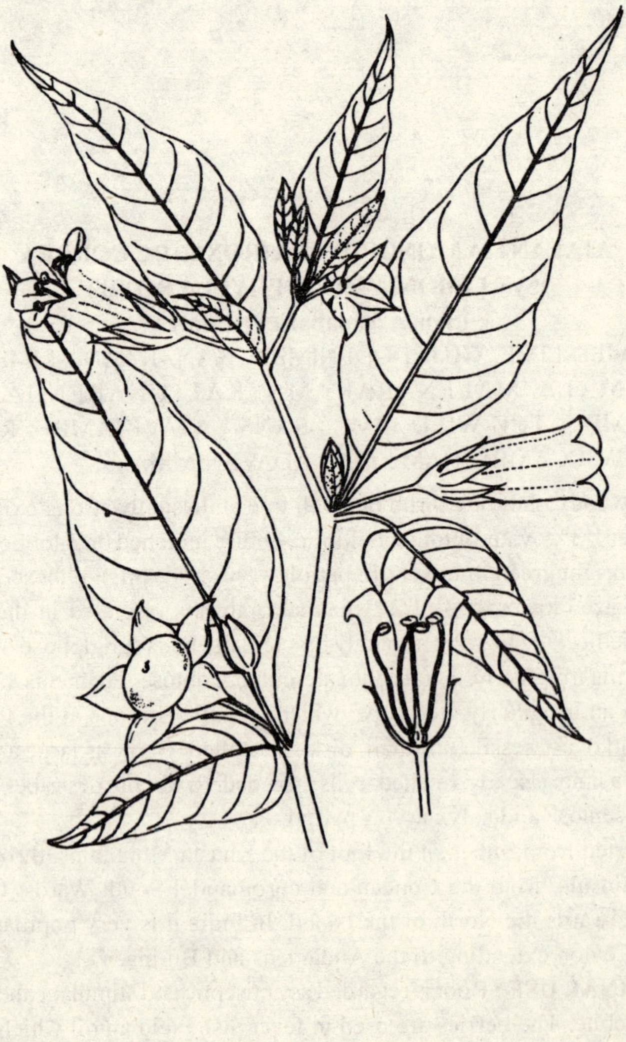

SOLANACEAE

ATROPA ACUMINATA ROYLE EX. LINDLEY
(A. BELLA-DONNA (NON L.) C.B. CLARKE)

BENG.- YEBRUJ., **ENG.**- INDIAN BELLADONNA., **HINDI.**- SAG-ANGUR., **KASH.**- MAIT-BRAND., **MAR.**- GIRBUTI., **PUNJ.**- BANTAMAKU.

It is popularly known as (Indian ATROPA' or INDIAN BELLA-DONNA). It is considered as one of the indispensable drug of plant origin. It is a tall, erect herbaceous perennial, about 3 to 5' high. The plant has got a large taproot with many lateral rootlets. The roots are woody; pale brown in colour, 6" or more in length and 3/8 - 3/4" in diameter. The roots have got small horizontal marks due to the folding of outer bark. The aerial shoots die every year in autumn and new ones arise in the following year and form a large crown. The leaves are entire, elliptic-lanceolate, stalked, acuminate, 3-6" long and 2-4" broad. The petiole is 1/2". Pedicels 1/2-1-1/2". The axillary flowers are large, bell shaped, solitary or many short-stalked, about an inch long and are dirty-purple or lucrid yellow. Calyx in flower 1/3-2/3". It is deeply 5-lobed, scarcely larger in fruit. Corolla widely tubular companulate; lobes-5, triangular and blunt imbricate in bud. Stamens attached near the base of the corolla, filaments linear hairy and swollen at base anthers oblong, dehiscing longitudinally. Ovary 2-celled; style linear, stigma obscurely 2-lobed. The fruit is a berry globular C. 1-3 cm., black purple, surrounded by the persistent calyx. Seeds many compressed embryo peripheric.

It is reported from Pakistan to Himachal Pradesh 1500-3000 m. Forests, shruberies, cultivated in Kashmir herb gardens. Flowering season January to August. The fruit is formed in October. It also occurs in Baluchistan. In general it is found from Western Himalaya, alt. 6-11000 ft. from Kashmir to Shimla, it is also distributed from Europe to the Caucasus and N. Persia.

MEDICINAL USE : The drug constitutes dried leaves, roots and other plant parts. The drug is collected when plant is in flowering. It brings about reduced sweat secretion and gestric and salivary glands. It is a very strong anti spasmodic in colic and other spasmodic indications. It is also used in asthma and whooping cough. Roots are prescribed for external applications and neuralgia, inflammations and rheumatism due to their poisonous contents. They are also used in manufacture of tinctures and plasters.

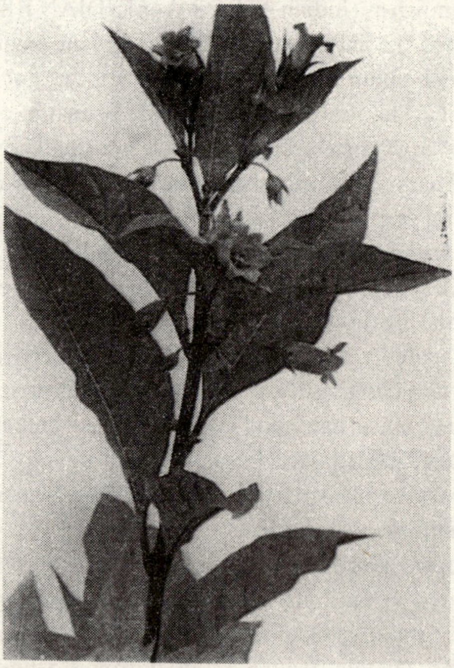

SOLANACEAE

ATROPA BELLADONNA LINN.

BENG.-YEBRAJ., **MARATHI**- GIRBUTI., **ENG.**- BELLADONNA., **ENG.**- DEADLY NIGHT-SHADE., **HINDI**- ANGURSHAPE-LUCKMUNEE, SAGNM., **PUNJ.**- SUCHI, BANTOMAKU., **KASH.**- MAITBRAND.

It is an erect herbaccous perennial with large ovate pointed leaves and pale purple dropping bell shaped flowers tinged with yellow or green flowers axillary one or many. Corolla short with fine broad blunt lobes; calyx with broad leaf lobes, filaments hairy and swollen at base. Leaves are stalked and entire, the upper ones are smaller. Fruit is a berry globular, black to purple surrounded by the persistent calyx.

It is reported from Pakistan to Himachal Pradesh 1500-3000 m. Forests, shrubberries; cultivated to a small extent in Kashmir at Baramulla, Darang and Yarikah.

MEDICINAL USE : Drug from A. ACUMINATE consists of dried leaves, roots and aerial parts of the Plant. It brings deerease in secretion of sweat gastric and salivary glands. It is used in asthma and whooping cough. Roots are used as application externally on inflamations and rheumatism. It is also used in making tinctures and plaster.

The roots of A. BELLADONA are known as Bi-radix and leaves as B. FOLIUM. Commercially and are used as tonic, antispasmodic and sedative. Preparations of Atropin from this plant is used for dilating eye pupil and for studying eye problems.

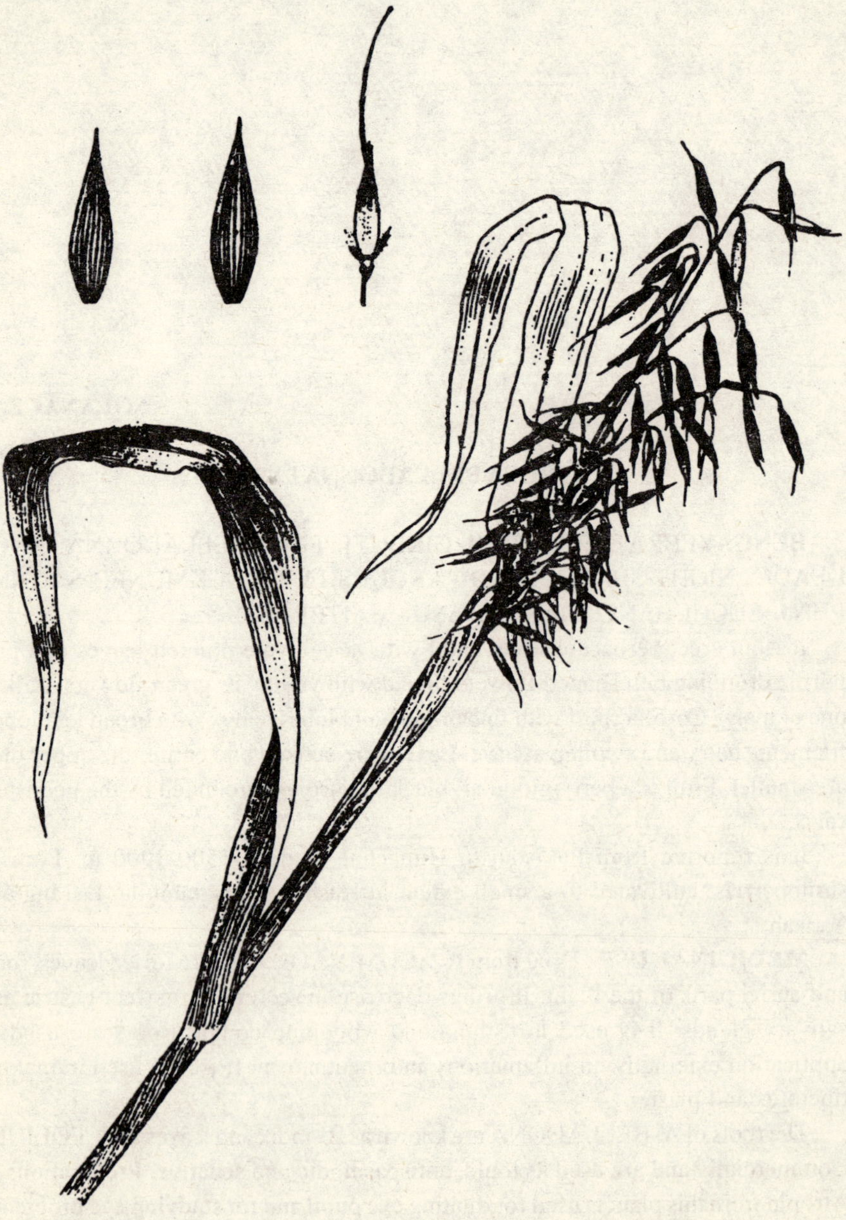

GRAMTNACEAE

AVENA SATIVA AUCT (NON LINN)
(Syn. A. STERILIS LINN. VAR. CULTA)
ENG.-OAT., **HINDI.**-JAI, JAVI

It is a large genus of annual or perennial grasses, Oats are largely self pollinated, natural crossing being negligent. Originally the crop was domesticated from the weed A. FATUA which was carried with wheat and barley. Basically it is considered as a fodder crop but oatmeal and rolled oats are used for human consumption also.

It is an erect, polished annual 1-3 ft. nodes hairy. Clums simple, moderately stout, fistular, branches equally spreading all round. Leaves: linear-lanceolate, 40-50 X 2 cm flat, scaberulous; sheaths smooth; ligule short, torn, prominent. Panicle : 6-10"; branches and pedicels scabrid. Spikelets : in large lax. terminal, open panicles, hanging from one side 25 X 33 X 4-5 mm; usually 2 to 3-flowered; rachilla hairy; top of rachilla like a peculiar "Suekermouth" shape. Florets all bisexual, one awn at the base and one or two awnless florets above or with all the florets awnless. Callus of glume III short, obtuse, Setulose; awnstout, longer than the glume; glumes I and II subequal 9- nerved, III and IV firm scaberulous, shortly 2-fid, clothed below with long fulvous hairs. Grain tightly enclosed by the floral glume and palea, free, silky.

In most of the Indian floras A. SATIVA is the most agreeable species. But Bose (1929) has pointed out that A. SATIVA of India is identical to A. BYZANTINAE C. Koch, grown in the mediterranean region. This species is now known as A. STERILIS Linn. var. culta. The flowering and fruting season is Jan-March.

It is cultivated during the cold season as pure or mixed crop. It is reported from Punjab, N.W. Himalayas and Western Tibet, in cultivated fields, ascending to 9000 ft. Sikkim, Himalaya, alt. 9000 ft; Gammie, Distribution: Temperate, Europe, N. Aftica and N Asia. Cutivated in North India from Bengal to the Indus and the Himalayas upto 12,000 ft.

MEDICINAL USE : Seeds are stimulant, laxative, antiseptie and nerve tonic. Whole grains contain vitamin B; particularly rich in fat and protein (Chopra et. al. 1956).

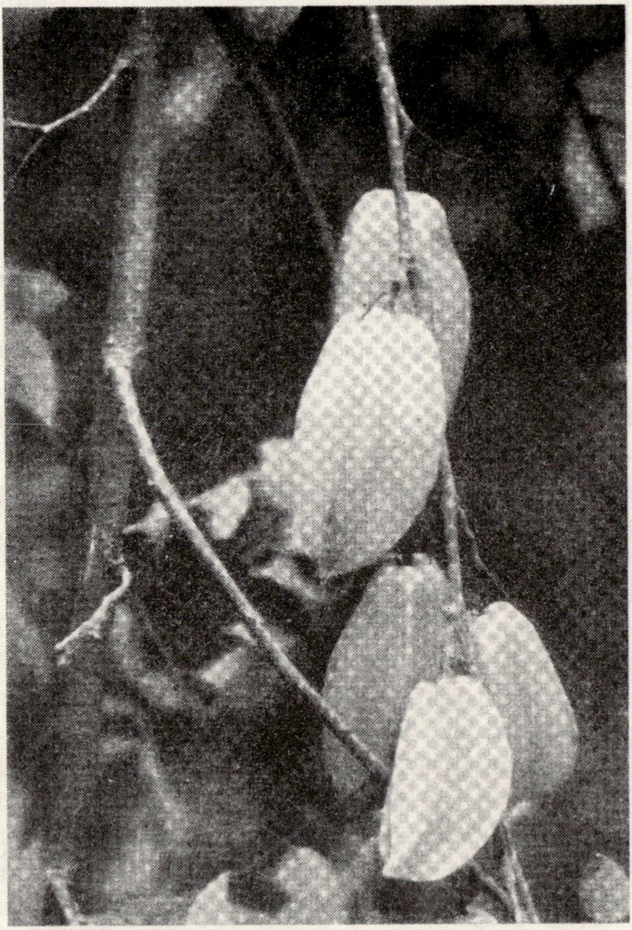

OXALIDACEAE

AVERRHOA CARAMBOLA LINN.

HINDI-KARMAL, KAMRALKH., **B.**-KAMRANGA, KARAMORA., **TAM**.-TAMARATTAI., **TEL.**-TAMATA.

It is a medium-sized tree, leaves are imparipinnate flowers are purplish borne in axillary cymes and also on main trunks and branches. Fruits are green when unripe and yellow when ripe, ovoid or ellcpsoid sacculant and acutely angled. Seeds are arillate, flowers bloom in summer and rainy season and fruits ripe in winter.

This plant is now cultivated all over India for its edible fruits. Also it is found wild in the Tropical parts of India.

MEDICINAL USE : Flowers and stems are good source of iron vitamin B and C fruit is astringent, stomachai and cooling; in the form of curry usuful in piles & scurvy.

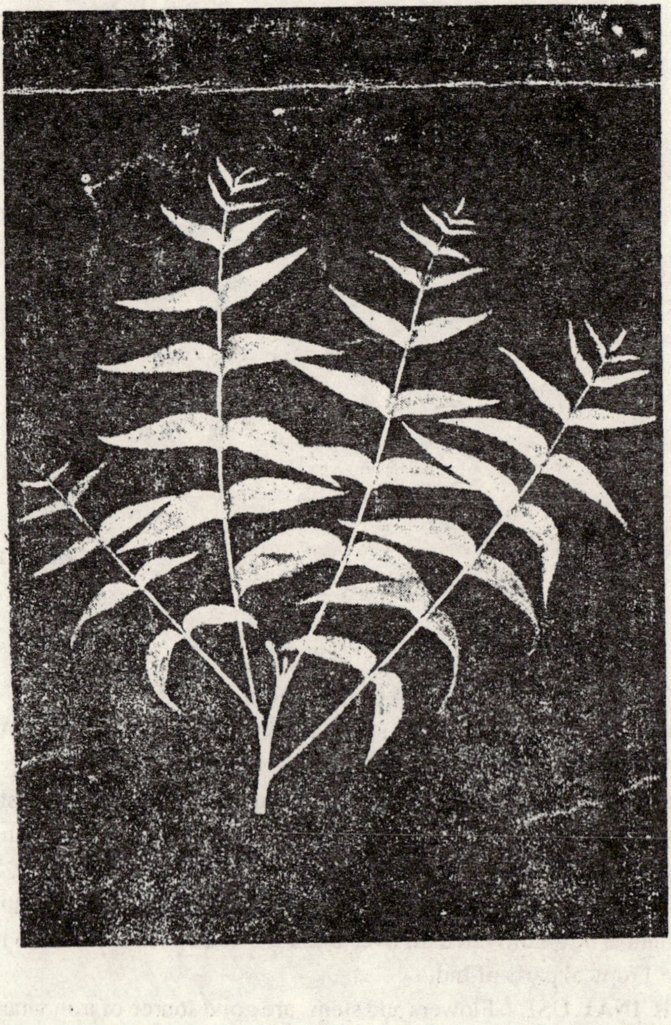

MELIACEAE

AZADIRACHTA INDICA A. JUSS
SYN. MELIA AZADIRACHTA LINN.

LOCAL NAME- BUKAIN., **BENG.-** BOMB., **HINDI-** NIM., **SANS.-** NIMBA., **GUJ.-** LIMBA., **TAM.-** VEMBU, VEPAMARAM., **TELGU-** VEPA, **MAL.-** VEPU, **PUNJ.-** NIMB., **KAN.-** BEVU, BEVINAMARA., **KON.-** BEVA-ROOKU., **ENG.-** MARGOSA TREE, 'PERSIAN LILAE', NIM or NEEM TREE., **LOCAL NAME-** NIM, NEEM., **PERS.-** NIB, AZAD- DARAKTHT., **MAR.-** KADUNIMBA

This is a genus of tall, evergreen plants. It is a large tree being 40-50 ft. high with a straight trunk and compound leaves. The stem is with a clear hole of 10-25' and a girth of 6-8'. The bark is moderately thick with longitlrdinal or oblique furrows on the outer surface. It is dark grey outside and reddish inside. Leaves. 6-15", crowded near the ends of the branches; leaflets, 1-3 by 1/2 - 1 1/2" leaf lets 9-15 opposite, subopposite or alternate laneeolate acuminate oblique or subfallcate, senate glaberous, shortly petiolate sometimes sublobed near the obtuse base. Flowers : White honey-cented, panicled axillary; pubescence often stellate-mealy; 1/6-1/5" long, 5 - mermo, calyx 5 - fid with obtuse or rounded lobes, imbricated petals shortly ciliate, anthars nearly equalling the obtuse teeth of the staminal tube, ovary 3 celled, fruit 1 - celled, 1- seeded. Drupe- oblong 1/2-3/4" long; globse, more or less dry, yellow and wrinkled at maturity. Flowering season is March-May and fruiting season is May-July. It is planted along road sides and gardens. It is referred to as "Pride of India". It is reported from all over India, often planted, as elsewhere in hot climates.

MEDICINAL USE : Almost every part of the tree has found application in indigenous medicine. The trees are planted near hospitals, especially near T.B. Sanitoriums as the air cleaned by these plants is specially benefitted to sude patients. The extract of fresh leaves is used in skin diseases and for cleaning ulcers and boils. The soft twigs of plants are used to clean teeth gums and Pyorrhoea. The bark is a good bitter tonic, astringent and antiperodic. The dry flowers are considered tonic and stomachic. The berries are regarded as Pungature, emollients and anthelmintic. The seeds give out an oil. This oil has got antisceptic properties and is popularly used in medicated bath soaps, toothpastes, lotions and creams etc. which are mainly used for skin infatrims and infections similar to it. The main constituent of neem oil is Nimbi which is very bitter. It is used for making several pharmacutical preparation including emulsions, liquors, ointments, medicinal cosmets such as Lotions, Shampoos, Creams, hair tonics and gargles. It is also used in leprosy, intestinal worms, piles and urinary diseases.

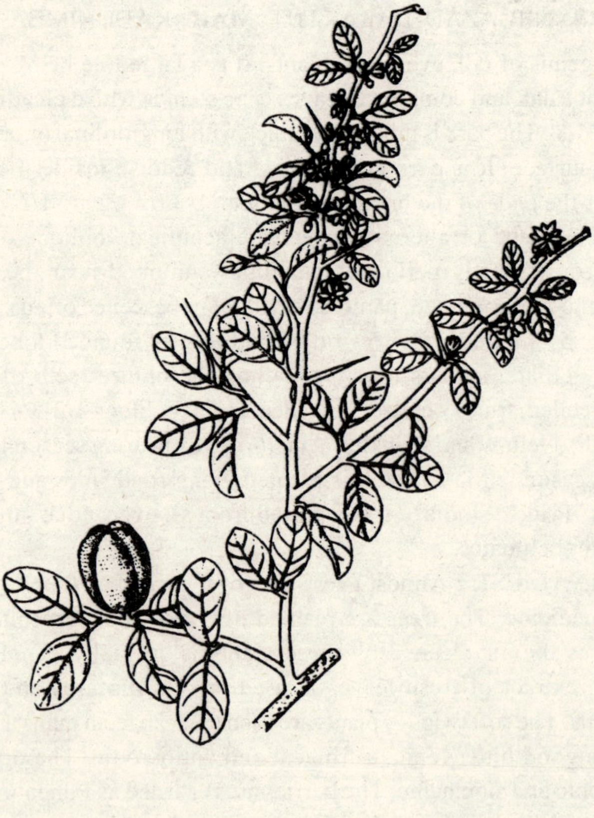

SIMAROUBACEAE
BALANITACEAE

BALANITES AEGYPTIACA (LINN) DELILE
(SYN. B. ROXBURGHI PLANCH.)

S.- INGUDI., **H & B.**- HINGAN., **BO.**- HINGANBET, HINGOT., **TAM.**- NANJUNDA., **TEL.**- GARI.

It is a small spiny evergreen tree. They are distinguished by their usually pinnate leaves and numerous small flowers in spike-like clusters or branched panicles. The fruit is a nut or capsule. Petal, and sepals 3 - 7. The stamens are twice as many as petals and a ring or cup like disk occurs between the petals and stamens. Ovary is superior 3 - 5 carpels, and united above by the style or stigmas.

Hingota flowers bloom twice, in April and October every year.

It is reported from drier parts of India. From South East Punjab and Delhi to Sikkim, Bihar, Gujarat, Khandesh and the Deccan.

MEDICINAL USE: Chemical analyses have shown that diosgenin, an important raw material for the production of oral contraceptives and steriod harmons are present in the roots, leaves, seeds and fruit pulp. The seed oil is used in the treatment of cuts and wounds and the seed extract as a hypotensive.

Hingota oil contains 31% linoleic acid which is responsible for preventing hardening of ateries (Artherosclerosis).

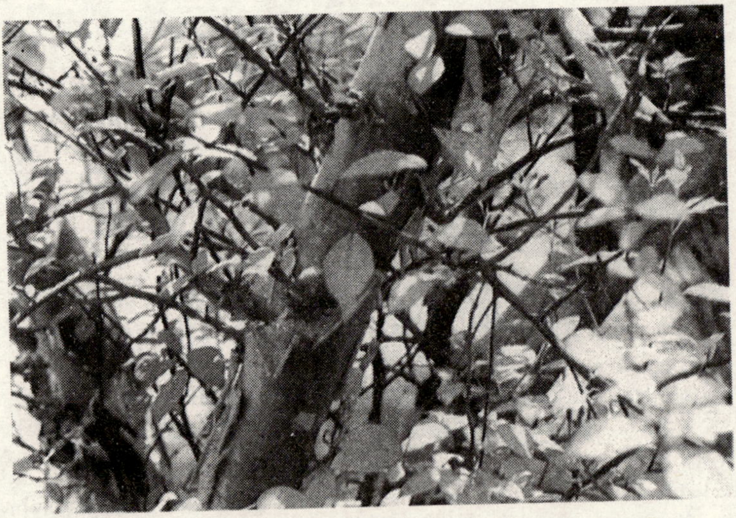

BARSERACEAE

BALSAMODENDRON MUKUL HOOK
SYN. COMMIPHORA MUKUL (HOOKER STEDOR)

BENG.- GUGUL., **HINDI**- GUGAL., **ENG.**- INDIAN BEDELLIUM., **KAN.**- GUGGULU., **TAM.**- KUKKULU, GUGGULU, GUKKULA., **GUJ.**- GUGANA., **TEL.**- GUKKULU, GUGGULU.

This is a perennial plant ranging between 4 ft. to 12 ft. From the stem and branches always brown coloured thin skin flakes keep on shelling and below the skin is green in colour. Branches keep on emerging unsystematically which are spiny. The leaves are thick, leathery and small arranged alternately. The margin of the leaf is serrate. The lower leaves are longer and upper leaves are smaller in size. The flowers are axillary and terminal, single, small and reddish in colour. The fruits are rust coloured (red and brown) shiny and glabrous.

The plant as a whole is aromatic. Any part of the plant emits pleasing smell. In winter this plant exudes a sort of gummy material which is known as Guggle in India and Loban in Africa.

It is reported from Bellary, Mysore, Deccan, Khandesh, Shatiwawar, Rajputana Desert, Sind and Baluchistan.

MEDICINAL USE: Gum-resin is astrin, antisep., expect., aphrodis, enriches the blood demulc, aper, carmin, altern, antisep, emmen in snake bite and scorpion bite. It is supposed to be a nontoxic drug and the only side effects reported are rashes and mild kidney irritation which disappear on withdrawal of the drug.

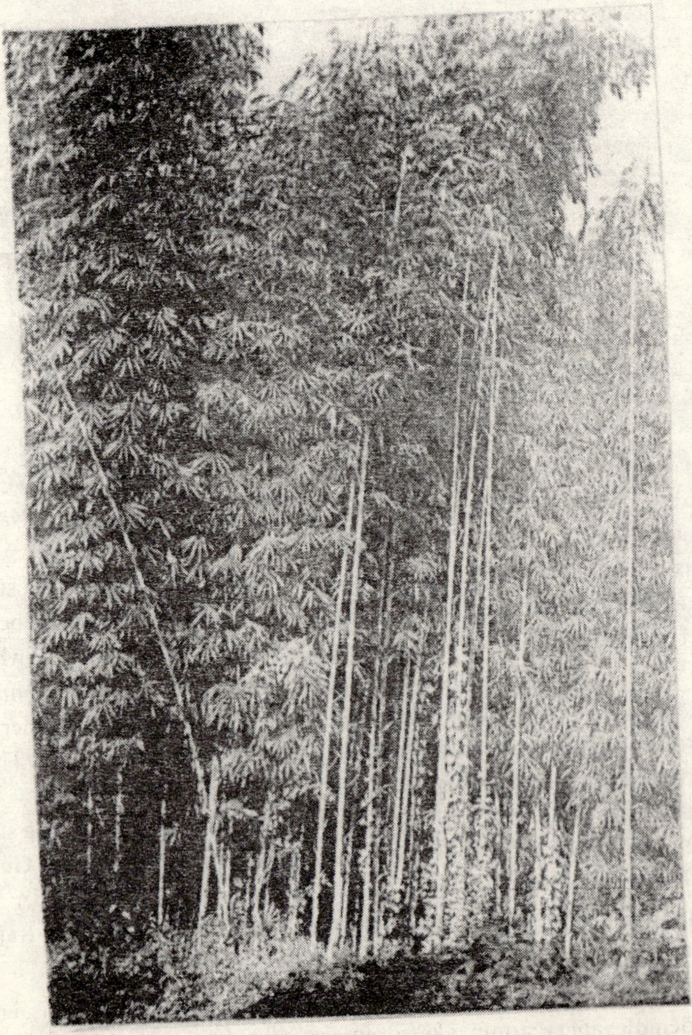

POACEAE

BAMBUSA BAMBOS DRUCE.

(Syn. B. ARUNDINACEA (RETZ.) WILID.)

(Syn. B. SPINOSA ROXB.)

SANS.- VANSH., **HINDI**- BANS., **GUJ.**- BANS., **MAR.**- BANS., **BENG.**- KETUA, KUTUAST., **TELGU.**- BONGU-VEDURU, PENTE-VEDURU., **TAMIL**- MUNGIL., **MAL.**- MUNGIL., **KAN.**- BIDURU., **ASSAM**-KOTOHA., **BURMA**- KYAKATWA.

Shrub or tree, usually large and coespitose, rarely climbing; plant thorny root stocks stout and central; culms terete bright green shining when young, becoming golden yellow with age, 80 - 100 ft. high and upto 6-7" in diameter. This plant blooms gregariously, once in about thirty years. Stems either graceful and curving or short and thickly branched), branched from the base; nodes prominent; lower with long horizontal shoots armed with 2-3 recurved spines; internodes upto 18 in; often subangular, the smaller flattened on one side, walls 1-2 in thick. Stem sheaths:- 12-15 by 9-12 in; coriaceous, young orange-yellow often strtiped green or red, top rounded, edges plaited, young thickly clothed with golden hairs; blade triangular, upto 4 in; acuminate, concave, glabrous margins involute, decurrent on the sheath, wavy long and thickly eiliate, hardly auricled; Leaves:- linear-lanceolate upto 8 by 1 in; articulated on the sheath; flat, many nerved tip sharp stiff, base rounded ciliate, subtessellate by pellucid glands, sheath glabrous or nearly so above and hairy beneath. Inflo:- usually a large leafless panicle bearing heads on spiciform branches, or of leafy panicles, or panicled spikes. Panicle enormous, often occupying the whole stem; rachis striate hard not shining, sometimes soft and angular, spikelets many shorter 4-6 fid; leaves glabrous above hairy beneath, sheaths hairy, then subglabrous ½-1 in; sessile lanceolate, acute, empty glumes 0-2 ovate-laneeolate acute or mucronate many-nerved, flower glumes 3-7 like the empty lower bisexual upper male with 2 or 3 upper most imperfect, 2 keeled palea ciliate, lodicules 2-3 small; stamens-6; anthers sometimes apiculate yellow obtuse, ovary elliptic, oblong or obovate, tip hairy; style long or short, stigmas 2-3. Flowers gregariously and in small clumps. *Flowers of the species B. SPINOSA are not known.

Found mostly at 3000-7000', but a few such as B. BALCOOA, are restricted to the plains. It is found throughout the plains and low hills of India and Ceylon, wild and cultivated. (Cultivated only in the lower Himalayan and in the valleys of the Ganges and Indus.

MEDICINAL USE : The young shoots contain 0.03% HCN and are lethal to living beings. Leaves : Emmenagogue; used in haemetemesis and vetanary practice. B. Manna is used as tonic, useful in fever, cough, and in snake bite etc., (Chopra, 1956). A compound white crystalline extracted from Bambusa sp. is known as Vansh Iochan. It reduces blood cholesterol in the body and prevents stone formation in kidney. Its use in pregnancy help the child in forming health, tissues and makes delivery easy as it effects directly in the uterine activity.

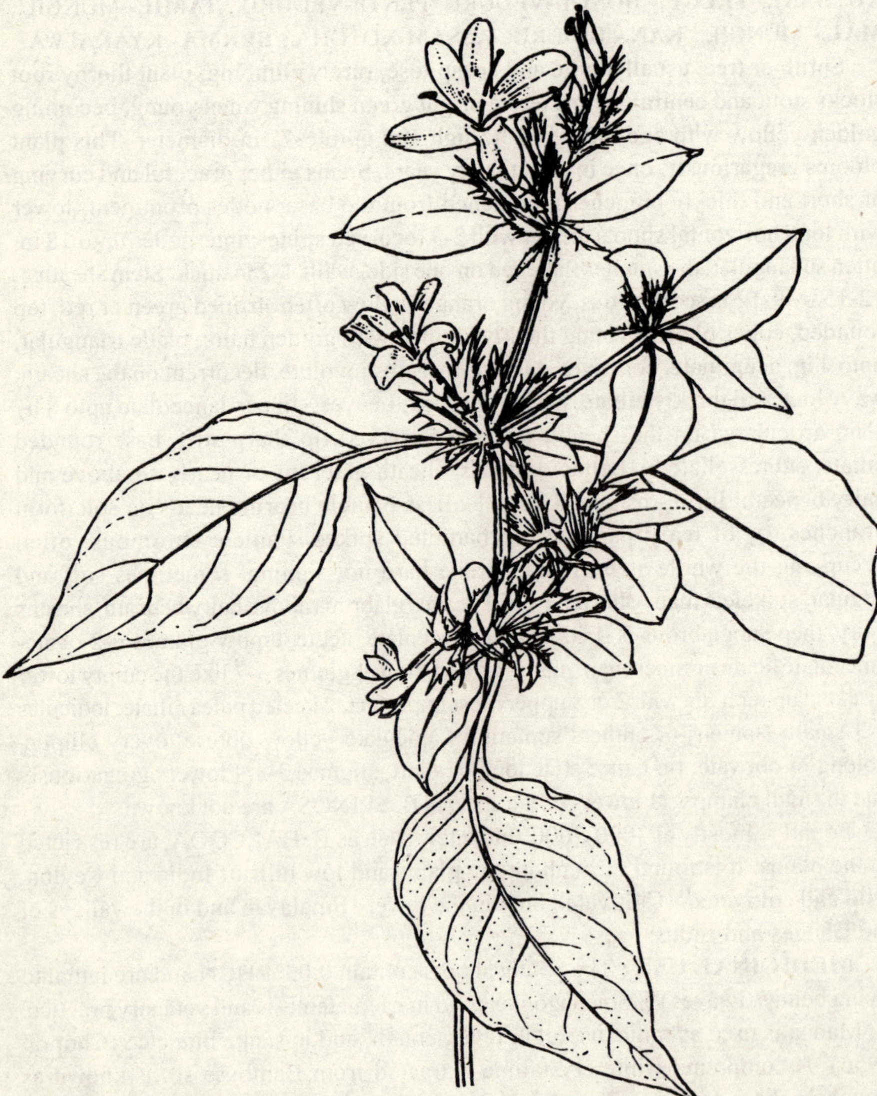

ACANTHACEAE

BARLERIA CRISTATA LINN
(SYN. B. CILIATA ROXB.)

S.- AND B.- JHINTI., **P.-** TADRELU., **TAM.-** UDAMULLI., **TEL.-** KODIKANNU., **ASSAM-** JHINLI.

It is an errect, stiffly hairy, busy perennial under shrub. Stem is branched profusely and leaves are narrow, elliptic and entire. Leaves are short stalked with fine bristly hairs. Bractoles shorter than the outer spinous sepals. Flowers are voilet with a white throat or pink in dense clusters either terminal or axillary in position. Calyx lobes unequal, the outer ovate, slender, pointed, toothed, the Inner awl - shaped entire. Corolla is funnel shaped with rounded lobes spreading, the fruit is capsule, ellipsoid and four seeded.

It is reported from Pakistan to Bhutan, India, Burma, S.E. Assia, Light forests; shrubberies and open slopes.

MEDICINAL USE: Roots and leaves are used to reduce swelling. Infusion is given in cough, plant is used in snake bite throughout India.

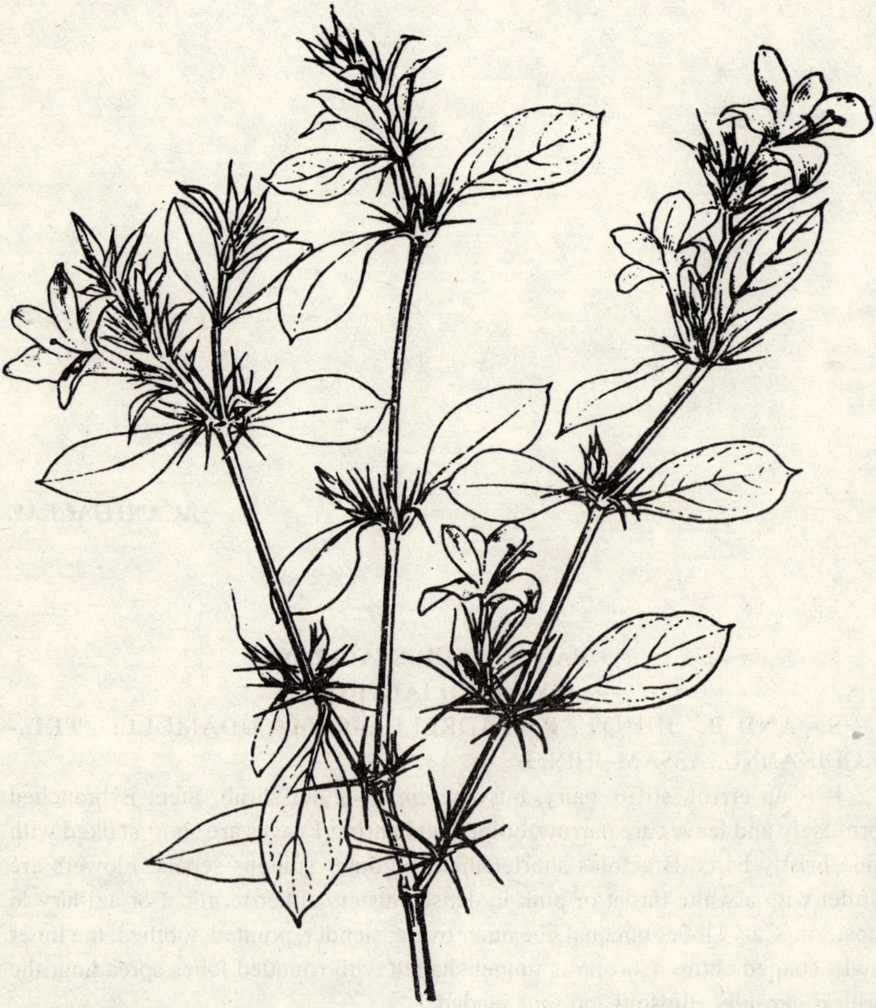

ACANTHACEAE

BARLERIA PRIONTIS LINN.

BEN.- KANTAJATI., **GUJ.**- KANTASHERIO., **HINDI**- CATSERINA., **KAN. & TEL.**- MULLU-GORANTI., **KON.**- GORTI., **MAR.**- PIVALA KORANTA., **SANS.**- AJRADANTI, KARUNTA., **TAM. & MAL.**- SHEMMULLI., **BO.**- VAJRA DANTI.

It is a bushy, prickly undershrub commonly grown as a low hedge plant branching from base. It reaches a height of 2 - 5'. Stems grey white, spines 3 - 4 or more in the axil of leaves, white. It is densely scabrid lineolate, sometimes puberulous. Leaves opposite, elliptic acuminate at both ends spine tipped glabrous or sometimes tawny sericeous beneath. Leaves are 4 by 1-½" entire; petioles of the lower leaves usually distinct. Sometimes ½ - 1 inch. It flowers in the cold season and bears orange yellow or cream coloured flowers. The flowers are in terminal spikes or axillary, 1 3 nate, uppermost spiked. Orange, yellow, or creamish bracts large elliptic spine-tipped, bracteoles very small bristles none or O. Bracts ½ - 1" entire. The lower larger foliaceous; sepals broadly lanceolate, acuminate, 2 outer 2/3 - 3/4 inch; 2 inner ½". Corolla 1 ¼ -1 3/4" glaborus or puberulous and spine tipped. Stamens 4, 2 minute or sterile. Disc-annular. Pistil glabrous capsule 3/4 - 1"; 2-seeded. Seeds 1/3 in diam much compressed, ovate black pointed and larger than calyx. The seeds have surface hairs which smell when wetted.

It is locally known as kala bansa or Piabansa the flowering season is October - March and fruiting season is March - June.

It is used as a hedge plant and found in waste places near gardens. It is reported from tropical India, from the Himalaya to Ceylon and Malacca, probably in most cases introduced.Distribution: tropical Asia and Africa.

MEDICINAL USE: The juice of leaves is slightly bitter and acid. It is mixed with honey or sugar and used in catarrhal affections accompanied with fever in children. This mixture is also useful for bleeding gums, toothache and in Otitis. The juice of leaves of white variety mixed with the Jeera is given in spermatorrhoea. The juice is also applied to the feet in the rainy season to prevent their cracking or laceration. Medicated oil is applied to unhealthy wounds and paste of root is applied to boils and glandular swallings. (Dymock, Warden and Hooper, III, 43.). The plant parts are used in catarrh, cough and anasarea.

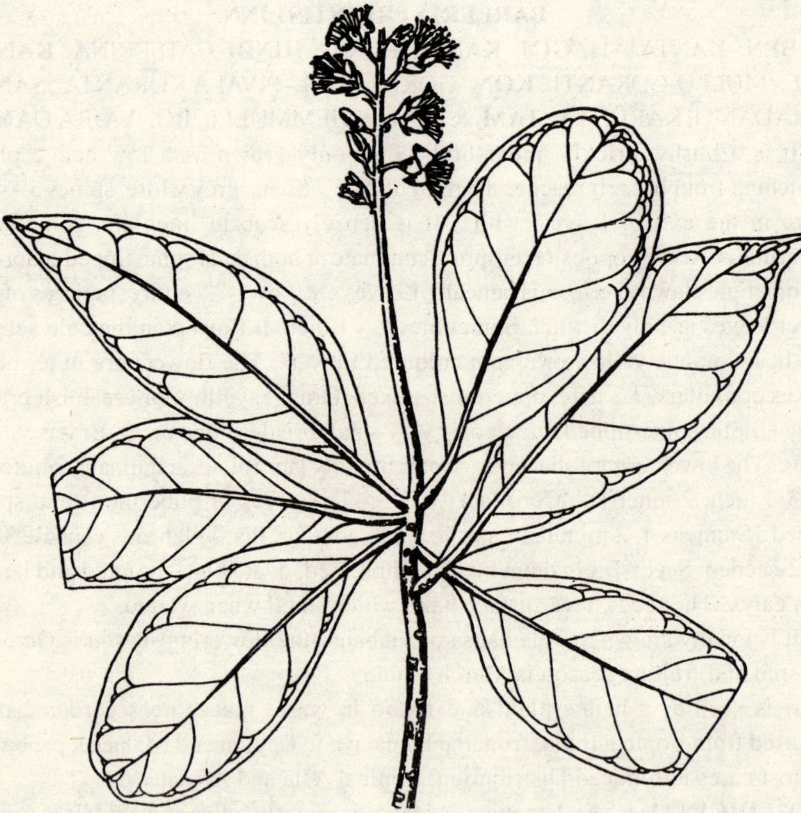

MYRTACEAE

BARRING TONIA ACUTANGULA LINN GAERTN

BENG.- SAMANDER., **MAR.**- PIVAR., **GUJ.**- SAMUDARPHAL., **TAM.**- KADAPPAMARAM., **HINDI**- HIJJAL., **TEL.**- KANAPA.

It is a small tree grown as an ornamental on account of its pretty flowers, which occur in conspicuous pendulous spikes. The leaves are glabrous, coriaceous, with serrate margin, broad petiole and flat upper surface. The cuticle is thick and the epidermal cells are polygonal in shape. Cuticular striations are present.

The roots have a tough bark, which can be peeled off easily. It is a dark brown externally with longitudinal wrinkles, inner surface is buff or yellowish in colour, fracture is fibrous and fractured surface is uneven and pale yellow.

It is common in the sub-Himalayan tracts, east of the Jamuna, in Bihar, Orrisa, Bengal, Assam. Madhya Pradesh and South India.

MEDICINAL USE : The juice of the leaf is used in diarrohea and dysentry and as bitter tonic, powdered seed emetic, expect. and as snuff in headache. Root has been found to be cooling, aperient, expectorant and also to possess properties similar to cinchona (Ahmed, 1969).

It is also used as an emetic and in liver infections in Himalaya Drugs.

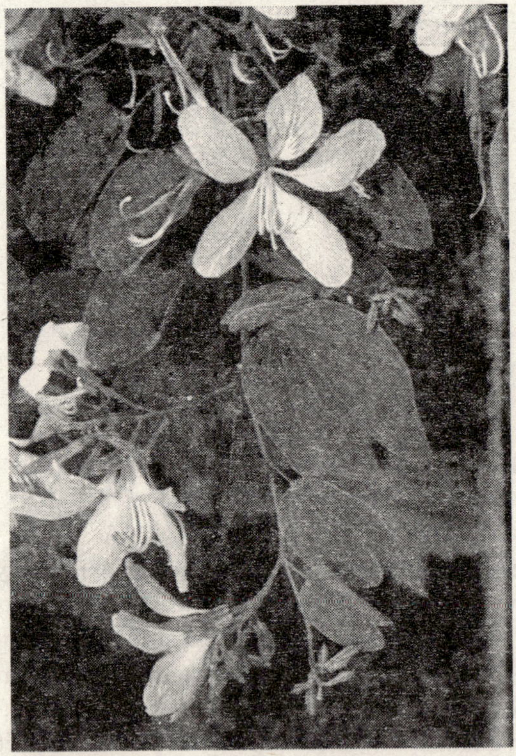

CEASALPINIACEAE

BAUHINIA PURPUREA LINN

B.- PURPUREA LINN., **S.**- VANARAJA., **H.**- KHAIRWAL, KALIARH, LAL KACHNAR., **BOM. & MARATHI**- RAKTAKANCHAN., **ENG.**- CAMEL'S FOOT TREE., **PUNJABI**- KOIRAL., **TAM.**- MANDARI., **TEL.**- KANCHANAM.

A middle sized erect tree, with moderately stout glabrescent branchlets. It is an evergreen ornamental tree. The bark is ashy to dark brown. Leaves are very distinctive by being deeply cleft at the apex into two rounded usually blunt lobes, 9 - 11 nerved. They are rigidly subcoriaceous, glabrous, shallowly cordate. Flowers in terminal and axillary short-peduncled few-flowered corymbs; bracts minute, deltoid; lower pedicles ¼ - ½ ; Calyx tube 3/4 to 1; wolly-haired, splitting into 2 recurved lobes; lobe cordateorate, remaining to the end spathaceous and entire. Flowers pink purple occurring with the leaves slightly drooping, few in terminal or axillary clusters. Petals 3 - 4 cm. lanceolate narrowed to a long stalk; veined red in colour. Fertile stamens 3 - 4 ovary grey downy, with a long stalk and style and moderately large obligue stigma. Pod ½ - 1 ft. by 3/4 - 1', firm, flat, glabrous, late in dehiscing, rather decurved, 12 - 15 seeded.

It is reported from Pakistan to Bhutan. India China to 1600 cm. Secondary forests, cultivated areas. Sept - October; fruiting Jan. - March. It is also reported from the foot of the West Himalayas and KHASTA Mts. (alt. 4000 ft.) to Ceylon and Penang. This tree is indigenous to the lower slopes of the Himalayas, and distributed in N. India, Assam, Khasi Hills and W. Penisula.

MEDICINAL USES:

Bark.- astringent in diarroea.

ROOT- carminative

FLOWERS.- Laxative.

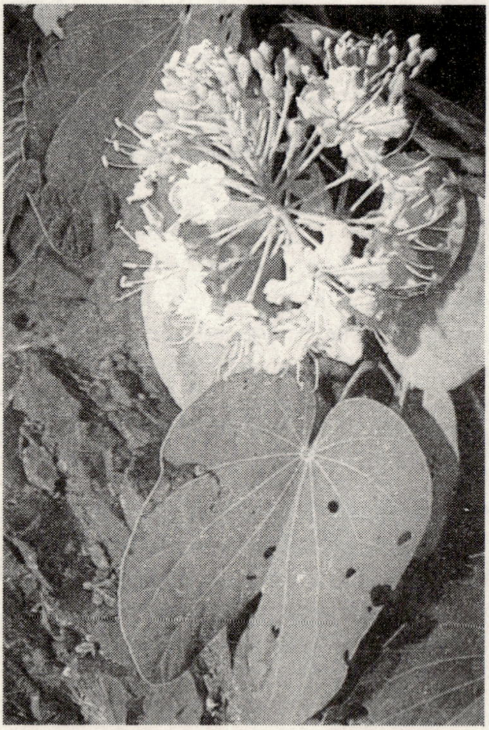

CEASALPINIACEAE

BAUHINIA VAHLII WAND A

H.- MALJAN, JALLUR., **B.-** SIHAR, CHEHUR., **TEL.-** ADDA., **ENG.-** CAMEL'S FOOT CLIMBERS.

It is a large woody evergreen climber with rusty brown and hairy leaves and shoots. Flowers are pale yellow in dense stalked flat topped with terminal clusters, Petals oblong, silky haired, on the ventral side, leaves rounded with heart shaped base. The cleft of the leaves is still deeper upto 1/3 of the total length, upto two rounded apices, dark green above, dawn beneath, branch lets with paired tendrils.

It is reported from Kashmir to Sikkim, India, Assam, Madhya Pradesh and Bihar.

MEDICINAL USE: The seeds are tonic, aphrodisiae; leaves demulcent, mucilaginous.

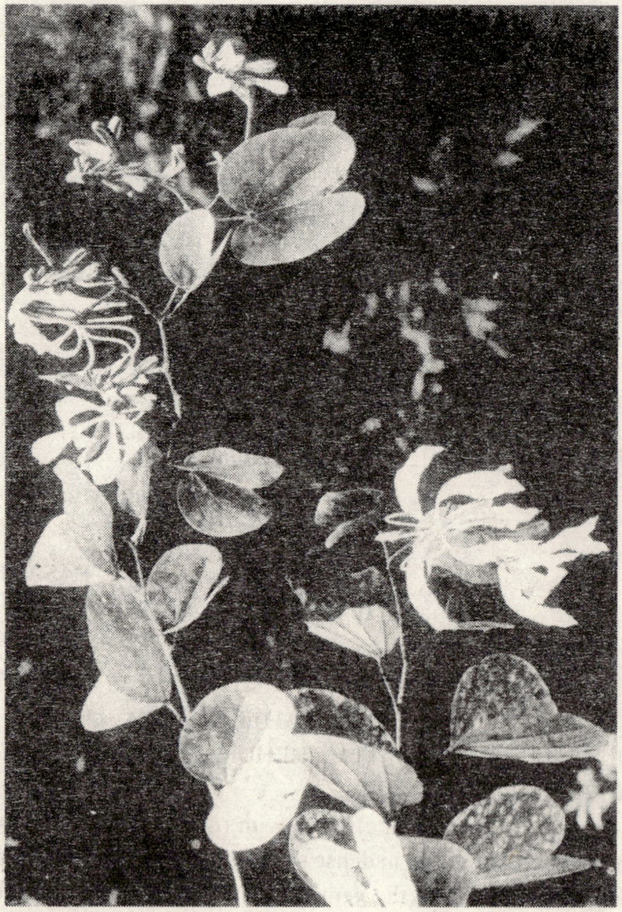

CEASALPINIACEAE

BAUHINIA VARIEGATA LINN

(SYN. B. CANDIDA ROXBA.)

S.- KOVIDARA., **H.**- KACHNAR., **B.**- RAKTAKANCHAR., **T.**- SPEGAPU - ΛANCHORI., **TEL.**- MANDARA., **ENG.**- MOUNTAINEBONY, VARIEGATED ;AUHINIA.

It differs from B. PURPUREA as follows. The flowers bloom in spring on leafless ranches. Leaf cleft goes deep down further till 2/3 of the distance and calyx tube iperseed the calyx limb. Flowers fragrant, petals white sometimes four petals are ale purple and 5th petal is darker with purple veins; fertile stamens five, calyx athe like and not splitting.

It is also found in dry forests of Eastern, Central and South India.

MEDICINAL USE: Bark is alterative, tonic, astringent useful in skin diseases, cers and scrofula. Dried buds used in dysentry and piles, diaorrhea and worms. ecoction of root - in dyspepsia and roots are antatid to snake poison.

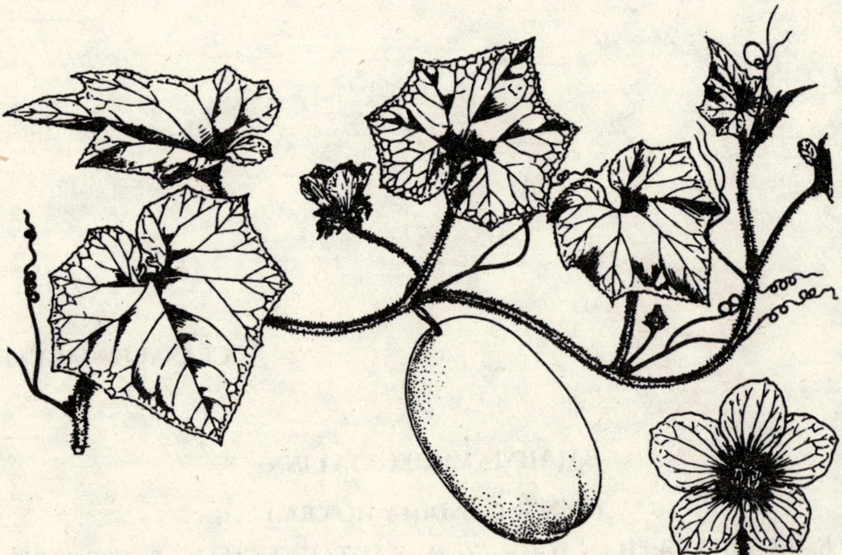

CUCURBITACEAE

BENINCASA CERIFERA SAVI

(SYN. B. HISPIDA (THUNB.) CONG

ENGLISH- ASH GOURD, WHITE GOURD., **ARABI**- MAJDHAB., **SANS.**- BRIHATPHALA., **ASSAMESE**- KUMURA., **BO.**- KOHALA., **BENG.**- CHAL KUMRA., **ORIYA**- PANIKAHARU., **TELUGU**- BUDIDA GUMMADI., **TAMIL**- SAMBOT, POOSARI., **MALAYALAM**- KUMBALLANGA., **KANNADA**- BUDUGUMBLA., **MARATHI**- KOHALA., **GUJARATI**- KOHALU., **PUN.**- PETHA., **LOCAL NAME**- PETHA.

It is a robust annual, climbing or trailing, gourd. Stem is stout, light green with scattered rough hairs and petiole is very long and leaves are 5 - 7 lobed and histrid, beneath. Flowers are large and yellow. Fruits fleshy, broad oblong or ovoid cylindrical with a waxy bloom. The pulp of the fruit is white. Flowering and fruiting takes place in rainy season.

It is cultivated largely in U.P., Punjab, Rajasthan and Bihar for its , fruit almost all over India.

MEDICINAL USE: The fruit is laxative, diuretic, tonic, aphrodisiae, antipyretic, specific for haemoptysis and other haemorrhages from internal organs. Juice of fruit given in insanity epilapsy and other nervous diseases, seeds are anthelmentic

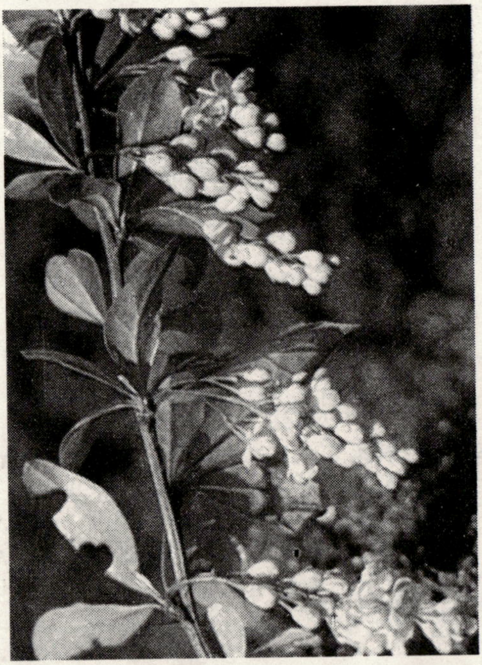

BERBERIDACEAE

BERBERIS ARISTATA D.C.
(VAR. FLORIBUNDA (G.DON.) HOOK AND B. THOMAS)

BENG.- DARHALDI., **MAR.**- DARUHALAD., **PUNJ.**- SAMLU., **ENG.**- INDIAN OPTHALMIC BURBERRY., **TREE.**- TUMERIC., **HINDI**- RASAUT DAR-HALD., **TAM. & MAL.**- MARAMANJAL., **KAN.**- DODDAMORADARISINA., **TEL.**- KASTURIPASPU., **SANS.**- DARUHARIDRA.

It is a shrub from 2 - 4 mtr. in height. The stem is yellow with 1 - 3 arching pale yellow branches. The leaves are elliptic and spineless, often present at nodes, opposite and in whorls. The flowers are regular and bisexual present in short stalked clusters, having numerous flowers of yellow colour in each cluster, much longer than the leaves. The fruit is dark red finally blue - purple style is very short.

It is distributed in N-W. Himalayas, Nilgiris, Kullu and Kumaon, Himachal Pradesh to Central Nepal, from Bhutan to Kunawer.

MEDICINAL USE : The plant is used as tonic, stomachic and astringent. A decoction of root bark is used in malarial fever.

Root bark, wood and extract made from root bark (Rasaut) rich in berbarine drug is alterative, deobstruent, used in skin diseases, menordiar, jaundice and affections of the eyes.

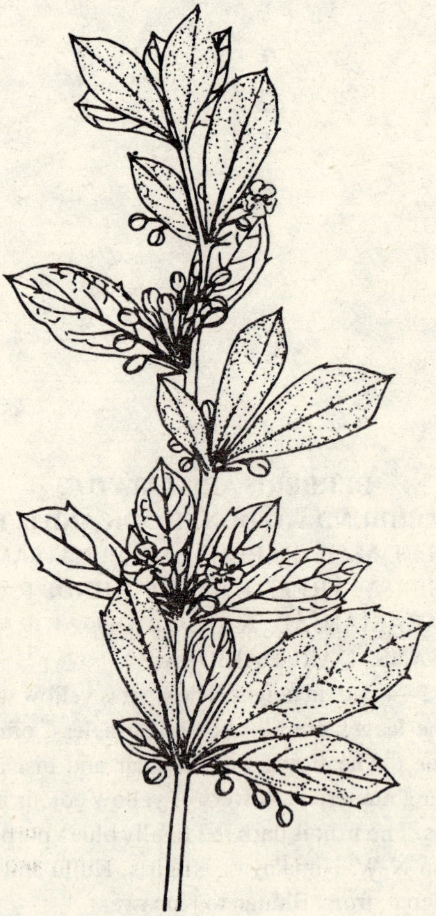

BERBERIDACEAE

BERBERIS ASIATICA ROXB, EX D.C.

H.- SUMLA., **KUMAON** - KILMORA., **GARHWAL**- KINGORA., **NEPAL**- CHITRA., **HINDI**- KILMORA.

It is a much branch shrub 2 - 4 m. in height. The branches are woody and yellow. Leaves are thick and rigid evergreen, with 2 - 5 spiny teeth, shining dark green above and greyish beneath. The flowers are pale yellow in flat - topped clusters shorter than the leaves with red hairless stalks; petals obovate, notched; leaves ovate to elliptic, stem spiny, fruit is ovoidal glaucous and dark purple.

It grows in dry valleys of the Himalayas in Bhutan, Garhwal, Bihar and on the Parasnath - hill, Afghanistan.

MEDICINAL USE: The root of this plant is considered as one of the chief source for extraction of Rasaut.

Plant contains barberine and oxyacanthine, roots used for healing ulcers, urethral discharges, in leucorrea; Opthalmia, jaundice; fever and soucces of Rasaut.

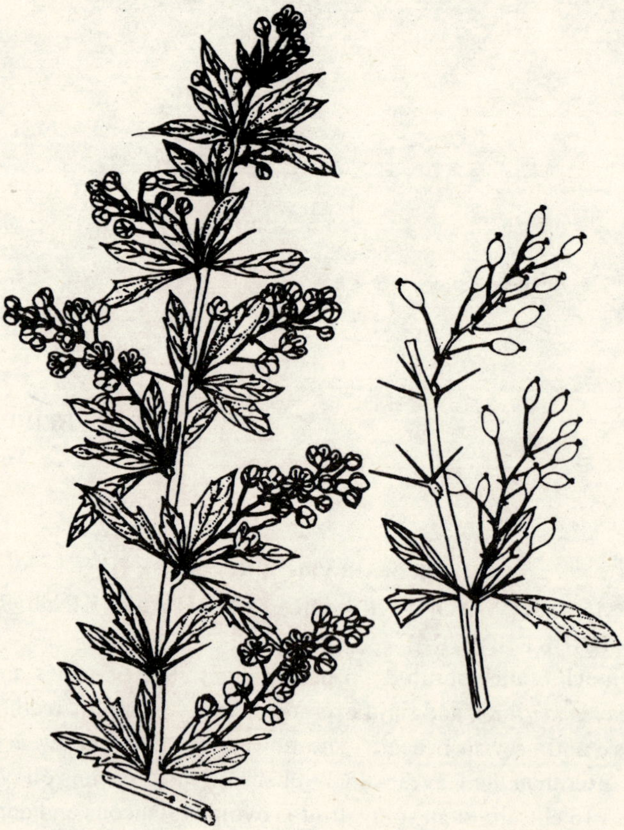

BERBERIDACEAE

BERBERIS LYCIUM ROYLE

H- KASHMAL., **BO.-** DAR HALD., **MAR.-** DARHALD.

It is a shrub 3 - 4 mtr. with white stems and narrow fine - pointed leathery leaves mostly without spiny teeth, glaucous beneath. Flowers dull yellow. borne in axillary clusters, longer than the leaves. Leaves oblanceolate, stems hairless, stem spines present; Fruit black.

It grows in dry hot places in western Himalayas from Garhwal to Hazara.

MEDICINAL USE : It is used in treatement of opthalmia, active principle being berberine. Also used for piles and as tonic and laxative. It is also used in chronic diarrohea and jaundice.

Interest has been arouosed in Barberine containing plants on account of its successeful use in the treatment of cutaneous leishmaniasis i.e. oriental sore.

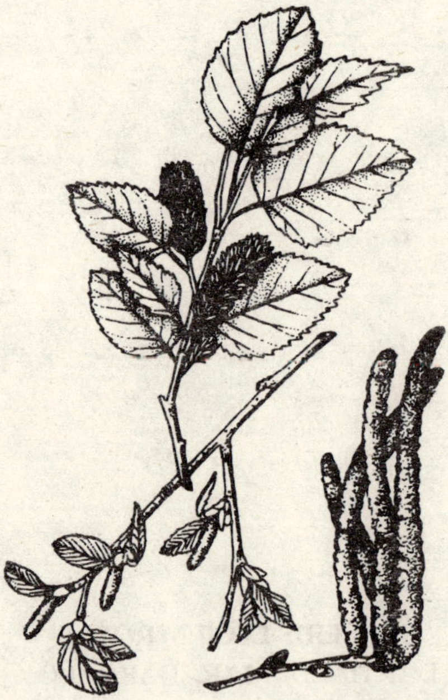

BETULACEAE

BETULA UTILIS D. DON
(SYN. B. BHOJPATTRA WALL)

BENG.- BHURJAPATRA., **SANS.**- BHURJAPUTRA., **HINDI.**- BHOJPATRA, BURJ., **BO.**-BHOJPATRA., **GUJ.**-BHOJAPATRA., **KAN.**- BHOJPTTRA., **TEL.**- BHUJA PATRI CHETTU.

It is popularly known as HIMALAYAN SILVER BIRCH or INDIAN PAPER BIRCH. It ranges between a shrub and a moderate sized tree up to 20 m in height usually the bole is irregular. The bark is very distintive which peels off in very thin pale almost transparent horizontal strips. The leaves are ovate, aeeuminate, irregularly serrate, finely hairy when young, 5-8 cms long flowers are in pendulous spikes. Male catkins mostly 5-10 cms, reddish, appearing on bare branches or with the young leaves. Fruiting catkins 2.5-4cm by 1.2 cm. broad. Nutlets c.2 mm. conspicuously winged with a 3-lobed much longer braet. Fruiting and growth period is from April to May.

It is met with throughout the main Himalayan range from Butan westwards as cending to an altitude of 4.200 m. It is also reported from Pakistan to S.W. china 2700-4300 cm. from forests at upper limit of tree growth.

MEDICINAL USE : The bark is aromatic and has antiseptic properties, an infusion of the bark is carminative in hysteria. The bark containing betulin is reported to possese antifertility activity.

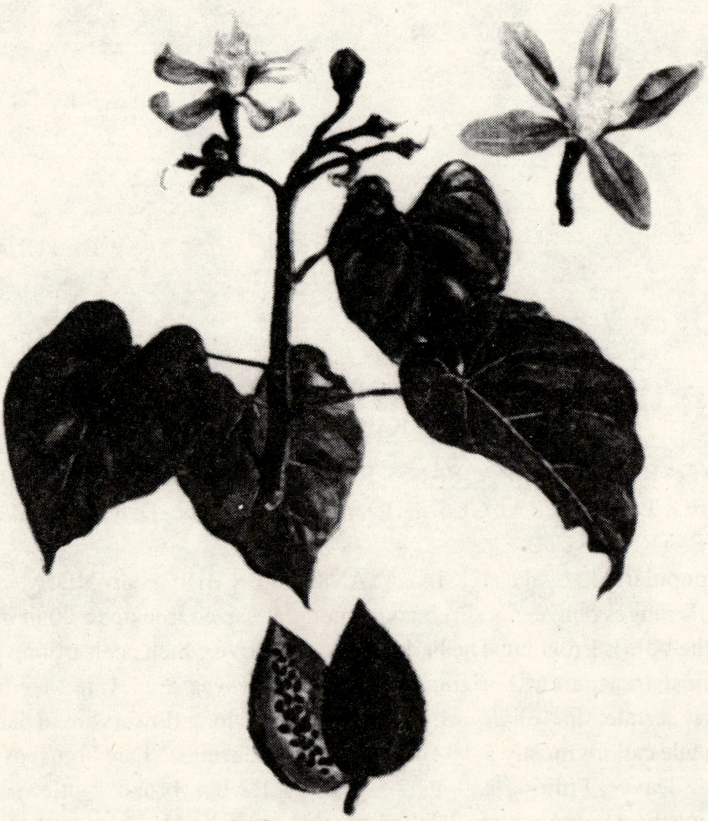

BIXACEAE

BIXA ORELLANA LINN

H & B.- LATKAN., **S.-** SINDURI., **BO.-** SHENDRI., **TAM. & TEL.-** JAPHARA., **ENG.-** ANNATTO, URUCU.

It is a shrub or small tree. It is native of Amemrica and West Indies but now completely naturalized in India. The stem is erect and leaves are chordate arranged alternately. Leaf venetion is reticulate. Flowers are found in terminal bunches. The petals are five, each petal is veined. The androceium and Gynecium are in a central cup like structure, the latter projecting out of the cup. The fruit is valvular and much hairy. The calyx is persistant.

It is cultivated to some extent in Mysore and is grown in Indian gardens as a hedge plant. It occurs as an escape in Travancore, coromandal and Malabar Coasts and in some districts of Bombay, Bengal and Assam.

MEDICINAL USE : Fruit is used as an astringent, purgative, Root bark - antiper, antipyr. Seeds - cordial, astringent febge good remedy for Gonorrea, antiper, antipyr. Leaves are used in jaundices and snake bite.

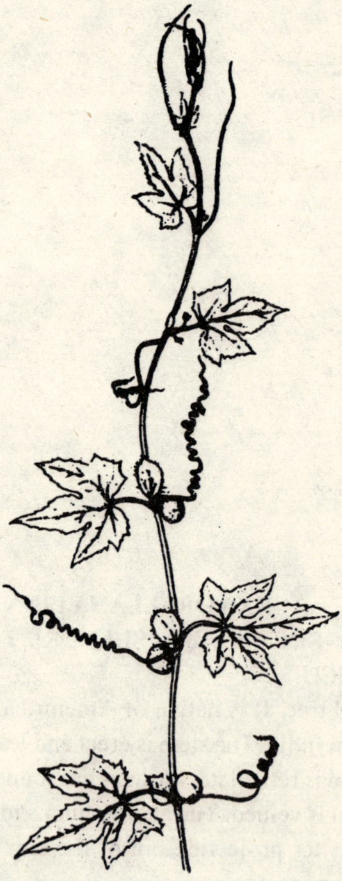

CUCURBITACEAE

BLASTANIA GARCINI (LINN) COGN.
(SYN. CTENOLETIS GARCINI (LINN) CL)
SICYOSGARCINIL INN

TEL.-GUDIMURALU.

It is a pretty, annual climber. Leaves are 5 lobed with serrate margins. Long coiled tendrils are present, nodular opposite leaves are five lobed. Stipuliform bracts ciliate. Flowers pale green, small. Fruits globose present in axils of leaves, red when rip. Flowers and fruits October-February.

It is commonl in the area climbing upon trees and shrubs. It is reported from N. Circars, Deccan and carnatic, extending west ward to the Ghats.

MEDICINAL USE : Fruits, seeds and roots used in medicine. The mucilaginous sap of the fruit is irritating to the eyes.

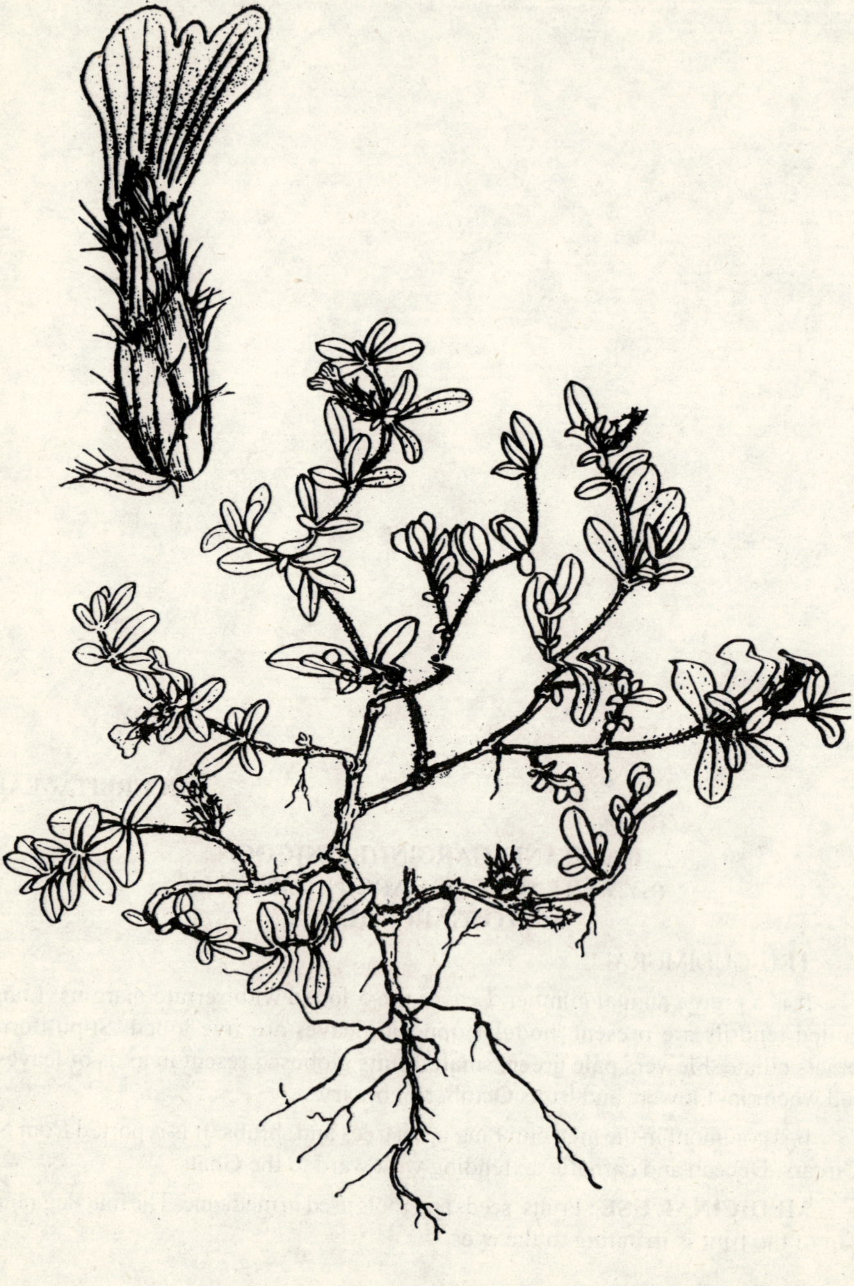

ACANTHACEAE

BLEPHARIS PERSICA (BURM.F.) KUNTZE (SYN. B.EDULIS PERS)

HINDI.- CHAUPATIA, UTTANJAN., **MAR.**- KARADU., **SANS.**- SHIKHI., **URDU**- UTINGANA, UTTANJAN., **BENG.**- SHASHANI., **GUJ.**- KHADOKATIRA, OTIGANA., **BOM & PUJN.**- UTTANGAN, RAJASTHAN, DAKHNI-CHAPPAR.

It is a small grey-pubescent or nearly glabrate perennial herb. Stem is short C 30 cms long rigid leaves in fours at the nodes, upper pair 5 cm x 1, an oblong narrow elliptic, lower pair smaller, flowers blue coloured in strobilate inflorescence orescence capsules one 5 or more clongated.

It is found in Punjab, western Rajesthan.

MEDICINAL USE : It is been identified as an aphrodis drug in Ayurveda. The leaves are useful in wounds, ulcers/nasal haemorrhage, asthma, throat, inflammation/ ascites and disorders of liver and spleen and a purgative. The root is considered as diuretic and is beneficial in urinary discharges & dysmenorrhoea. The seeds are diurtic, aphrodisrae expectorant and deobstruent and useful in strangury and conjunctivites. They yield a bitter ghueoside blepharin ($C_{14} H_{17} No_7$, mp 226-27^{0})

Its another variety B. SINDICA Stocks ext. Anders. G. The seeds are used as tonic when boiled in milk. The plant or the seeds are used as a cure for ear-ache.

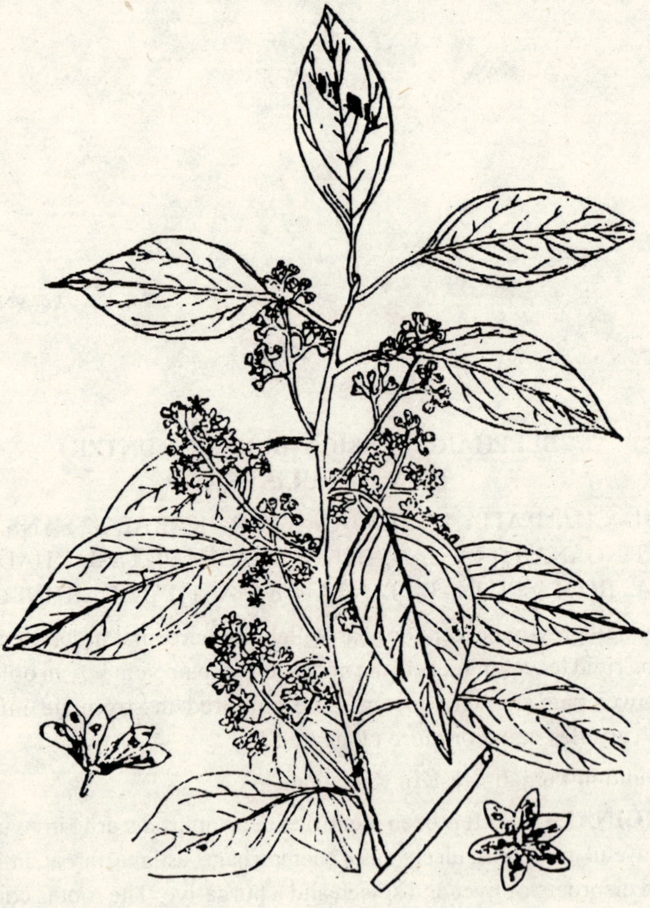

COMPOSITAE

BLUMEA BALSAMIFERA D.C.
(Syn. CONYZA BALSAMIFERA L)

(The most arboreous of all the species, smelling strongly of camphor).

HINDI-KAKARONDA., **ENG**.-NGAI CAMPHOR., **MAR**.-BHANGARUDA., **GUJ**.-KALAHAD

Annual or perennial, glandular pubescent or woolly herbs; tomentose or villus or silky woolly, stem tall corymbosely branched above; Leaves: alternate, usally toothed or lobed; 4-8 in coriaceous elliptic or oblong-lanceolate usuallysilky above serrate sometimes pinnatifid narrowed into a usually auricled short petiole. Heads 1/4-1/3 in, sessile or peduncled in rounded clusters on the stout branches of a large spreading or pyramidal corymbose panicle; rarely racemed, heterogamous, disciform, yellow, outer florets serrate, ♀, fertile, filiform, 2-3-toothed; disk florets, few, fertile, tubular, slender, limb 5- toothed, involuere: ovoid or campanulate, bracts, tomentose, narrow, acute, soft or herbaceous, outer smaller; receptacle glabrous; flat; naked; anther-base sagittate, tails small, slender. Style-arms of female, flattened or almost filliform rarely connate with the adjoining anthers. Achenes small, subterete or angled 10 ribbed silky; pappus 1-serriate, slender rib often caducous. The flowering and fruiting season is March to May.

About 60, species tropical and subtropical Asiatic, African and Australian. In India it is reported from Tropical Himalaya: Nepal and Sikkim, alt. 1-4000 ft. Assam, Khasis Mts. Chitta Gong, Pegu, Burma and the Eastern Peninsula, to Singapore and Penang. Distribution Java.

MEDICINAL USE : Warm infusion of the plant is sudorific. Decoction of leaves is expectorant. Leaves yield crystalline essential oil containing a camphor known as Nagi-camphor and a glueoid, Injection of extract lowers blood pressure; used in the treatment of excitement, in Isomnia and hypertension.

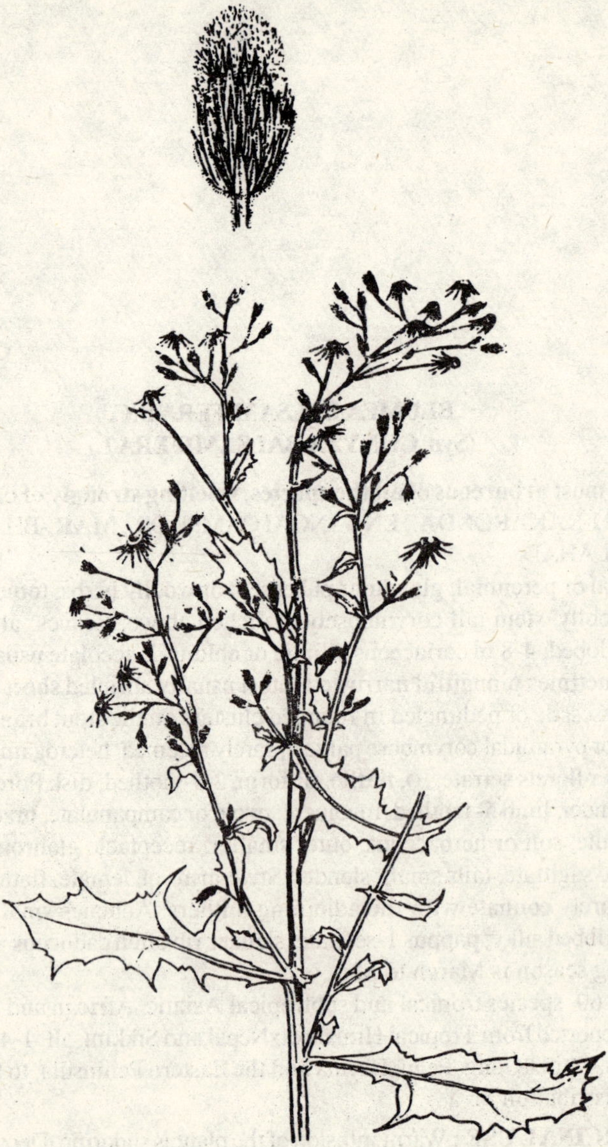

COMPOSITAE.

BLUMEA LACERA D.C.

SANS.- KUKURADRU., **HINDI**-KAKRANDA., **BENG**.- KUKURSUNGA., **MAR**.- BURANDO., **BOMBAY**- NIMRUDI., **TAM**.- NARAKKARANDAI., **TEL**.- KARUPOGAKU.

An erect annual herb with a strong odour of turpentine.

Many characters are similar to B. BALSAMIFERA. The characters which are different are given below. Hairy villous or glandular, rarely glabrescent, stem erect simple or branched very leafy, leaves petioled obovate toothed or serrate rarely lobulate, heads 1/3 in, in short axillary cymes and collected into terminal spiciform panicles rarely corrymbose, involucre bracts narrow acuminate hairy, recept. glabrous, corolla yellow, lobes of hermaphrodite nearly glabrous, achenes sub - 4 gonous not ribbed glabrate.

It is reported throughout the plains of India, from the N.W. ascending to 2,000 ft. in the Himalaya, to Travancore and Singapore and in Ceylon. Also from Malay Islands; China, Tropical Africa.

MEDICINAL USE : Juice of leaves is anthelmintic diuretic, stimulant and febrifuge. (Kanny Lall Dey, 1986; The Indigenous Drug of India.).

The herb gives 0.085% of essential oil, containing Blumea camphor (Wehmer, loc. cit.- Die P f lanzenstoffe, by C. Wehmer (Gustay Fischer, Jeno, 2 Vols., 1929 - 1931; Suppl. 1935. Plant as a whole is bitter and antipyretie. Root is used in cholera.

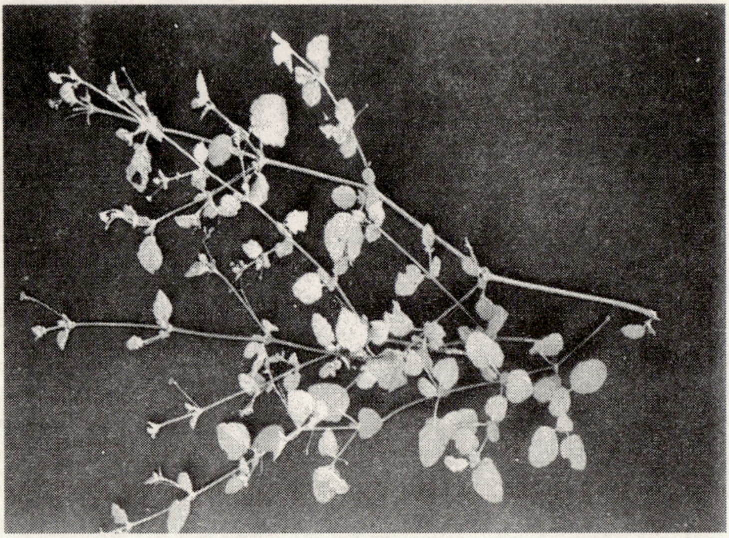

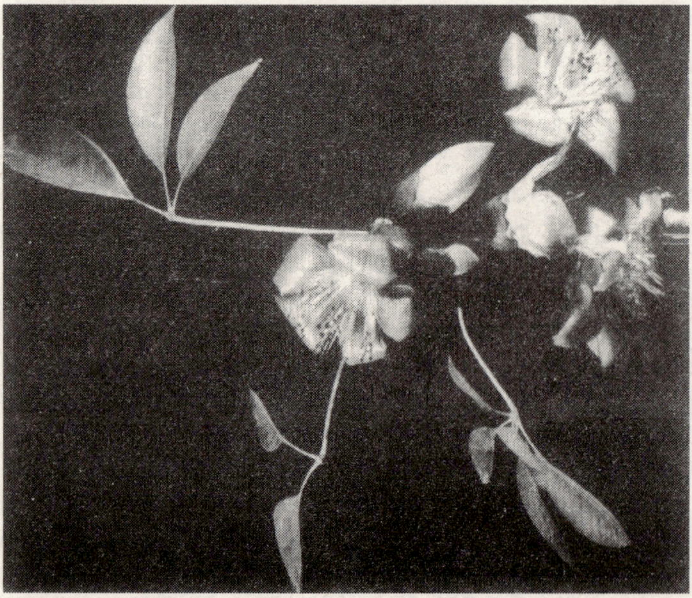

NYCTAGINACEAE

BOERHAVIA DIFFUSA LINN.
(Syn. B REPENS DELILE). LINN.)
(Syn. B. PROCUMBENS ROXB.)
its popularlyknown as PUNARNAVA.

ENG.- SPREADING HOG-WEED, HORSE-PURSLANE, NDHAPURNA, PUNARNAVA., **GUJ**.- VAKHAKHAPARO., **HINDI**- BESHAKA PORE, SANT, SANTHI, PUNARNAVA., **KAN**.- SANADIKA, KOMME., **MAL**.- TAMILANA., **PUNJ**.- ITSIT., **TAM**.- MUKKARATTA, SAATTARANAI, MUKARATTEKIREI., **TEL**.- ATTATAMAMIDI, PUNARNAVA., **SANS**.- PUNARNAVA, RAKTA PUNARNAVA., **BOMB**.- GHETULLI., **LOCAL NAME**: SANTHI, SANTH, BISKHAFRA., **MAR**.- PUNARNAVA, TAMBADI VASU, **BENG**.- GANDHAPURNA, PUNARRAVA.

A diffusely branched spreading parenial creeping herb, some times prostrate or ascending along walls. The root is taproot and fusiform, very stout, root stock woody. Diffusely branched, 6-24 in, more robust, long stout glabrous pubescent or viscous; Leaves: opposite and in unequal pairs; ½-2 in, thick; ovate, obtuse or acute usually cordate green beneath; petiole as long as blade or shorter. Inflorescence chiefly axillary; flowers pink or whitish capitate minute, in small, bracteate umbels of 4-10, arranged in long and slender-stalked, axillary and terminal panicles. Bracteoles small, rarely forming a minute involucre. Perianth red; tube long or short; limb funnel-shaped 5 lobed. Stamens 2-3, exserted. Ovary oblique, stipitate, Stigma peltate. Fruit 1/8" long shortly clavate, 5-ribbed; viscidly glandular on the ribs all over, top rounded.

A genus consisting of 40 species of herbs distributed in tropical and sub-tropical regions. Six species are found in India. Throughout India, from the Punjab to Assam and South to Travancore and Singapore; ascends in the hot Himalayan Valleys to 7,000 ft. Ceylon-distribution Tropical and Subtropical Asia, Africa and America. Locally it is common and abundant used in all parts of Delhi, in the unused lawns, and in crevices of ancient walls.

MEDICINAL USE : The root is diuretic, laxative, expeetorant in asthma, Stomachics; in Oedema, anaemia Jaundice, ascties, anasarca, scanty Urine and internal inflammation, antid to snake venam. The plant as a whole constitutes the drug punarnava which possesse an active constituent punarnavine. It has got diuretic properties, and is used in dropsy; dropsy associated with bright disease (Koman 1919, 141, 920, 3 & 40). Also recommended for asthma. (Surange, S.R. and Pendse, G.S. 1972.) Pharmaeognostic study of root of BOERHAVIA REPANDA Willd. (Punarnava) J. Res. Ind. Med. 7, 1. The Ayurvedic drug Punarnava is known as B. DIFFUSA in some parts of India and as TRIANTHEMA PORTULA castrum (Aizoaceae) in others Chakravarty (J. Ind. bot. Soc., 1942, 21, 87). B. DIFFUSA should be called RAKTA-PUNARNAVA, due to its pink flowers and T. portulacastrum with its white flowers SWEET PUNARNAVA. Though they belong to different families.

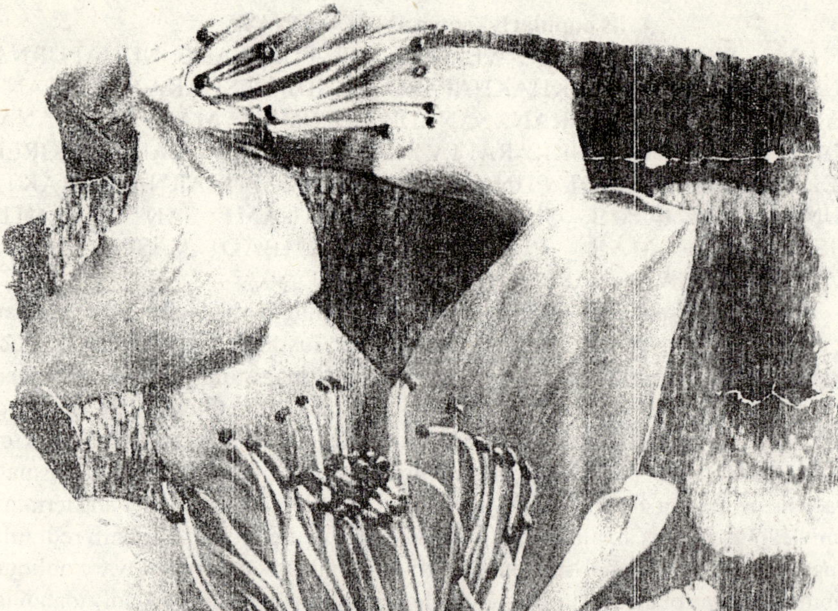

BOMBACACEAE

BOMBAX MALABARICUM DC.
(SYN. BOMBAX CEIBA. L.)
(SYN. SALMALIA MALABARICA (DC.)SCHOTT & ENDL.)

ENG.- RED SILK COTTON., **LOCAL NAME**- SEMAL., **BENG.**- ROKTOSIMUL, SEMUL-TULA, SHEMBAL, SENUR, PAGUN., **BOMB.**- SEMUL., **HINDI**- SIMUL, SEMUL, SHEBAL RAKAT-SENBAL, KAANTISENBAL, PAGUN., **SANS.**- SALMILI, RAKTA-PUSHPA, KANTAKADRUMA., **MAL.**- MOCHA, KALILAVAU, MULLILAVAU, MULLILA-PULA, PULAMARAM., **TAM.**- PURANI., **KAL.**-ILAVU, ELAVAM, MULLILAVU, PULAI., **TEL.**- SALMALI, BOORUGA., **KONDA-** BOORUGA, MUNDLABOORUGA CHETTU., **MAR.**- SEMUL, SARU, SIMLO, SAMAR, KANTESAVAR, SHEVARI., **KAN.**- BOORUGA, KEMPUBOORUGA, MULLUBOORUGA, MULLELAVA., **GUJ.**- SAWAR, SIMALO, SHEMOLO., **ORIYA**- BOURO, BUROH., **GARO.**- BOLCHU, PANCHU., **MUNDARI**- EDELSONG.

A tall lofty deciduous tree forming a spreading crown with stout hard conical prickles at the base, attaining a height up to 40 m. and a girth up to 6 m. or more, having a clear bole of 24-30 in; but tresses are present only in trees of about 30 yrs age or over. Branches spreading and prickly. Leaves digitate, deciduous; leaf lets 5-7 quite entire cuspidate, base tapering; 6-12", glabrous; petiole longer than the leaflets; secondary petioles 1"; stipules small, caducous. Peduncles axillary or subterminal, solitary or clustered, 1-flowered. Flowers: Large bright red appearing before the leaves; numerous, fasciled at or near the ends of the branches. Bracteoles O. Calyx: leathery, truncate or 5-7lobed; 1" smooth externally, silky within, margin slightly lobed, ultimately irregularly left, deciduous with the corolla and stamens. Corolla: Obovate; 5; oblong bright red, recurved, fleshy, twice the length of the stamens. Stamens: Pentadelphous bundles opposite the petals, and divided above into numerous filaments; anothers reniform, 1-celled; filaments ligulate half the length of the petals, staminal-tube short, filaments numrous, pluriseriate, 5 innermost forked at the top, each with an anther, 10 intermediate shorter, outer very numerous. Ovary: 5-celled; style clavate style longer than the stamens. Stigmas 5; ovules many in each cell. Capsule: Woody, oblong obtuse; 6-7", ovoid, downy, 5-valved, valves silky within seeds-numerous obovate, smooth woolly, enveloped in copious floss. The blooming season is Feb.-March. Fruits April - May.

B. MALABARICUM is found in tropical Eastern Himalaya and throughout the hottor forest regions of the India, to Burma and Ceylon.

MEDICINAL USE : Root and Bark emetic. Root stimulant tonic, form the chief ingredient in the musla-semul, a medicine which is aphrodisiae; given in impotence. Gum-aphrodisiac, demulcent; haemostatic, astringent, tonic, asterrative used in diarroea, dysentry and menorrea. Flowers and fruits used in snake bite.

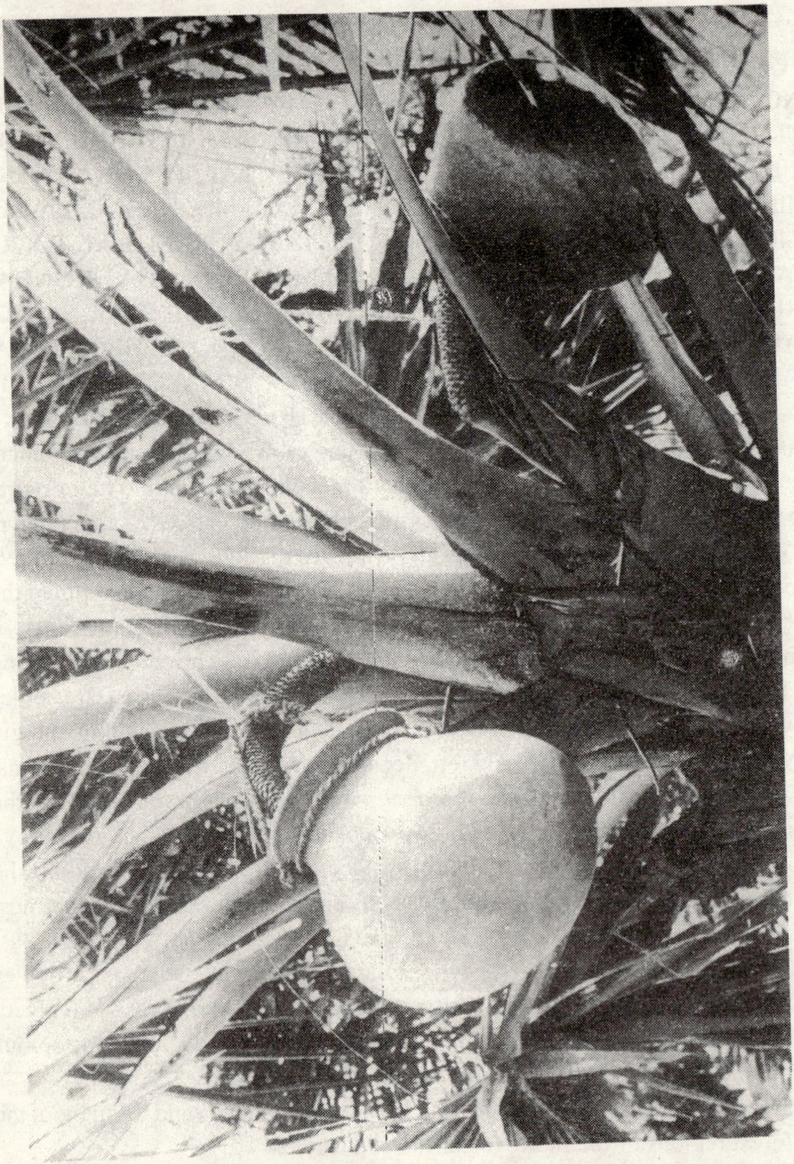

PALMAE

BORASSUS FLABELLIFER LINN
(SYN. B. FLABELLAFORMIS ROXB.)

ENG.- PALYMRO, PALM., **HINDI-** TAR, TAL (PALMAE)., **S & B- TAL.- H.-** TAR., **MARATHI & GUJARAT-** TAD., **TAM.-** PANAI, TALAI., **TEL.-** TADI - CHETTU. **MAL.-** PANA., **PERSIAN-** DARA KHTERTARI., **MALAYALAM-** PANNA.

It is 1 - 18 m. high and occupies an area of 3.1/2 ft. to 7 ft. It bears a cown of 30 - 40 leaves. The leaves are quite broad in width. The leaf stalks are long, strong and fibrous. The stem is dark black and consists of a hard outer portion mainly compressed stiff longitudinal fibres. The central portion or pith is soft and stoney. The plants are dioceious. The fruit is large and fibrous containing three nuts and each nut encloses a seed.

It is a tall palm plant distributed along the costal areas of Bengal, Bihar and West and East Peninsula. It is more or less common all over India. It is also reported from Sri Lanka and Malaysia.

MEDICINAL USE : Root restore cooling. Juice of plant is diur, stin, antiphlegm, useful in inflammatory infections and dropsy, Pulp is demulc, nutritive.

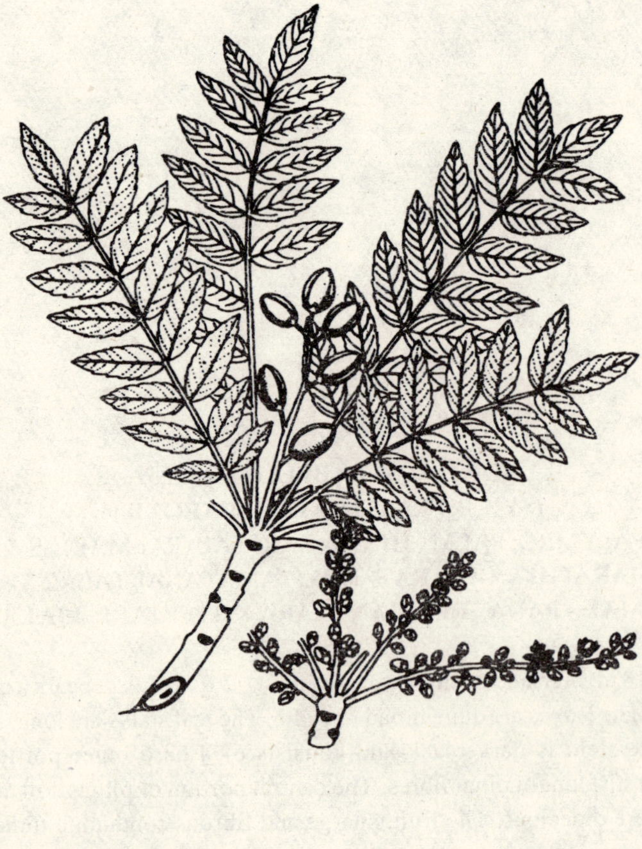

BURSERACEAE

BOSWELLIA SERRATA ROXB.

LOCAL NAME: SALAI, SALHE, GUNJ., **S.**- SHALLAKI., **H & B.**- LUBAN, SALAI., **ENGLISH.**- INDIAN FRANKINCARSES., **TAMIL & TEL.**- PARANGISAMBRANI., **KAN.**- MADDI.

It is tree commonly available in the drier parts of Peninsular India. A moderate sized deciduous tree with a spreading, flat crown. Leaves crowded near the ends of the branches. Leaflets many, variable, serrate and pubescent, flowers white from april to May. Drupes trigonous, fruits from July - August. The tree occupies an area of 90 - 150 centimeter.

It is reported from Madhya pradesh, Bihar, Orissa, Rajasthan, Maharashtra and Gujarat.

MEDICINAL USE : The plant exudes a type of gum which is diaphoretic, diuretic, astringent, emomen. Used in rheumatism, nervous and skin diseases.

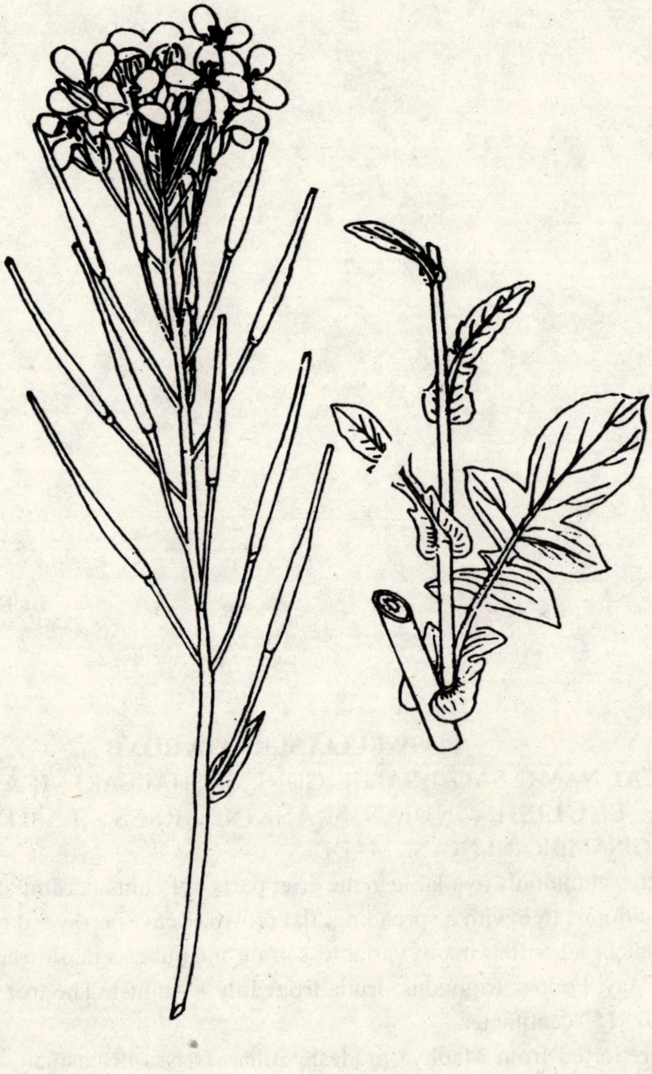

CRUCIFERAE

BRASSICA CAMPESTRIS LINN.
(Syn. B. RAPA (LINN.) HARTM.)
(Syn. B. DICHOTOMA WATT.)

BENG.- KALI SARSON., **HINDI**- KALI SARSON., **SANS.**- KALA-SARSHAPA., **MAL.**- KARUPAKATUKA., **TAM.**- KARUPPUKK ADUGU., **LOCAL NAME**- SARSON. **TEL.**- NALLAAVALU.

In India it is represented by the varieties Sarson and toria.

An erect, stout, simple or branched, glabrous or slightly hispid annual, 1 - 3 ft. high. Root stock often woody or tuberous. Leaves large, petioled, more or less pinnatifid upper oblong or lanceolate, lower leaves lyrate, upper auricled. Flowers bright yellow, in corymbos elongating into racemes. Pedicels 3/4", ascending or spreading. Sepals 4, free, 2 lateral (opposite the placentas) oten large and saccate at the base, imbricate. Petals: 4, free, hypogynous, placed crosswise, imbricate, persistent till the corymb lengthens, stamens 6 (rarely 1, 2 or many 3) 2 outer opposite the lateral sepals; 4 inner longer, in opposite pairs. Disk with usually 4 glands opposite the sepals. Ovary 2 - celled by a placental memberane, or 1 - celled or with superimposed cellules, style short or O; stigma simple or with 2 lobes opposite the placenta; ovules 1 - 2 or as 2 - serrate on two parietal placentas, rarely solitary and erect; Fruit is a pod 1 - ½ - 3", glabrous suberect, valves with midrib and flexuous veins, elongate, terete or angular often with an indehiscent 1 - seeded beak (sometimes) beak of pod is flat and seed less). Valves convex, 1-3-nerved, lateral nerves flexuose, style beaked or ensiform. stigma truncate or 2 lobed. Seeds 1-serriate, globose or sub compressed; cotyledons incumbent, concave or condullicate, the radicle within the longitudinal fold.

Species about 80; temperate regions of the old World. It is cultivated throughout India. Locally it is a cold seasoncrop and is common in Timarpur, Najafgarh, Shahadara and those near Ghaziabad. It is grown in rotation with many summer and rainy season crops. The crop is harvested in April and May and flowering and fruiting seasons is Jan,-April.

MEDICINAL USE : Seeds mix with hot water form an efficient counter iritant poultice. Oil combined with camphor forms an efficacious embrocation in muscular rheumatism and minar skin infections and eezema, stiff neck, etc., it is used in dengue fever with benefit, and is rubbed on the chest in bronchities. Roots and leaves are used as stomachic in the form of infusion acting as a tonic. Pure oil is often used in hairs for massage and is considered very good for luxurious hair growth.

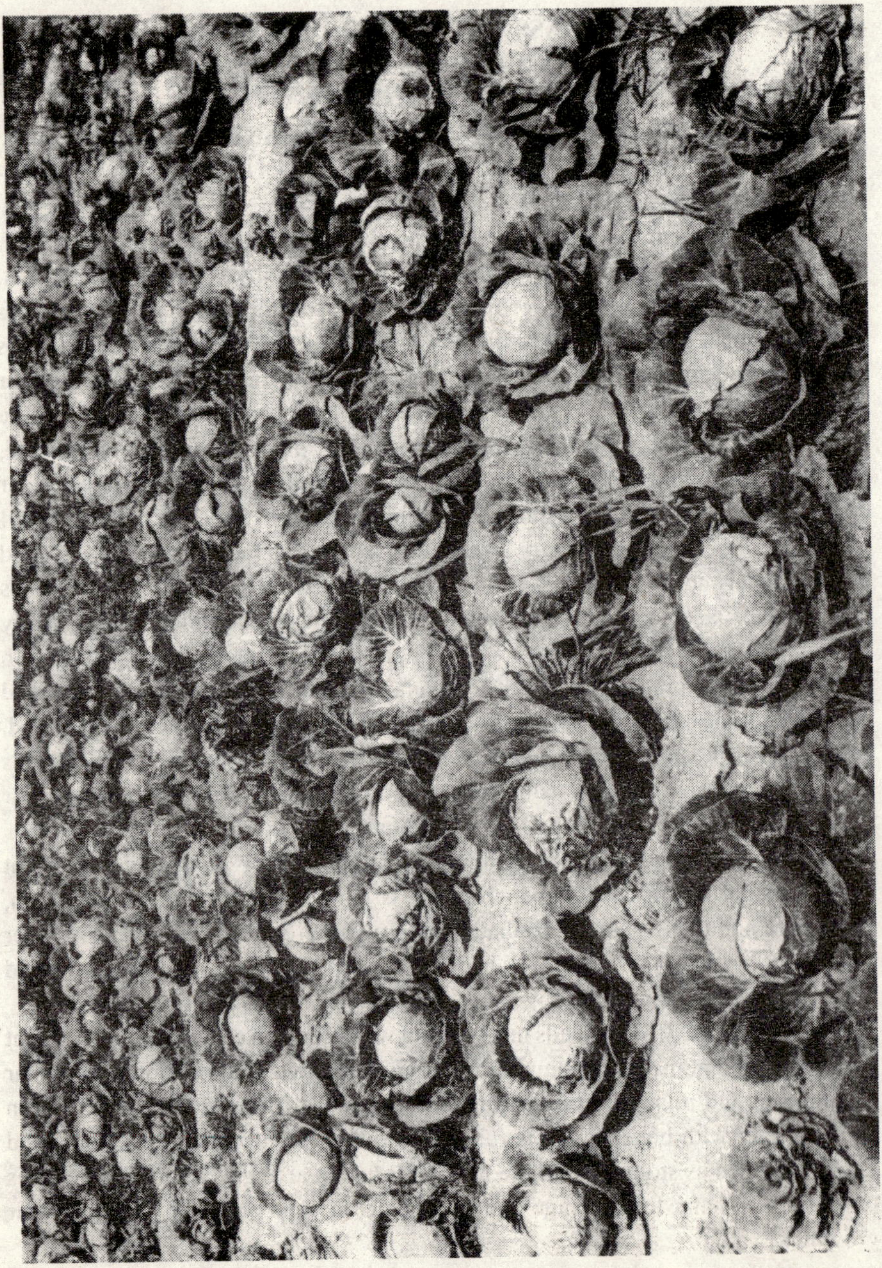

CRUCIFERAE

BRASSICA OLERACEA LINN

PUNJABI- BANDHA GOBI., **ORIYA**- BANDA GOBH., **BENG**.- KABI., **ENG**.- CABBAGE, CAULIFLOWER., **MAR**.- KNOLKHOL., **GUJ**.- PANGOLI., **TAM**.- KOSHIPOO., **HINDI**- BANDH GOBHI, PATA GOBHY., **TEL**.- KOSUGUDDAE., **KAN.**- KOSUGADDE., **ASSAMESE**- BANDHA KABI., **GUJARAT**- KOBIJ.

It is one of the most popular winter vegetable in India.

It is a biennial crop, grown as an annual. The growing point being surrounded with overlapping expanded leaves. Leaf colour, form, shape and size are variable. A few varieties have sunken leaf veins. others have a red pigment in the leaves.

MEDICINAL USE : Leaf extracts are used in gastric disorders, cardiac irregularaties, constipation, chronic cough bronchial asthama, biliousness, fever, urinary discharges piles and warts. It is also applied on blisterd surface to promote a free discharge. Its leaves are known for its calcium content and are found very useful to old people in the disease osteoporasis.

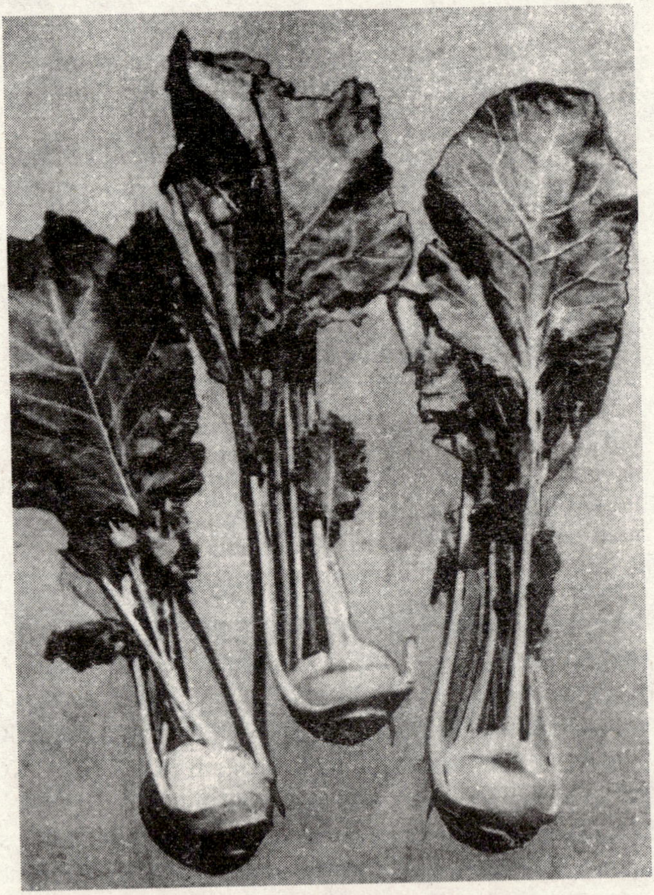

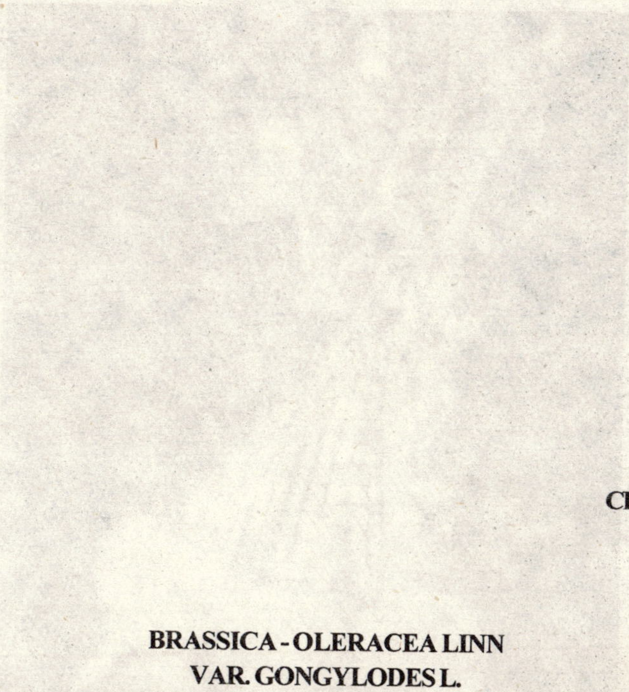

CRUCIFERAE

BRASSICA - OLERACEA LINN
VAR. GONGYLODES L.
(SYN. VAR. CAULORAPA PASQ.)

ENG.- KOHLRABI., **KNOL.**- KOHLI., **HINDI**- GANTHGOBBI., **H.**- KARAM KALLA., **S.**- DALAMALINI., DEC, KARAM **B.**- KOPI. **TAM.- & TEL.**- GOJ.

The popular name for Knolknol is kohl rabi. It exist in two varieties, one is white Vienna and the other one is purple Vienna, white Vienna is globular, light green, smooth, tender medium sized knobs while Vienna purple - the knobs are purplish and the flesh is greenish white. The portion is an enlargemnt of the stem which develops entirely above ground. It is a cool season crop, when the swollen stems reach a diameter of 5 - 7 cm. the plants are pulled out.

In its varieties cultivated all over India.

MEDICINAL USE : Leaves bitter, stomach, cardiotonic, application in gout and rheumatism. Seeds - diur., lex. stomach anthalm.

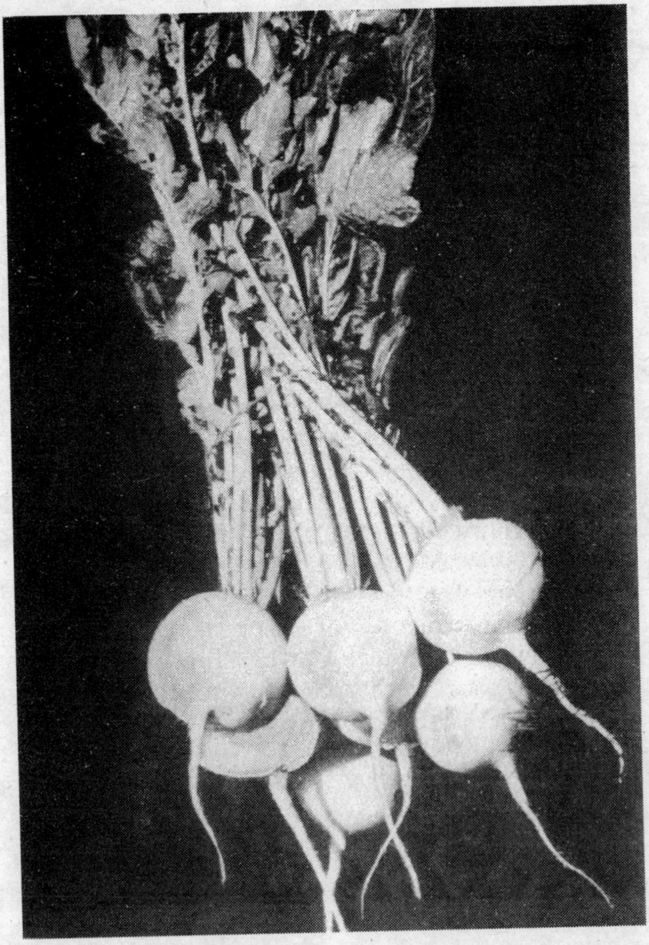

CRUCIFERAE

BRASSICA - RAPIFERA (METZG.) SINSK.
THE TRUE OR COMMON TURNIP, RAPE

ENG.- TURNIP., **HINDI-** SHALJUM., **KAN. & TEL.** - JAM., **BENG.-** SHALJAM., **MAL.-** SEEMAMULLANKI., **MAR. & ORIYA.-** SALGUM., **ASSAM-** SALGOM., **PB.-** GONGLU, SHALGAM.

Turnip is a popular light fleshed root vegetable with a swollen root and green leaves, distinctly hairy and is known as a biennial crop. The root is flat or globular, soft white fleshed with a slender taproot beneath it. Leaves are green lyrate and bristly; redical leaves 30-50 cm. long soft, prickly, lyrate-pinnatifid, petiole slender, cauline leaves are hairy with a clasping base; flowers bright yellow, those in anthesis close together and drup down overtopping the unopened buds. The fruit is siliqua on divaricate-ascending pedirel, 3.8 - 6.5 cum long with a slender beak seeds are blackish or reddish brown.

It is distributed all over India and widely cultivated in northern India, particularly in Delhi, Punjab, Jammu and Kashmir. It is also reported from Southern and Western India.

MEDICINAL USE : Turnip is a good source of ascorbic acid and calcium. The root contains a chemical called rapine which is antifungal and prevents the growth of bcocteria, fungi and yeast. The plant as a whole is sufficiently rich in protein and B-complex and to some extent can be subsituted for their deficiencies. The plant possess stomachic properties and is given in heamorrhage. It is also used for the treatment of tumours and carcinoma. The seed oil in dengue fever and rubbed on chest in bronchitis, with camphor the oil is used for muscular rehumatism and stiff neck.

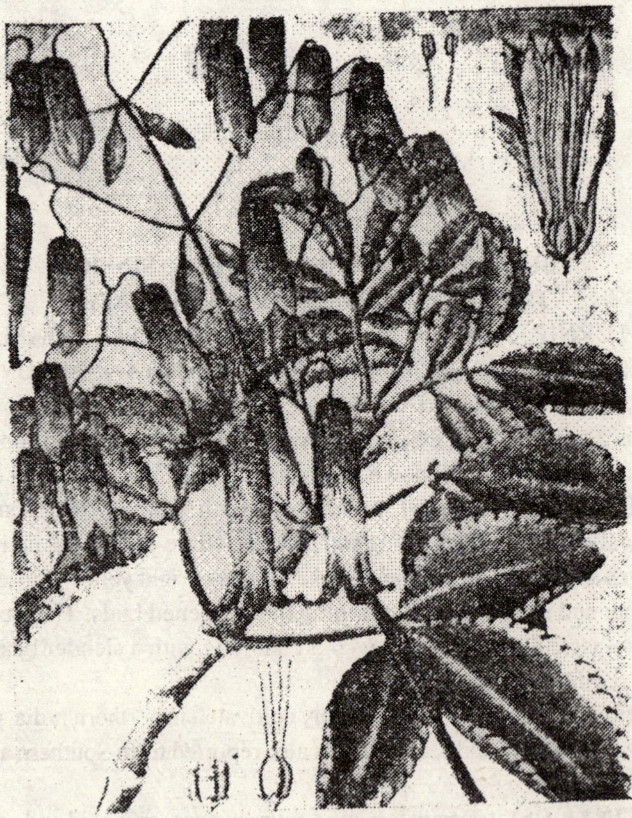

CRASSULACEAE

BRYOPHYLLUM CALYCINUM SALISB.
(SYN. KALAN CHOE PINNATA (LAMK.) PERS.)

BEN.- KOPPATA., **TAM.-** RANAKALLI., **HINDI-** ZAKAMHAIYAT., **TEL.-** SIMAJAINUAL., **MAR.-** GHAYAMARI.

It is an annual cultivated herb often grown in pots. The stem is almost straight and jointed. At nodes bilateral branch arise and each branch bears five to seven leaves. The margin of the leaf is serrated and venation is reticulate. Leaves are highly flashy and massive.

The flowers are pink to red and arise in bunches.

One notch of the leaf on sowing gives rise to a new plant. It grows throughout the hot and moist parts of India. It is most common in Bengal.

MEDICINAL USE : Leaves are bitter and contain mallic Isoçytric and citric acids, slightly warm leaves are used against Insect bite and small bruises, wounds and boils, warmer leaves are also used for different kinds of swellings and spraines. A fine paste of leave when applied to broken parts of bones regularly, the broken parts are joined and repaired without leaving a sign of illness.

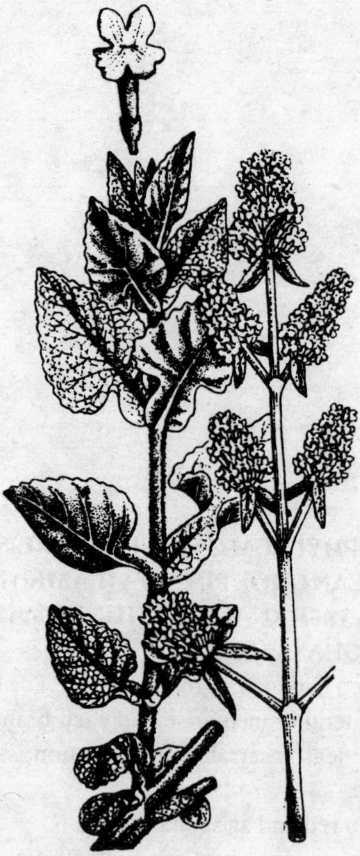

LOGANIACEAE

BUDDLEJA - ASIATICA LOUR.
KUMAON: BANA. SIMLA- NEWAR PATI.

It is ever green large shrub or small tree, with white fragrant flowers in long dense cylinderical terminal and axillary drooping panicles. Flowers tubular, four lobed. Corolla tube at least twice as long as the densely hairy Calyx. Branches, under sides of leaves and inflorescence are covered with a dense grey felt of star shaped hairs. Leaves lanceolate, accuminate, fluffy white beneath, entire or minutely toothed; usually hairless above. Capsule is hairless.

Grown commonly in hedges, shrubberies and gardens for its fragrant blooms. Flowers and fruits are found from February to June.

It is reported from sub-Himalayan tracts from Indus East wards, upto 1330 m. Common in Bengal and South India.

MEDICINAL USE : Used for skin complaints and as abortifaciant.

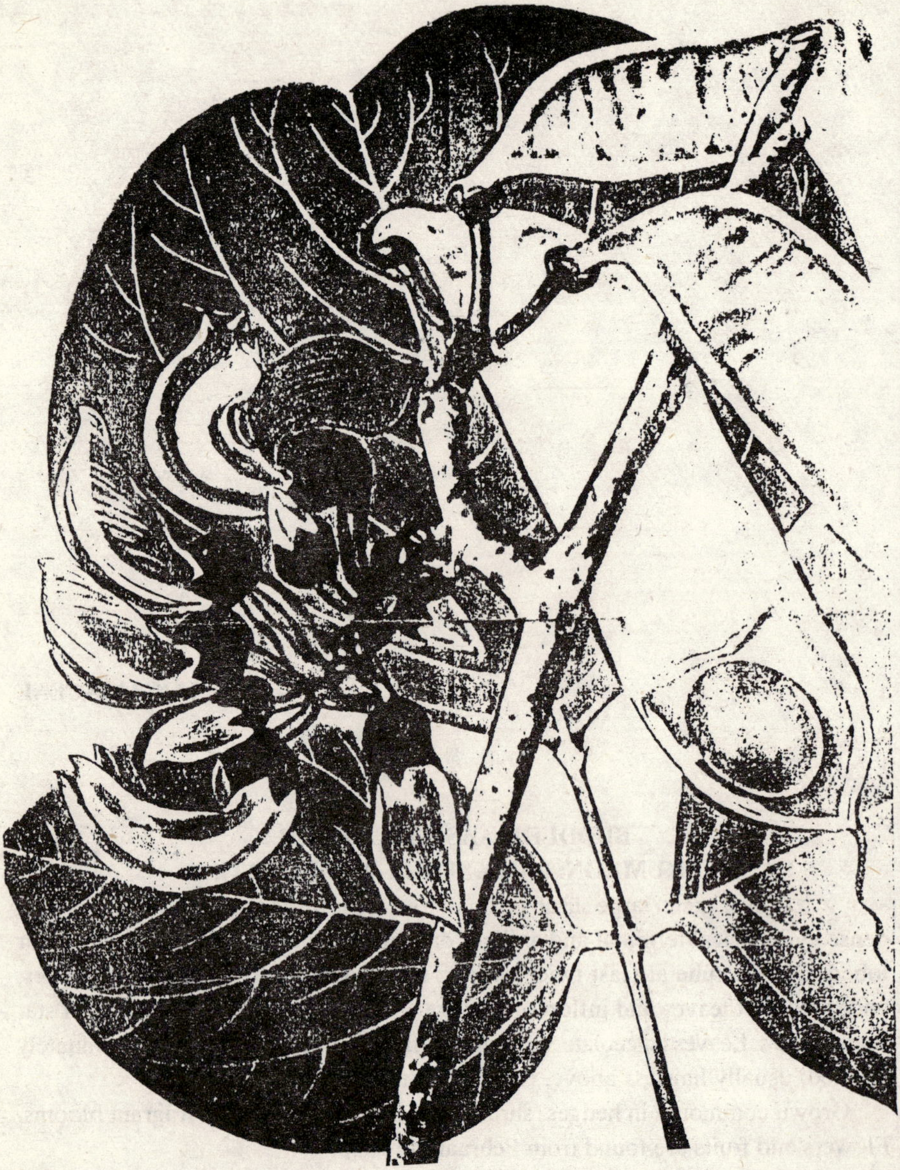

PAPILIONACEAE

BUTEA MONOSPERMA (LAMK.) TAUBERT
(Syn. B. FRONDOSA KOENIG EX. ROXB.)
(Syn. ERYTHRINA MONOSPERMA LAMK.)
(Syn. PLASO MONOSPERMA KUNTZE.)
Commonly known as Flame of the Forest.

ENG.- FLAME OF THE FOREST, BENGAL KINOI, BASTRD TEAK., **HINDI.**- DHAX, PALAS, TESU., **SANS.**- PALASHA., **MAR. & BENG.**- PALAS., **TAM.**- PARASA, MURUKAMARAM, PALASHAMARAM., **TEL.**- MODUGA, PALADULU., **MAL.**- PALASINSAMATHA, PILACHAM., **GUJ.**- KHAKRA., **KAN.**- MUTTHUGA., **LOCAL NAME.**- DHAK, PALAS, KESU, FLAME OF THE FOREST.

It is an erect medium sized deciduous tree, reaching a height of 40 - 50 ft. and 5 - 6 ft. in girth. Trunk is often crooked and latex is red. The bark is bluishgrey or light-brown and yields a gum. Shoots covered with grey or brown silky pubescence. The leaves are large stipellate and three foliate. Petiole ¼ - ½ ft.; leaflets 4 - 6 in long, coriaceous, glabrescent above, densly finely silky and strongly veined below; one end roundish with a rhomboid base, obtuse, often emarginate. The flowers are bright orange - red 5 - 8 cms long, bloom in great profusion at the begining of the hot season before the appearance of new leaves. Flowers densely fascicled, large, showy, in axillay racemes or terminal racemes or panicles. Calyx: ½" long, valvety; broadly campanulate; teeth short, delfoid. Corolla: much exserted, bright orane - red, equal, thickly clothed on the out side with silvery tomentum, the standard in broad, the keel semicircular, beaked. Stamens dia-delphous; anthers uniform ovary sessile or stalked, 2-ovuled, style filiform, curved, beadless, stigma capitate. Pods pendulous, silky-tomentose, firm, ligulate, splitting round the single apical seed, the largest part indehiscent, 6 - 8" by 1-½ - 2", argenteo-canescent, narrowed suddenly into a stalk longer than the Calyx. Blooming period is from April to May every year.

It is reported from the Himalayas to Ceylon and Burma, ascending to 4,000 ft. in the North West. Locally it is of common occurance on the ridge. This is abundant in the hilly tracts near Faridabad and Gurgoan.

MEDICINAL USE : Butea gum or Bengal kino is a powerful astringent and is given in may forms of chronic diarrhoea (Dymock, Warden & Hooper, I, 454). The seeds are valued as anthelmintic. Bird Wood (1936) prescribes them for round worms and tapeworms. Chopra (1956) also supports this view. With lemon juice the seeds act as powerful rubifacient and they have been sucessfully used in curing a form of herpes, known as dhobie's itch. The leaves are astringent and act as tonic. Flowers are astringent, diuretic, aphrodisiac and depurative. Bark mixed with seeds is used in snake bite.

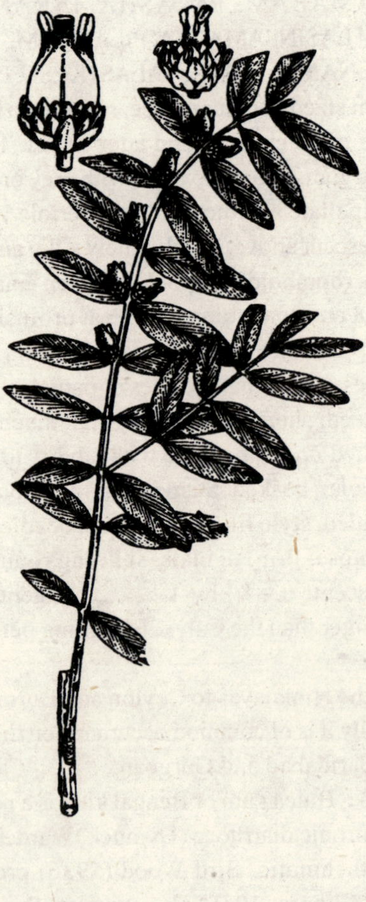

BUXACEAE

BUXUS WALLICHIANA BAILL
(SYN. B. SEMPERVIRENS LINN) (IN PART)

HINDI- CHIKRI, PAPRI., **KASH**.-CHIKRI., **P.**- PAPRI, SHAMSHAD.

It is a dense leafy evergreen shrub to a small tree. Branchlets are four sided with soft corky yellowish grey bark fissured into crocodile scales on old stems. Flowers yellowish in dense rounded axillary clusters female flowers are on the apex. Leaves entire leathery, liner lanceolate to elliptic-oblong, with a blunt or notched apex, shining above and hairless. Capsules ovoid with 3 valves and three diverging styles.

It is reported from Western and central Himalayas from Kumaon to Simla and Bhutan and on the Salt Range in West Punjab.

MEDICINAL USE : Wood of the plant contains a drug buxine. It is diaphoretic, bark is febge, leaves bitter purg. Diaphoretic, useful in rheumatism and syphilis.

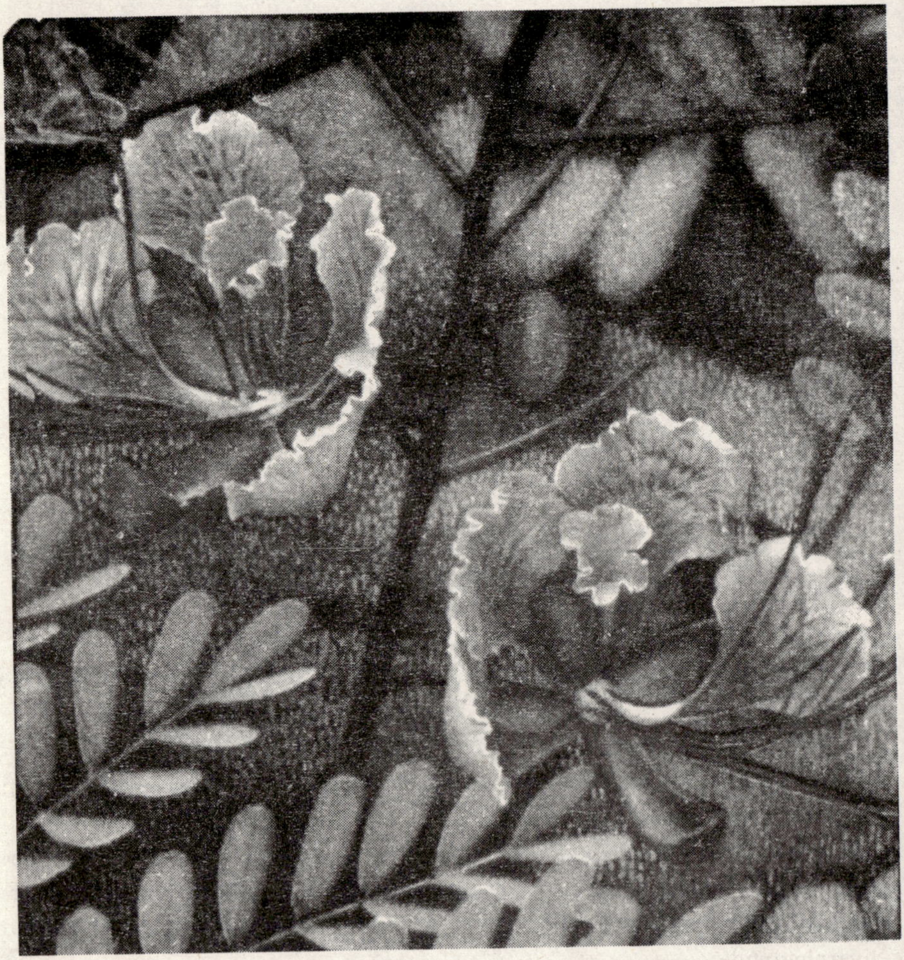

CAESALPINIACEAE

CAESALPINA PULCHERRIMA SWARTZ
(Syn. POINCCHANA PULCHERRIMA LINN.)

(popularly Known as Peacock Flower; Barbadoes Pride and Paradise Flower)

BENG.- KRISHNACHARA., **HINDI.**- GULETORA., **SANS.**- RATNAGANDHI., **GUJ.**-SANDHESHARP., **TAM.**-MAYURAM, MAYIKONNOI., **MAL.**-SETTIMANDARAM., **TEL.**- PAMIDITANGEDU., **BARM.**- DAUUNGSOP.

It is shrub or small robust erect tree upto 3 mts. tall with woody prickly climbers. Branches prickly and lenticellate. Leaves large abrubtly bipinnate. Leaflets sessile, close, membranous 1/2-3/4' long. Pinnae 12-18 leaflets 20-24 small oblique-oblong. Flowers variously coloured in red and orange, long-peduncled, in large, loose, terminal or axillary recemes. Reacemes very broad, the lower pedicels 3-4' long. Calyx 1/2-5/8' glabrous, Petals round, erisped reddish yellow, with a very distinct claw, the largest and most showy of all the species. Filaments bright red 3-4 times the length of the corolla, stamens much exserted. Pods thin ligulate flat glabrous 6-8 seeded, nearly straight, 2-3' long, the narrowest and thinest of that of any of the species.

It is said to have been introduced from America. Cultivated for hedges and in lawns and gardens shruberries. It is locally known as Gul-mohar. Flowering and fruiting period is April-December.

It is universally cultivated throughout India and elsewhere in the tropics; the native country not clearly known.

MEDICINAL USE : The leaves and bark are emmenagogue, purgative and tonic. Fresh leaves in post seeding stage contain HCN (onder-stepport J. Vet. Sci., 1941, Chem. Abstr, 1944, 1029). The bark is used as an abotifacient. An infusion of the flowers is said to be pectoral and febrifuge (Kirt and Basu, II 848; Burkill, I, 390) and is used in bronchitis, asthma and malarial fevers. (Dict. of Eco. Plants in India by Umrao Singh et. al. 1983). The flowers contain gallic acid, resins, benzoic acid, tannins, and a red colouring matter (Wehmer, I 511). The fruits are rich in tannins. A red dye has been isolated from the flowers. (Chem. Abstr. 1931, 25, 595). This species used commercially in the production of capyna compound, Geriforte lukol and Pilex.

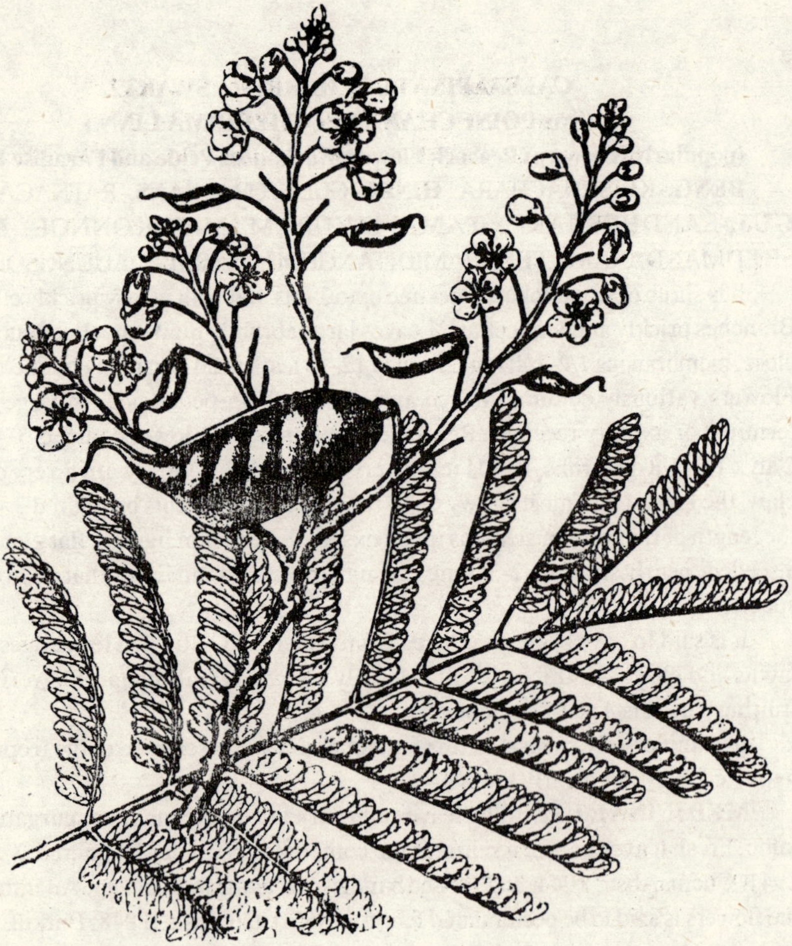

CAESALPINIACEAE

CAESALPINIA SAPPAN LINN

S.- PATANGA, PATTRANJERKA., **H. & B.**- BAKAM, PATANG., **MARATHI**- PATANG., **TAM.**- PATANGANI., **TEL.**- BAKAMU., **MAL.**- SAPPAN-NAU., **ENG.**- SAPPAN WOOD., **HINDI**- PATANG, BAKAM or SMALL TREE-NATIVE to INDIA & MALAYSIA.

It is a scrambling shrub or small tree-native to India and Malaysia with twice-pinnate leaves, with radius and branches with prickles, and with large erect spike-like clusters of bright yellow flowers. Flower cluster 30-40 cm. long. Flowers 2-3 cm across with rounded unequal petals; Calyx lobes ovate, I cm or more, stamens 10, free with filaments, which are woolly haired below; Leaves 23-28 cm with 5-10 pairs of pinnae, each with 8-12 pairs of oblong blunt leaflets 1.5-2 cm long and glaucous beneath. Pod 6-12.5 cm by 2.5 mm beaked woody.

It is reported from Pakistan to Bhutan, India, China, Japan S.E. Asia to 2200 mtr. shruberies, stony open slopes, from March-April. In India it is found chiefly in South and Bengal. Usually cultivated as a hedge plant.

MEDICINAL USE : Decot. of wood-considered emmen useful in diarroea and dysentry, given internally in certain skin diseases. It is commercially used in the preparation of cystone medicine.

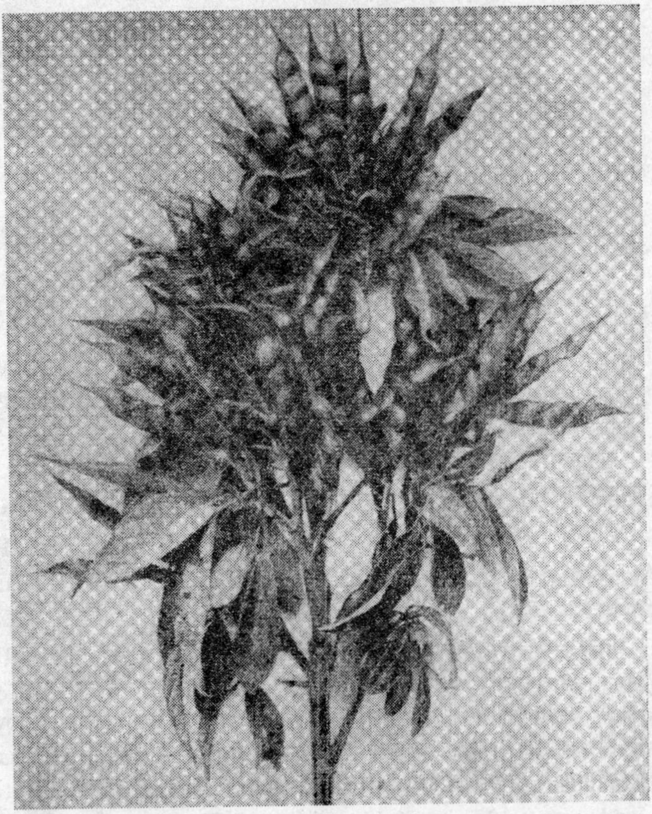

PAPILIONACEAE

CAJANUS CAJAN (LINN) MILISP.
SYN. C. INDICUS SPRENGEL.
CYSTISUS CAJAN L.

SANS.- ADHAKI, TUVARI, TUVARIKA., **HINDI**- ARHAR, TUR., **BENG.**- ARHAR, TURR, TURVER., **PUNJ.**- ARHAR, **BOMB.**- TUVER., **TAM.**- THOVARY., **TEL.**- KANDULU., **MAL.**- THUVARA., **MAR.**- ARHAR, TUR, TUVER., **KAN.**- TOGARE., **ENG.**- CAJAN PEA, PIGEON PEA, RED GRAM., **LOCAL NAME**- ARHAR, THUAR.

An annual or perennial erect shrub with slender suleate grey-silky branchlets, 4-10 ft. high, cultivated nearly throughout India as a pulse crop. Stipules minute, lanceolate; leaflets 3, minutely stipulate oblong-lanceolate, entire, subcoriaceous thinly silky above, densely beneath, indistinetly gland-dotted. Flowers in sparse distincly-peduneled corymbose racemes, often forming a terminal panicle; pedicels downy, 2-3 times the Calyx. Calyx: ¼" calyx tube companulate; teeth short, corolla much exerted, its petals equal in length; keel turncate; three times the calyx; yellow; or beautifully veined with red. Stamens:- diadelphous; anthers uniform. Ovary subsessile, few ovuled; style long, filform, much up-curved, stigma, capitate. Pod:- linear, straight, narrowed at both ends; 3-5 seeded, torulose with oblique linear depressions between the non-strophiolate seeds; 2-3" by ¼-½"; finely downy, tipped with the lower half of the style. The flowering and fruiting season is from November to July every year.

MEDICINAL USE : Seeds & leaves made into a paste, which is warmed and applied over the mammae to check seretion of milk. Seeds are used in snake bite.

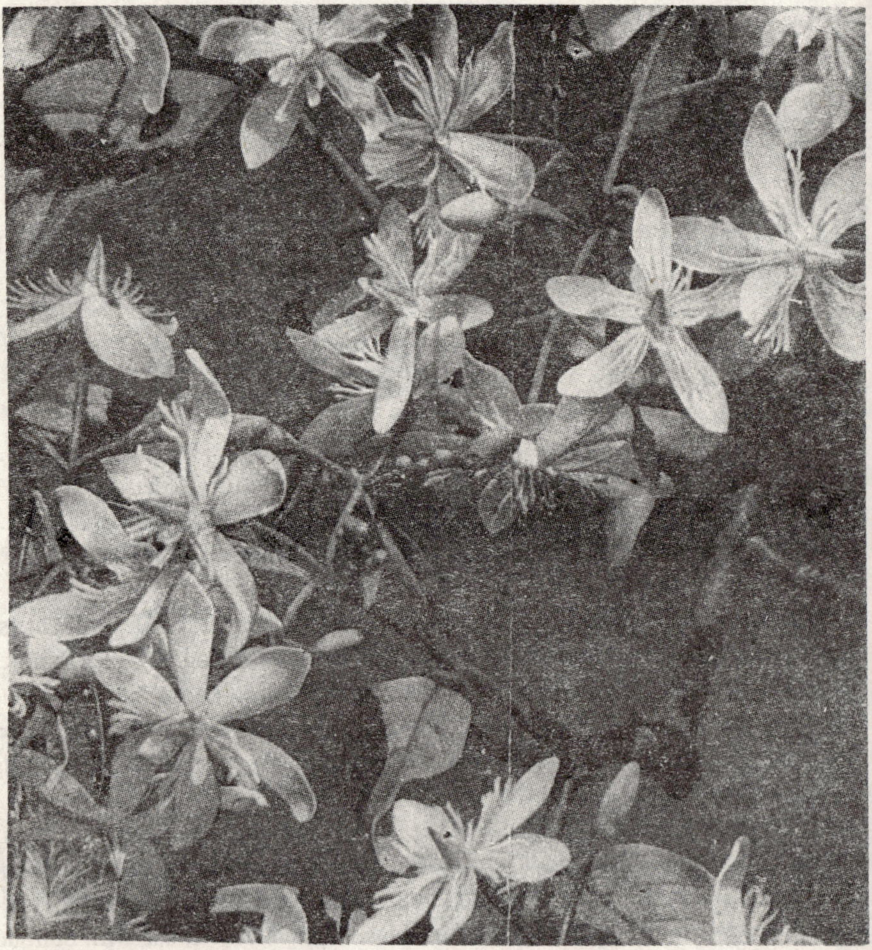

ASTERACEAE

CALENDULA OFFICINALIS LINN.

PUNJ.- ZERGUL., **HINDI-** SURAJ MUKHI., **ENG.-** MARIGOLD., **TEL.-** CHANDRAKANTAM.

It popularly known as pot Marigold is an annual hairy, erect hispidly pubescent, 1-2 ft. high plant. Leaves alternate, lower leaves spathulate quite entire, upper lanceolate, base cordate-amplexicaul toothed or subentire. Heads terminal; peduncled, hetrogamous rayed, yellow or organe; ray fl. female, 1-2 seriate, fertile, ligules entire or 3-toothed; disk-fl. hermaphaodite, sterile, tubular, limb dilated shortly 5-fid. Involucre broad; bracts 1-2-seriate; linear, acuminate, sub equal, margin often scarious; receptacle flat, naked. Anther-bases sagittate, auricles acuminate or tailed. Style-arms are undivided. Achens glabrous, of the ray, incurved, 2-3-8-eriate, heteromorphous, outermost often empty, the next broader often winged, inner shorter of the disk slender, empty pappus 0. Achenes all curved boat shapped dorsally muricate not beaked, outer larger ventrally crested scarcely beaked. (Clarke Comp. Ind. 210; Bot. Mag. t. 3204). Stem 12-18", corymbosely branched above. Leaves 1-3", acute, often hispid on both surfaces. Heads terminal 2", diameter and under involucre bracts 1/4"; incurved and appressed to the ripe achenes; ligules many, bright orange yellow, 3-toothed, tube hairy. Achenes longer than the involucre.

It is found wild in the N.W.F. Province, Punjab and Sind and cultivated in many parts of India as an ornamental garden plant. It is distributed upto Afghanistan and Westward to S. Europe.

MEDICINAL USE : The plant contains salicylic acid and inulin is present in the roots (Wehmer, loc. cit.). Marigold is a mild aromatic with diaphretic, diuretic, and stimulant properties. A tincture of the dried flowers is administered in treatment of amenorrhoea, and after dilution, as a lotion of sprains and bruises (B.P.C., 257). It may also be regarded as chloeratic (Chem. Abstr; 1944, 38, 5598). The present source of using calendula as a drug is now becoming obsolete and it is used to adulterate saffron and arncia flowers. (Irease, 547).

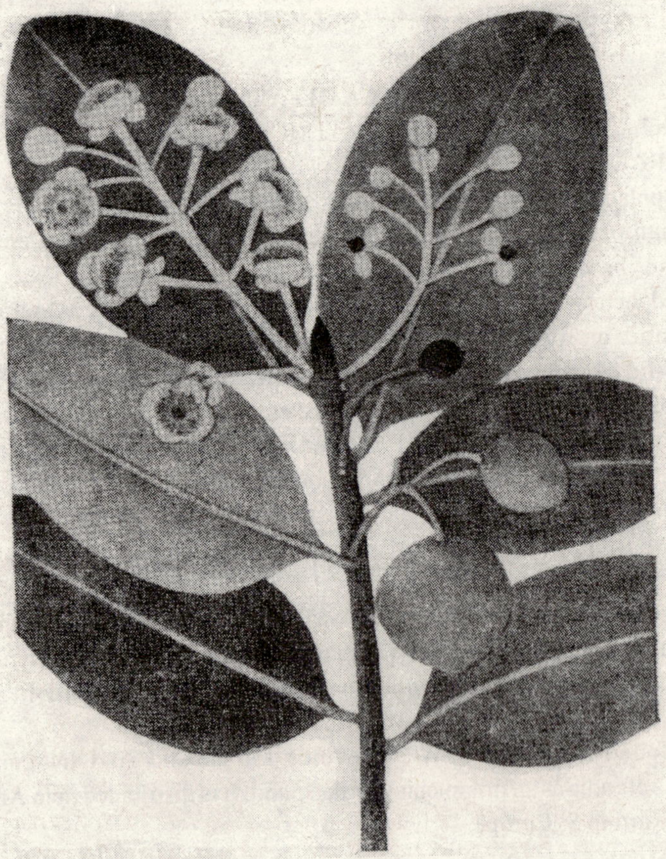

GUTTIFERAE

CALOPHYLLUM INOPHYLLUM LINN.

SANS.- NAGACHAMPA, PUNNAGA., **ENG.**- INDIAN LAUREL, LAUREL WOOD, ALEXANDRIAN LAUREL., **HINDI.**- SULTANACHAMPA, SURPAN., **BENG.**- PUNNAG, SULTANCHAMPA., **MAR.**- UNDI, SURANGI, UNDAG., **TEL.**- POUNA, PUMAGAMU., **TAM.**-PUNNAI, PINNAY, PUNNAGAM, PINNAIMARAM., **KAN.**- VUMA, HONNE, SURA HONNE., **MAL.**- PUNNA, CHERUPUNA., **URIYA.**-POONANG., **BURMA.**-POONNYET., **CEYLON.**-DOMBA., **TRADE**- POON., **BOMB.**- UNDI., **KON.**-UNDEE-PHAL.

It is a medium sized tree; evergreen and sub-maritime with fragrant flowers occuring on the coastal regions of India. The wood is reddish white to brown and heavy coarsed and grained the bark is grey and smooth. Leaves : Opposite, quite glabrous oblong or obovate-oblong obtuse or emarginate, on both surfaces shining with innumerable parallel slender veins at right angles to the midrib; 4-8 by 3-4 in; coriaceous; petiole 1/2 - 1 1/4", Flowers in short racemes, racemes sometimes panicled and terminal, usually axillary, racemes in the upper axils, loose, 4-6" long, shorter than the leaves, lax, few flowered. Flowers : Polygamous, in numerous axillary or terminal panicles. 3/4" in diameter, pure white fragrant; pedicles slender 1-2 in. Sepals 4, imbricate in series; inner sepals petaloid; petals 4, sometimes 6-8; like the inner sepals. Stamens-numerous, filaments filiform often flexous connate below; in four bundles; anthers erect, 2-celled, dehiscence vertical; ovary : globose, stipitate; style much exceding the stamens, stigma peltate lobed. Fruit 1 inch diameter, globose, smooth, yellow and pulpy. Seed erect, ovoid or globose, testa thin or thick and spongy.

It is reported from Western Peninsula; from Concon and Orissa, Southwards; Ceylon; Eastern Peninsula; from Pegu Southwards; Andaman Islands. E. African Islands, Malay Archipelago, Australia, Polynesia-cultivated throughout India.

MEDICINAL USE : (i) The leaves contain saponin and hydrocyanic acid, and are poisonous to fish (Burkill, I, 411). Pounded bark is applied in Orchitis and its juice is used as purgative. A decoction of it is employed as lotion for indolent ulcers. A yellowish-green aromatic resin, possessing emetic and purgative properties, is obtained as an exudation from the bark. (Dymock, Warden and Hooper, I, 174).

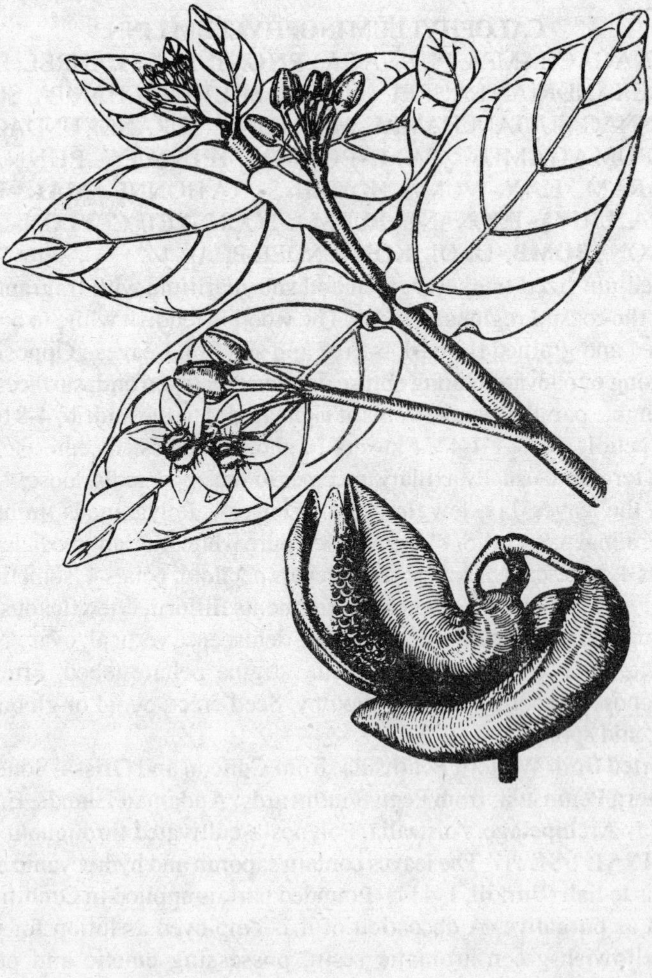

ASCLEPIADACEAE

CALOTROPIS GIGANTEA (L) DRYANDER
(Syn. ASCLEPIAS GIGANTEA WILLD.)

BENG.- AKANDA., **ENG.**- SWALLOW-WORT, MUDAR., **GUJ.**- ARADO., **HINDI**- MADAR, AK., **KAN.**- EKKA, ARKAGIDA., **MAL.**- ERIKKA., **MAR.**- RUVI, RUI., **TAM.**- AERUKKU, ARKKAM., **TEL.**- MANDARAMU, JELIEDU., **SANS.**- ARKA, MANDARA., **BOMB.**- AKANDA., **ARAB.**- ASHUR., **PERS.**- KHARK., **SIND.**- BIJALOSHA., **LOCAL NAME**- AK, AKRA, ANKTA, MADAR.

An erect perennial, glabrous or hoary shrub or small tree reaching a height of 8-10 ft. Trunk is stout; bark is pale and shoots are woolly. Young foliage hoary. Leaves opposite, broad, subsessile thick, ovate-oblong or elliptic sub amplexicaul, 4-8 by 1-3 in; may be euneate-obovate; base cordate, axils beareded, smooth above, cottony beneath. Flowers are in simple or compound axillary and terminal corymbose cymes. The flowers are strong smelling; pale silvery outside, dull mauve, purple or white internally. Inflorescence white cottony; umbels peduncled, simple or compound; bracts oblong. Calyx: Campanulate or bell shaped, Calyx teeth five; greenish colour outside; purple white inside; sepals glandular within. Corolla pale purple; broadly companulate; lobes broad, naked valvate; 1.2-2.5 cm. across, with reflexed ovate-lanceolate corolla lobes 1-5 cm. hairy on the outside; horns of corona hairy up curved. (Corona of 5 fleshy laterally flattened horns radiating from the stamen tube). Anther tips memberanous, inflexed; pollen masses one in each cell, pendulous flattened, waxy, stigma depressed, 5 angled or lobed. Carpels paired, curved, 8-10 cm. by 2 cm. broad. Follicles short thick, recurved 3-4 inch. Seeds ¼ inch., broadly ovate; flattened with long bright silky white coma. It bears a five, soft, gloosy and resilient floss of cream colour.

India, China, S.E. Asia, Throught Himalaya to 1200 mt. Wasteland, river graval; common in lower Nepal valleys. March - October. In India it is reported from Punjab to Asam, Ceylon and Singapore. Malay Islands and S. China. Locally it is of common occurance in open, waste, sandy, dry places.

MEDICINAL USE : Its latex is a voilent purgative and initant to skin. (Sharma, Indian J. Vet. Sci., 1934, 4, 63, Chopra, loc. cit.). A tincture of the leaves is used in the treatemnt of intermittent fevers. Powdered flowers in small doses are useful in the treatment of colds, coughs, asthma and indigestion. Powdered root bark gives relief in dysentry (Koman, 1919, 1915). The root bark is said to be similar to ipecacuanhar in its action. In small doses (0.2-.6gm) it is diaphoretic and expectorant, and in large doses (2-4 gm.) it is an emetic (B.P.C. 259). The root bark, in the form of a paste, is applied in elephantiasis (Chopra, loc. cit.).

In CALOTROPIS poisoning cases, demulchant and mucilaginous drinks, milk, rice-gravel, etc. should be given, and morphine and atropine administered to allay pain. Skin irritation can be allayed by the application of cold water followed by soothing preparations like glycerine belladonna.

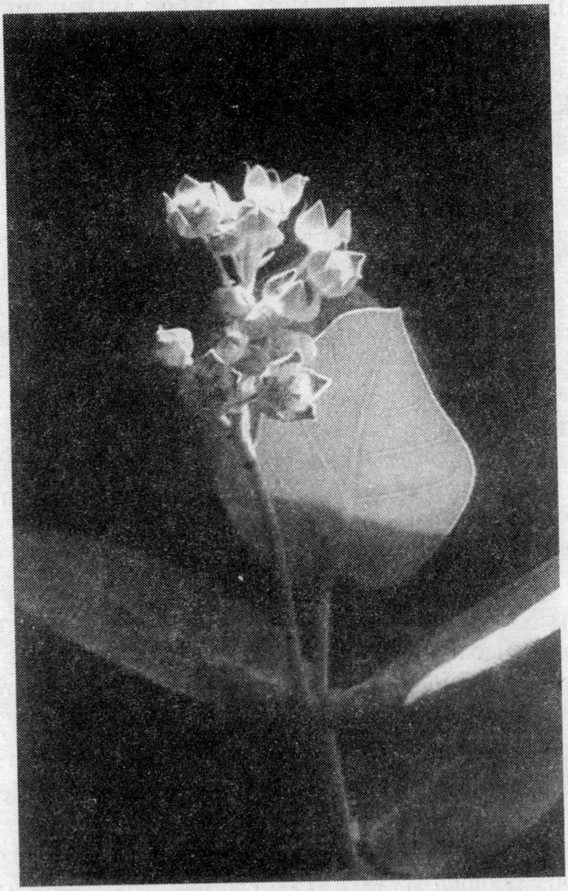

ASCLEPIADACEAE

CALOTROPIS PROCERA R.BR. DRY AND EX. W. AIT.
(SYN. ASCELEPIAS PROCERA WILLD)

BENG.- AKANDO., **MAR.**- MANDORA., **HINDI**- SAFED AK, MANDORA., **PUNJABI**- SHAKAR-AL-LIGBAL., **ENG.**- AKODA, AKUND., **TAM.**- VELLAEUKKU, SWALLOW-WART., **LOCAL NAME**- AK, AKRA, ANKTA, MADAR.

An ever green erect shrub. Young foliage hairy fleshy and sticky, leaves thick ovate-oblong or elliptic sub amplexicaul, Flowers purplish red, pale silvary outside, strong smelling, in terminal and axillary, corym-bose cymes. Follicles recurved smooth. Seeds flat with a silky white dot. Flowers and fruits March to July.

Found in north, western and central India from Sind and in Punjab Bengal, Bihar and Bombay and in the drier climate of the Deccan. This is the smaller white flowers variety.

MEDICINAL USE : The leaves and latex are used in various body troubles such as pain, swelling etc.

Root Bark is used in Dysentry, it is used as diaphoretic expectorant and emetic. Powdered flowers are used in cold cough and asthma.

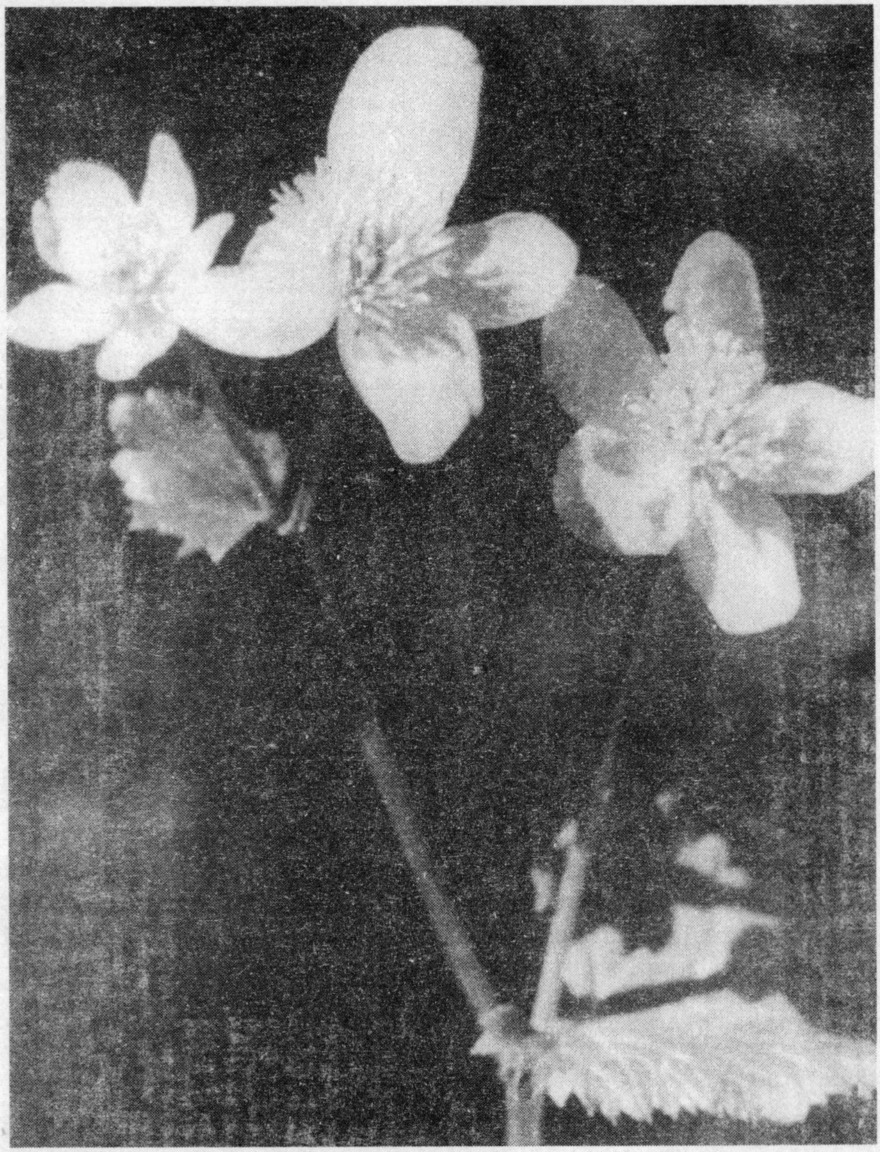

RANUNCULACEAE

CALTHA - PALUSTRIS L.
VAR. HIMOLENSIS (D. DON) MUKERJEE

ENGLISH- MARSH MARIGOLD., **PUNJABI**- MAMIRI, MUNNINI, BARINGU.

It is a fleshy - looking hairless plant found in damp and marshy places. Hence also known as Marsh Marigold. It is distinguished by its large shining rounded or heart shaped leaves. The flowers are found in clusters containing few in nos. situated terminally. The flowers are usually yellow or white coloured, cup shaped. Flowers are 2.5-4 cm across with 5-8 ovate petals; and numerous stamens and carpels. Leaves are generally basal. Long stalked, blade 3-15 cm across, finely toothed, Fruit is a cluster of beaked follicles each one is nearly as broad as 1 cm.

It is reported from Pakistan to Bhutan, 2400-4000 in open slopes, damp places on grazing grounds, very common, March- May- August.

MEDICINAL USE : Roots - acrid and poisonous.

Roots contain helleborin and veratrin.

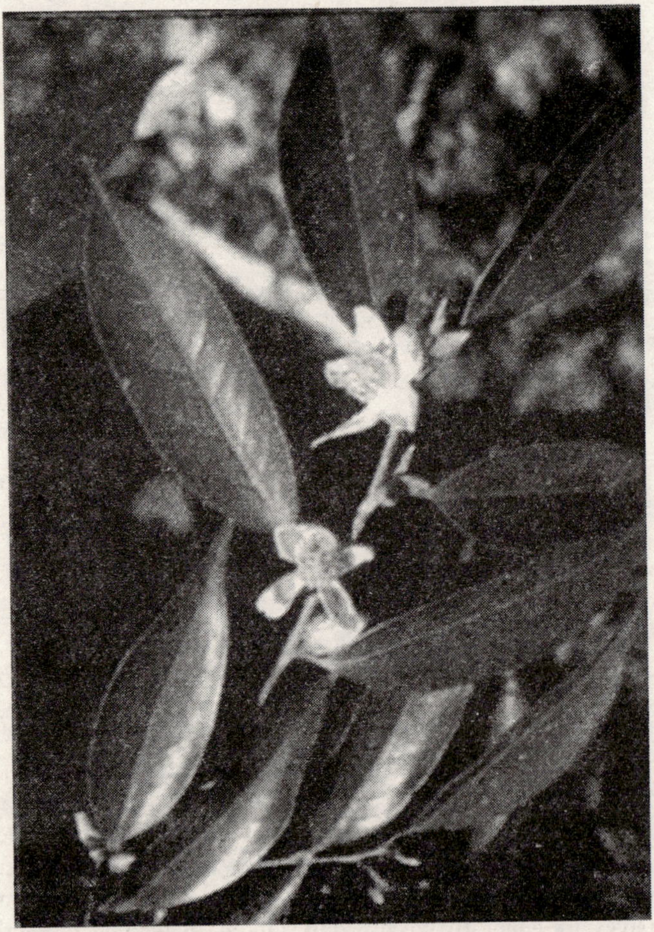

THECACEAE

CAMELL IA SINENSIS (LINN.) KUNTZE
(Syn. C. THEA LINK.), (Syn. C. THEIFERA GRIFF.)
(Syn. THEA SINENSIS L.)

HINDI.-CHA, CHAI., **BENG.**-CHA, CHAI., **PUNJ.**-CHA, CHAI., **BOMB.**-CHA, CHAI., **TAM.**-THAYALAI., **TEL.**-THEYAKU., **ENG.**-TEA.

It is evergreen tree or shrub reaching to a height of 30-50 ft. normally. But under cultivation it is usually pruned down to a height of 3-6 ft. and is generally maintained in the form of a bush. Branchlets glabrous; buds silky. The leaves are evergreen, elliptic, oblong acute or cuspidate-acuminate puberulous on the nerves beneath; 4-8 by 1-1/2-2 -1/2 inch. tapering at either end, more or less senate membranous; the young leaves are more or less pubescent, while mature leaves are bright green in colour, leathery and smooth varying in length from 2-12 inch; petiole is 1/6 inch; Flowers axillary, solitary, or aggregated, sessile or shortly stalked; 1 1/4" in diameter and white. Peduncles 2-3 bracteate, short Sepals : 5-6 unequal, graduating from the bracts towards the petals orbicular, glabrous, with membranous ciliate edges. Petals : slightly coherent at the base, broadly obovate; 5; all equal; stamens-numerous, the outer most in many rows, slightly or almost wholly monadelphous, adherent to the base of the petals, the inner most 5-12 free. Stamens glabrous. Ovary 3-5 celled; styles short; are united for 2/3 part of their length. Ovules 4-5 in each cell, pendulous. Capsule woody, usually short, loculicidal, leathery, trigonous; cells 1-rarely 2-seeded. Seeds 3/4" in diameter nearly globose or obtusely angled, smooth, pale brown; mostly solitary in each cell.

The flowers are noddling, sepals persistent. There appear to be two main axes of geographical distribution. The two axes roughly correspond with the valleys of Brahmaputra, Irrawaddy, Salween, Mekong and Yaugtse Kiang. It is considered as native of China and cultivated there for centuries. Possibly also native in E. Himalaya; extensively cultivated in Assam and Darjeeling since the nineteenth century. In E. Nepal, it is cultivated near and around Palampur in Kangra in the West Himalaya to 2,300 ft. December-March. It is also extensively cultivated in Darjeeling, Assam, Travancore, the Nilgiris, Malabar, N. Bengal, Dehradun and Kumaon.

MEDICINAL USE : Tea leaves are astringent stimulant, gently excitant and diuretic. It is an accepted wholesome and stimulating beverage; more strimulating to muscular system than to brain and it relieves bodily fatigue. It contains vitamins, such as niotinic acid; pantothenic acid riboflavin and ascorbic acid in fresh state.

Infusion of tea leaves are used in conjunctivitis because of their astringent character. Black tea water mixed with salt and lime juice (No milk and No sugar) is a good remedy and precautionary measure for malarial patients.But protection against tooth decay is not the only oral hygienc benefit of tea drinking. Japanese research has also suggested that a regular intake of tea can help to prevent the build-up of plaque, the scaly substance which contributes so much to gum disease in later life. For centuries in Japan, green tea has also been used as a folk medicine to prevent halitosis (bad breath). Green tea extracts are also used in some tooth-pastes to give a lasting "just brushed" sensation. Green tea also contains chemicals called cathechins, thought to have cancer-fighting properties.

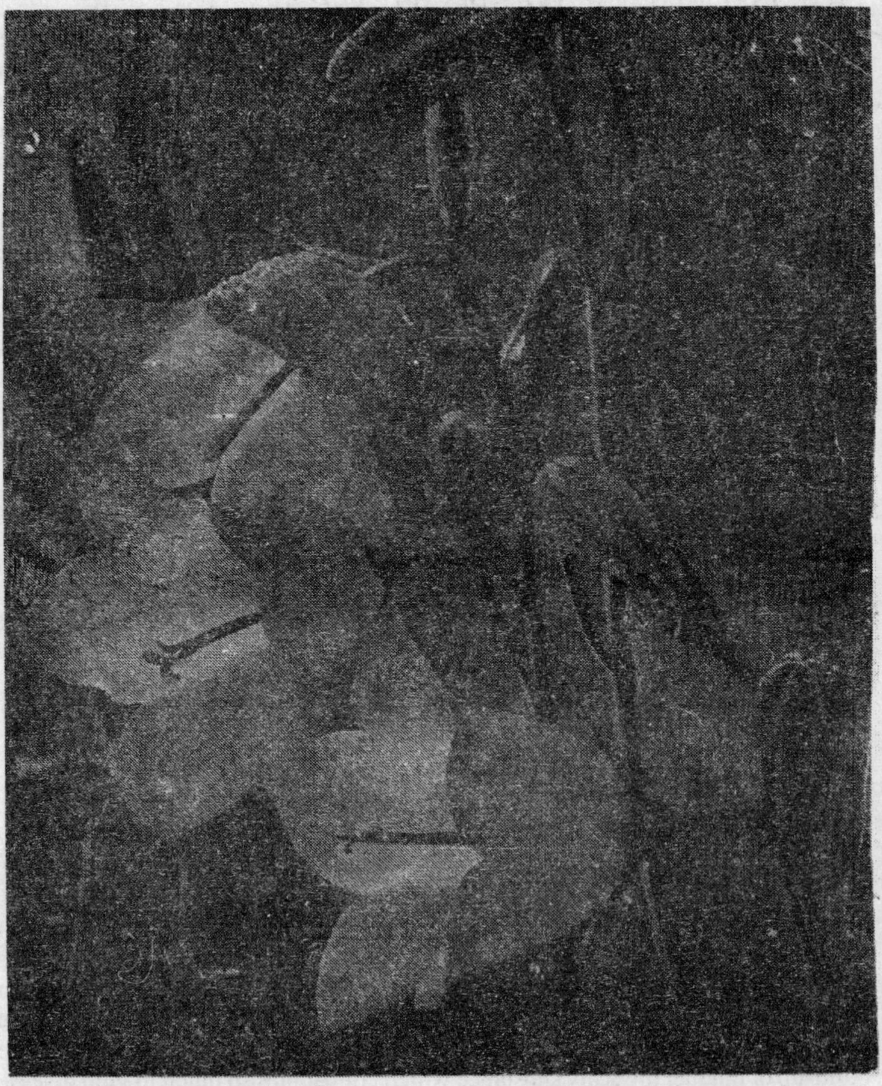

CAMPANULACEAE

CAMPANULA ROTUNDIFOLIA L (SYN. C. LATIFOLIA L.)

In English it is popularly known as large (bell flower or Chimney, bell flower).

It is an ornamental robust leafy perennial with large nodding dark blue-purple bell shaped flowers, 4-5 cm. long, borne in a long spike-like terminal cluster on stems 60-200 cm. Flowers axillary, short-stalked, the stalk down-curved in fruit, corolla lobes triangular lanceolate, calyx tubes narrow lanceolate, much shorter than corolla. Stem leaves mostly stalkless, 5-12 mm ovate, or lanceolate with rounded base, margined toothed, hairy leaves becoming progressively smaller above capsule globose.

It is reported from Pakistan to C. Nepal, W & M Asia, Europe 2100-3600 m. Forests, shrubberies. July-August. It is reported from West, Himalayas from Kashmir, to Garhwal, 8000.

MEDICINAL USE : Its related speies known as CODONOPSIS OVATA Banth, also known as Ladut, Its leaves and roots are used as poultices used for bruises, ulcers and wounds.

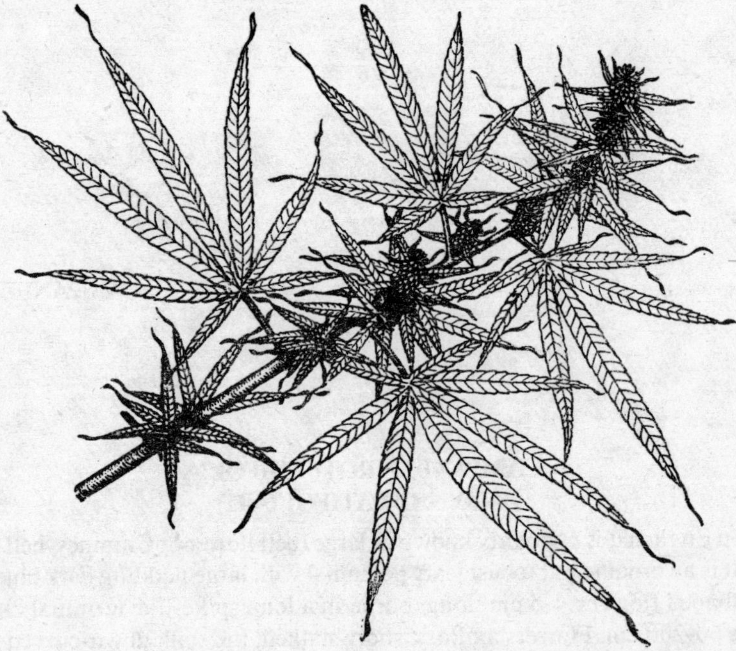

CANNABIDACEAE

CANNABIS SATIVA LINN.
(Syn. C. INDICA LINN.)

ENG.- HEMP, INDIAN HEMP., **HINDI**- GANJA, BHANG, CHARAS., **SANS.**- BHANGA, GANJIKA, VIJAYA., **BENG.**- BHANG, GANJA, CHARAS, SIDDHI, JIA., **BOMB.**- BHANG, GANJA, CAHRAS, SIDDHI, JIA., **PUNJ.**- BHANG., **TAM.**- BHANGI, GANJA, KANJA., **TEL.**- GANZAI, KALPAM-CHETTU, GANJAYI., **GUJ.**- BHANG, GANJA, CHARAS, SIDDI, JIA., **KAN.**- BHANGI., **KON.**- BHANGI., **MAR.**- BHANG., **MAL.**- KANCHA., **LOCAL NAME**- BHANG.

It is a erect, tall, robust annual dioecious herb, 4-16 ft. high with angular stem being 4-8 ft. strictly, sub-simple; bearing palmately divided or digitate leaves with narrow coarsely toothed leaflets. Leaves are 4-8 inch. in diameter; 3-8 foliate; long petioled. alternate or the lower opposite, upper 1-3; lower; 5-11 partite serrate all leaves long-stalked, gland dotted, pale, very finely downy beneath; leaflet variable in size 3-10 cms. Stem palmatclinerved; stipules lateral. The palnt is dioecious or rarely monocious. Flowers greenish yellow grooved finely, hairy with slender branches. Small, axillary diocious 4mm long; males facicled in short pendulous panicles; females crowded under leafy convolute bracts. Male flowers with 5 lobed perianth imbricate and 5 stamens with yellow anthers and with thread like filaments; pistillode O; Female flower. Perianth hyaline, embracing the ovary; ovary sessile; style central, arms 2 filfiform caducous; ovule pendulous. Fruit; 4mm. membranous, subglobose, not oblique, laxly clothed with the persistant sepals. Seed globose

Originally this plant is considered as native of Western and Central Asia, but it is naturalised in the Sub-Himalayan tract in India and is abundantly met within waste lands from Punjab East-wards to Bengal and Bihar and extending southwards to Decan. It is cultivated in temperate and tropical regions. In India the drug being a monopoly of the Government, it is grown in some areas such as Bengal, Karnataka and Tamil Nadu by license holders. Flowering and fruiting is in the cold season.

MEDICINAL USE : The intoxicating drugs "ganja" and 'Charas' are obtained from the resinous exudations of the stem, young leaves and flowers. 'Bhang' or 'Pot' consists of the larger leaves mixed with some fruits. All these are best for medical use (Nadkarni, 1954). All parts of the plant are considered to be intoxicating, stomachic, antispasmodic, analgesic, stimulant aphrodisiac and sedative. In large doses for a prolonged period it causes lassitude, indifference, lack of productive activity, insomnia, headache, hystomgus, increased susceptibility to infactions, gestro-intestinal disturbances, sexual impotence and personality changes. Mortality at very high doses was due to respiratory arrest.

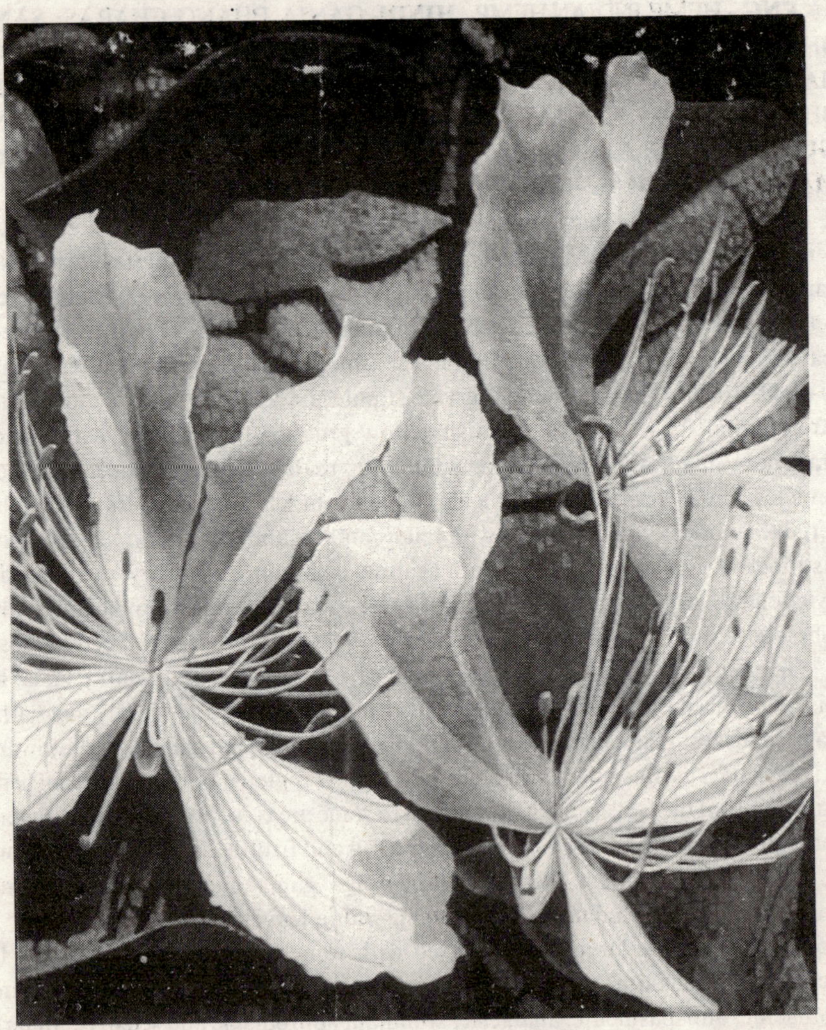

CAPPARIDACEAE

CAPPARIS SPINOSA. LINN
THE CAPER BUSH

HINDI-KABRA., **GUJ**.- KALO, KANTHARO, KANTHARO., **KAN.**-KATRIMULLINAGIDDA, MARATTAMAGGU, MULLUKATTARI., **BO.**-KABAR., **KUMAON**-BUSAR., **TEL.**-KOKILAKSHAMU., **LADAKH**-KABRA., **PUNJAB**-BARAR, KAUR.

A straggling spreading shrubby plant, glabrous or hoary, branches prostrate or trailing. The branches are spiny. the leaves are leathery, simple or rarely rounded. Leaves variable, orbicular ovate to elliptic, 1-4 cm. mostly spine-tipped; pale green not shining acute; obtuse or retuse; stipules of 2 hooked brown or yellow spines. Flowers large 3-8 cm. across, long stalked borne in the axils of the younger leaves. The flowers are white with purple filaments; pedicels equalling or exceeding the leaves. Sepals 4, free imbricate in 2 series, or 2 outer subvalvate, Petals 4, sessile, imbricate or obovate, 2-5 cm.; stamens indefinite, inserted on the torus at the base of the long gynophore. Ovary stalked, 1-4 celled; stigma sessile; ovules many, on 2-6 perietal placentas. Fruits fleshy, oblong ellipsoid 2-5 cm., long stalked with red flesh and brown seeds rarely bursting by valves. Seeds many, imbedded in pulp, testa crustaceous or coriaceous; cotyledons convolute.

It is reported from Afghanistan to E. Nepal, West Asia, Europe. 2,000-3,000 cm. stony slopes, in dry valleys. North Africa, Australia, Sandwich Islands, Flowering May-September. It is also reported from rocky and Hilly localities in the Ocean peninsula, Rajputana and North-Western India, Hot Western Himalayan Valleys Eastward to Nepal, West Tibet, ascending to 13,000 ft. Sindh; Punjab and Western Peninsula in the Mhableshwar Hills. It is known as native of the Mediterranean region. It is also reported from Rajasthan and Peninsular India.

MEDICINAL USE : The bark is bitter aperient, diuretic, expectorant, emmenagogue and tonic. It is used in rheumatism, paralysis, tooth ache, infections of liver and spleen, and tubercular glands. The bruised leaves are used as poultice in gout. (Kirt and Basu, I. 196).

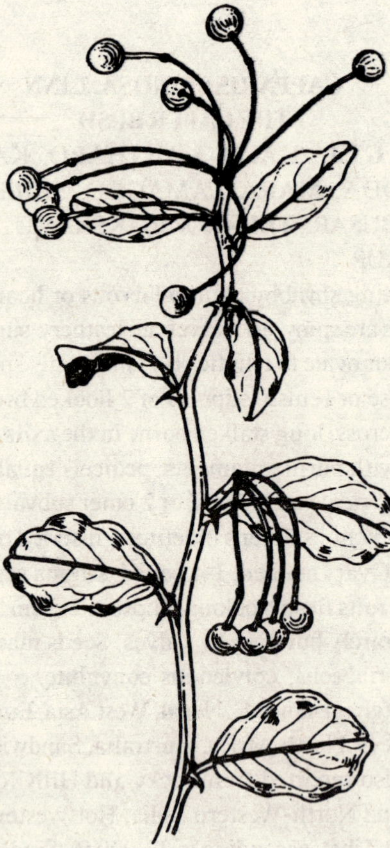

CAPPARIDACEAE

CAPPARIS ZEYLANICA LINN.
(Syn. C. HORRIDA LINN.)
C. ACCUMINATA ROX B

BENG.- KALO-KERA., **HINDI**- GOVINDAPHAL, ARDANDA, GITORAN., **MAR.**- WAG., **BOMB.**- WAG., **PUNJ.**-KARVILA., **TAML.**- ADONDAI, TONDAI. **TEL.**- ADONDA.

A rigid, wiry glabrous, armed much branched shrub; shoots sometimes puberulous. Leaves : 1 1/2 -3 by 1/2 -1 1/2 inch; coriaceous, shining above, sometimes pubescent beneath; broad ovate to lanceolate usually acute and mucronate reticulate beneath. The flowers are solitary, usually regular; 2 inch in diameter; white; or 2-3 on a short shoot (racemes), Pedicels 1-2 inch, slender. Sepals 4, free, inbricate in 2 series, or 2 outer sub-valvate. Petels-4, sessile imbricate. 2 lower petals yellowish changing to red-brown stamens indefinite, inserted on the torus at the base of the long gynophore. Ovary pubescent, oblong stalked superior, of 2 fused carpels; 1-4 celled with many ovules on 2-6 parictal placentas. Stigma sessile. Fruits : fleshy; 2 inch; ovoid; smooth usually a capsule splitting by valves, sometimes a berry; Seeds many inbedded in pulp, testa erustaceous or coriaceous; cotyledons convolute.

It is found commonly in the carnatic and Malabar Hills; occasional in the Western Deccan; dry parts of Ceylon. It is also reported from Afghanistan to E. Nepal W. Asia to Europe. 2,000-3,000 m. Stony slopes, in dry valleys. May-Sept. It is reported from all parts of India.

MEDICINAL USE : The root bark is bitter, Sedative stomachic Cholagougue, anti-hidrotic (Kirt & Basu, I, 201), and is used in Cholera.

Leaves : Counter-irritant and as cataplasm in boils swellings and piles.

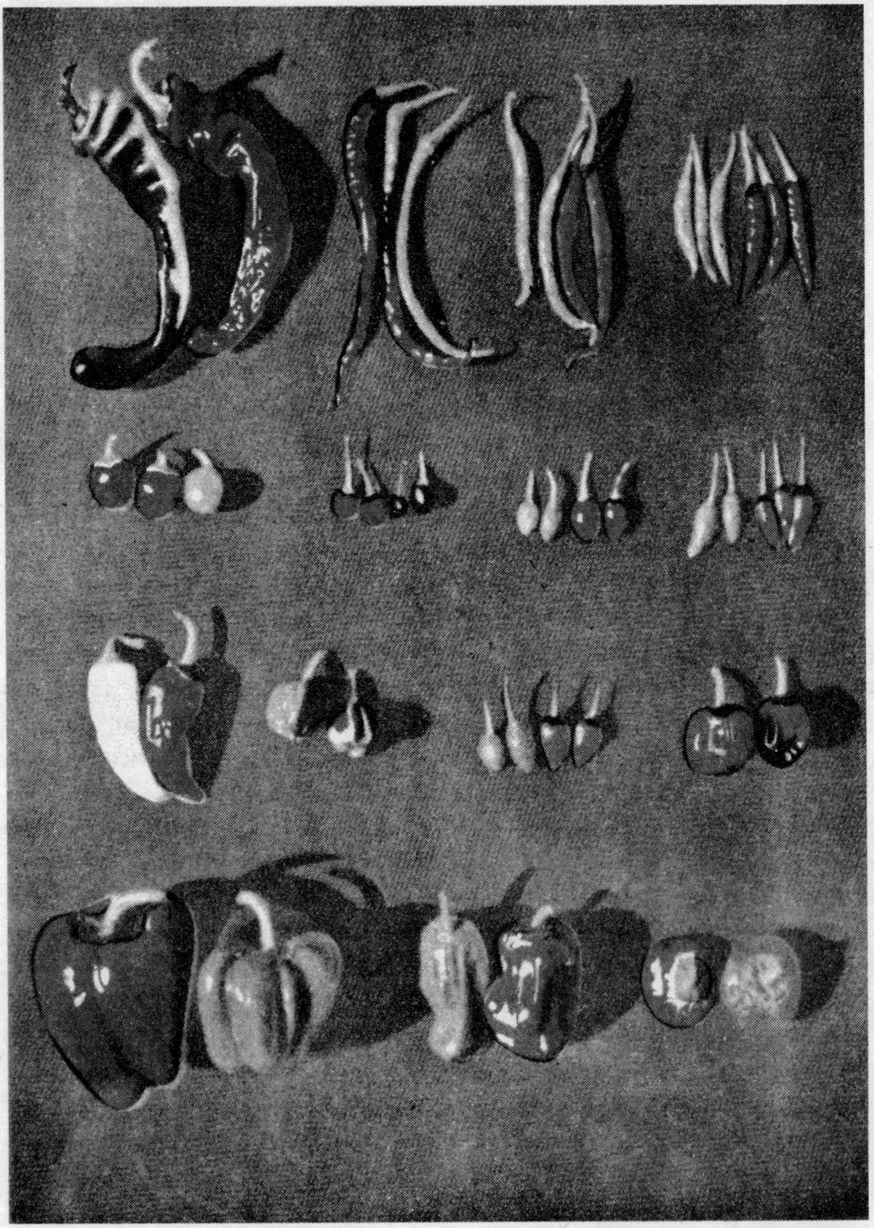

SOLANACEAE

CAPSICUM ANNUUM LINN. (VARIETY ACCUMINATUM)

ARAB.- FILFILIAMHAR., **HINDI**- LALMIRICH, GACHMARICH., **TEL.**- MIRAPAKAYA., **KAN.**- MENSINA KAI., **MAL.**- MULAKU., **ENG.**- RED PEPPER, CHILLIES., **LOCAL NAME**- MIRCH., **PUNJ.**- LAL MIRICH., **TAM.**- MILAGAY., **BENG.**- LANKAMORICH, LALMORICH.

A cultivated crop. There are two to three crops in a year. Numerous varieties, differing in habit and mode of growth and in size, shape and colour of the fruits have evolved in the course of time in different environments. Broadly speaking, all of these varieties are considered under two categories.

a) CAPSICUM ANNUM :

b) C. FRUTESCENS:

Out of these two the former is more important some people however do not cosider them as two different species. These plants are annuals with a short growing season. They are small and busy reaching a height of 1 to 3 ft., glabrous or nearly so. Leaves : Entire or repand, oval and dark green in shape and colour. The flowers are white in colour and droping, and fruits are borne singly in the axil of leaves; Pedicels-single and axillary or sometimes 2-3 together. Calyx : Campanulate, subentire or minutely 5-toothed, much shorter than the fruit. Corolla rotate; lobes 5, valvate in bud; stamens 5, attached near the base of the corolla, anthers not longer than the filaments, dehiscing longitudinally. Ovary 2-rarely 3-celled; style linear, stigma subcapitate, Berries 5-10 cm. long, much longer than broad, reflexed, red or yellow, many seeded, mildly pungent. Seeds discoid, smooth or subscatrous; The flowering and fruiting season is from June to October every year.

Species 20, native in America, some cultivated in all warm countries. It is grown in many parts of India, especially in Madras, Bihar, Hyderabad and Bombay, and to a lesser extent in the plains of North India. It is grown also in the hills up to 6,500 ft. Today peppers are grown in each and every tropical country of the world and have become the most important spice in a number of countries. Andhra Pradesh, Maharashtra, Karnataka and Tamil Nadu, M.P., Bihar and Rajasthan account for about 75 per cent of the annual production.

MEDICINAL USE : Capsicum is given internally as powerful stimulant and carminative, especially in flatulent dyspepsia. Tincture of capsicum is something added to gargles for pharyngitis and relaxed sore throat. Externally it is used for lumbalgo, neuralgia and rheumatism. In the form of ointment it is applied to painful joints & in rheumatoid arthritis.

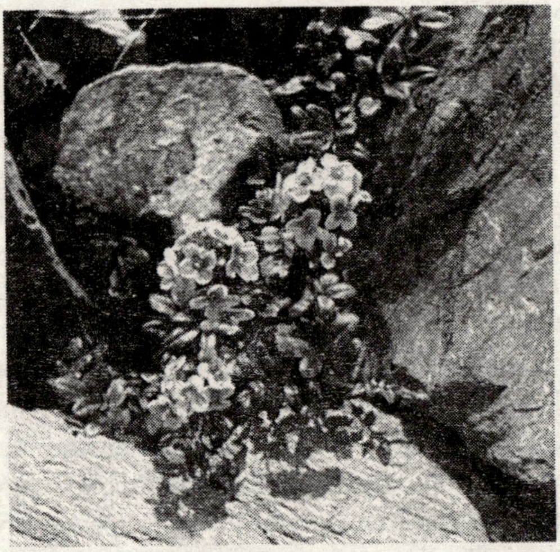

CRUCIFERAE

CARDAMINE LOXOSTEMONOIDES O.E. SCHULZ

It is a small delicate ornamental perennial, with relatively large lilae or pinkish flowers borne on flexuous spreadings stems, and with small pinnate leaves. Flowers 1-15 cm across petals strongly veined, 3 times as long as sepals. Leaves with 4-7 pairs of rounded to narrow oblong leaflets, usually 5-15 mm the terminal leaflet similar, entire or 3 lobed Stem 10-20, Rhizome creeping with bulbils. Fruits 2.5-3 cm. long with a style 2-3 mm flattended strongly compressed, hairless valve of fruit coil up suddenly from the base ejecting the seeds.

It is reported from Pakistan to Bhutan, Tibet 3000-5000 mtr. rocks, scored May-July. Its other specis C. LOXOSTEMOMOIDES U.E. Schulz and C. MACROPHYLLA_wild are found in Pakistan to South West China. 2100-3600 m. Forests, streamsides, common in West Himalaya. May-August.

MEDICINAL USE : Plant-Stim, diaphor, diur, Flowering tops, in Epilepsy. Seeds contain myonic acid and an oil. Similar to mustered oil (U.S.D. 1385)

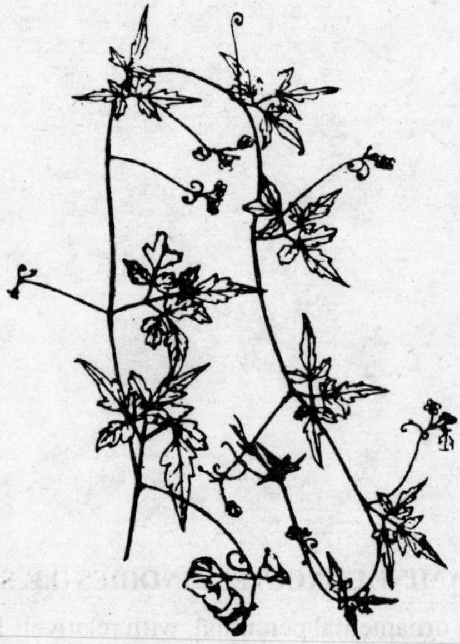

SAPINDACEAE

CARDIOSPERMUM HALICACABUM LINN

ENG.- NAYAPHATAKI., **MAL.-** UZHINSA, PALLOOLAVAM., **MAR.-** KANPUTTI., **ENGLISH-** BALLOON VINE, WINTER CHERRY., **MAR. & PUNJ.- HABUL** - KALKAL., **GUJ.-** KAROCHO., **TAM.-** VALALAVAE, MUDAKKITTAAN., **HINDI-** KANPHATA., **TEL.-** BUDDAKAKARA.

An erect herb or climbing by tendrils. Leaves bipinnate Leaflets pinnately lobed. Flowers white. Capsules trigonous, bladderlila winged at the three angles. Seeds black.

Common during the monsoon period on the waste land and the nearby hilly tracts, often climbing on shrubs and trees in shady places or depressions. Fruits and flowers- August and October.

It is found chiefly in Bengal and Uttar Pradesh.

MEDICINAL USE : Root and leaves are diuretic, laxative, stomachic, alterative and emetic, externally used as rubifacient (Nadkarni, 1954).

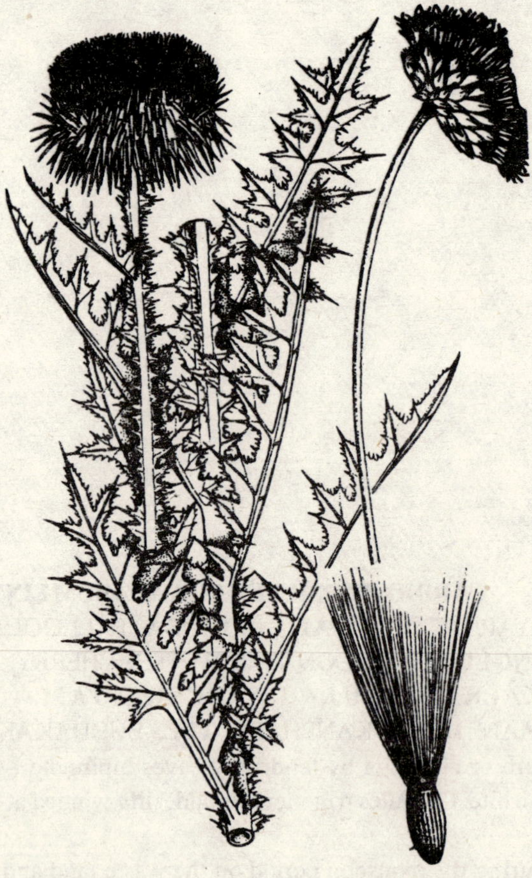

COMPOSITAE

CARDUUS NUTANS LINN (C)
(SY. C. RAMOSA (ROXB)
C. EDELBERGII RECH. F. VARI LUCIDUS D.C.)
SYN. VOLUFARELLA DIVARICATA BENTH

KASH.- GULIBADAWARD, **P.**- BADAWARD, KANCHHARI., **LOCAL NAME**-RISSA.

An erect perennial, with pinnately lobed very spiny-margined leaves and spiny stems and with large globular or ovoid, solitary or clustered, crimson or rarelywhite flower heads, 2.5-4. cm across, flower heads usually slender stalked in a lax inflorescence, or short stalked and densely clustered with many overlapping spine tipped recurved bracts with reddish tips. Stem leaves alternate, mostly 4-10 cm, lanceolate in outline with triangular long spinned lobes and blade prolonged into spiny wings down stem; stem 30-120 mm.

It is common in dry, waste places; comes up annually on the university grounds, locally. It is found in West Himalayas from Kashmir to Shimla 6000-12000 ft. Afghanistan to S.W. China, 1500-4000 mtr. cultivated areas, grazing grounds common June-August.

MEDICINAL USE : Flowers febge, used to purify blood. Seeds contain 41-44% oil.

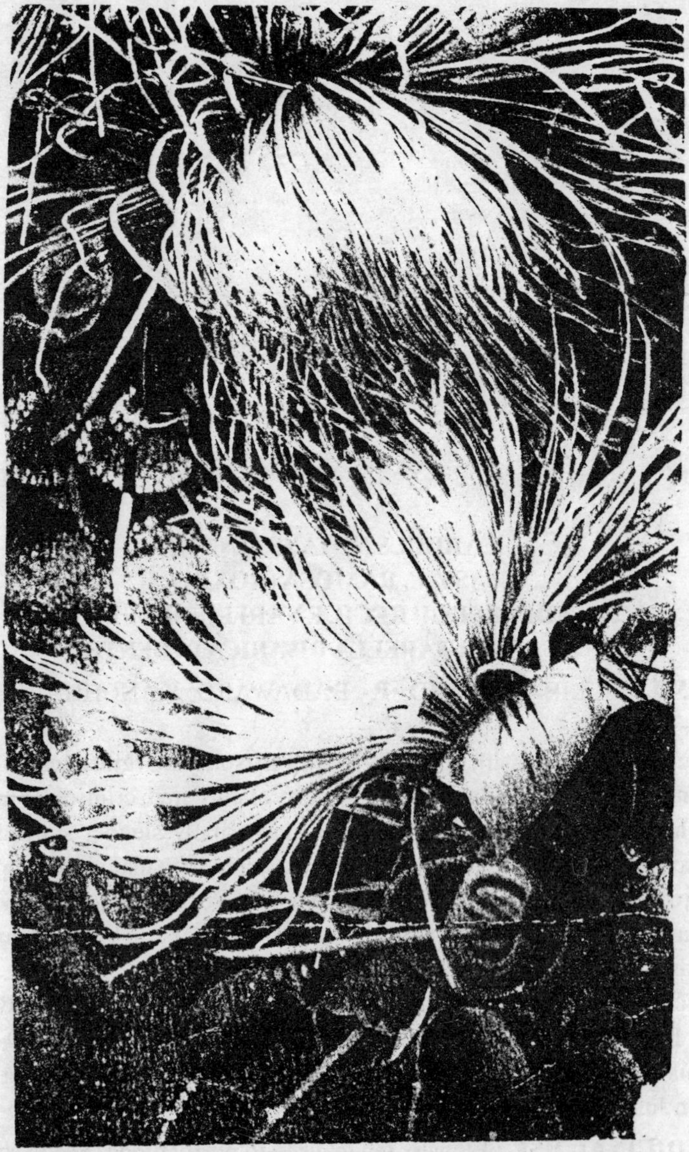

BARRINGTONIACEAE (LECYTHIDACEAE)

CAREYA ARBOREA (ROXB.)
IT IS POPULARLY KNOWN AS PATANAS IN ENGLISH

S., H., & B.- KUMBHI or VAKUMBHA, **MUMBI.**- KALIKATBHI., **KAN.**-)ADDALA., **MAL.**- ALAM or PEELAM or PELU., **TAM.**- ACIMAMARAM or \YMA., **TEL.**- DUDIPPI or ARAYA.

A large decidous tree 30-60 ft. high Leaves 12 by 6', oblong or orbicular, obtuse f shortly acuminate, narrowed at the base, crenate denticulate, glabrous; petiole -1'; spikes 3-8'; flowers usually few, sessile; bracts 3, unequal. Calyx total length /4-1' terete; campanulate, obscurely pubescent; lobes ovate, obtuse, petals 1 3/4; vhile elliptie filaments red. Ovules in two rows in each cell of the ovary (Kurz For. 'l. i. 499. Fruit 2 1/2 by 2'; globose, surmounted by an enlarged mouth having a epressed pit at the vertex within the Calyx-teeth. Seeds 3/6-1/4'; ellipsoid. issepiments; of the fruit permanent, at least sometimes.

It is distributed throughout the sub-Himalayan tract from the Kangra district astwards, Bengal Central Western and Southern India, upto 5,000 ft. distributed iroughout India up to an altitude of 5,000 ft.; from the Himalaya to Travancore nd Tenasserim : Willis, 1973 stated that C. ARBOREA Roxb. as patanas was lmost the only tree on the grassy expaure known as patanas in Ceylon. However, enthem and Hooker (1979) stated that no example from Ceylon has been reported.

MEDICAL USE : Bark and fruit astringent and demulcent. The fruit is edible id aromatic. It contains an astringent gum. A decoction of the fruit is given to omote digestion (Wealth of India, II, 76). The leaves are used for ulcers. The eds are reported to be poisonous.

The bark is used as a demulcent in coughs and colds; in the preparation of an nollient embrocation, and as antipyretic and antipruritic in eruptive fevers, rticularly small pox. The calyces of the flowers contains mucilage and are used demulcent (Kirt & Basu, 11, 1061).

The leaves contains 19% tanin. Kumbi is a fish poison. Its inner bark rubbed shoes keeps off leaches (Chopra and Badhwar, Indian J. agric. Sci.,)40, 10, 26).

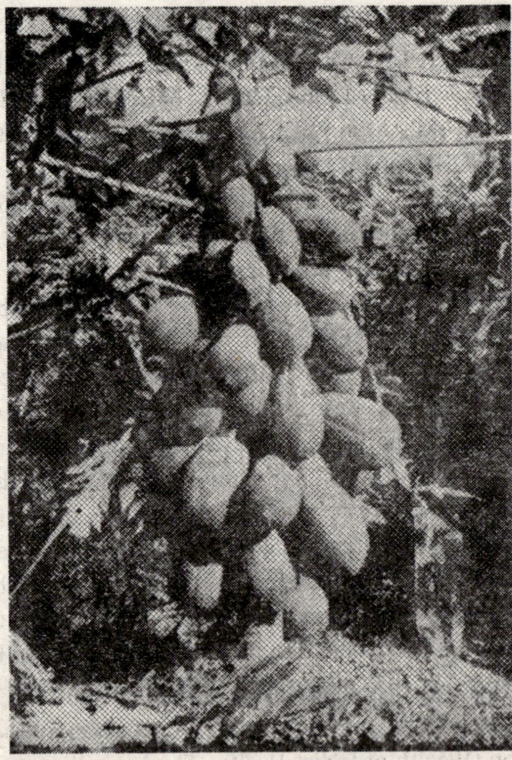

CARICACEAE

CARICA PAPAYA L.

ENG.- PAPAY, PAPAW TREE., **HINDI**- PAPAYA, PAPEETA., **BENG.**- PAPAIYA, PAPEYA., **MARATHI**-PAPAY., **BO.**-PAPAI., **GUJ.**-PAPAYI., **TAMIL**- PAPPALI, PAPPAIYI., **MAL.**-PAPAGAM.

The papaya is a tropical plant with ornamental foliage. Laden with dark green fruits, pale green leafless trunk and bright foliage at the crown. The fruit can be used raw as a vegetable and when ripe as dessert. It is a rich source of Vitamin A. It is 3-4 m tall latex containing tree. The stem is unbranched with terminal crown of leaves. The leaves are palmate or digitate. Alternate and exstipulate. Flowers are regular dioceious and unisexual rarely bisexual. Inflorecence is a loose axillary panicle. Calyx-5, small, partially open corolla 5, united contorted or valvate, female flowers with a short corolla tube and male flowers with a long corolla tube. Stemens 5 in two whorls of 3 and 2, gynoceium-5 synearpous, hypogynous with a short style and 5 stigmas ovules numerous with anatropous parietal placentation. Fruit a berry.

It is cultivated throughout India. Sri Lanka, Philippines Hawai and Austrialia.

MEDICINAL USE : The ripe fruit is digestive, carminative and stomachie. It is used in curing spleen and kidney disorders and haemoptysis, bleeding piles, skin diseases and psoriasia (Ayurveda and Unani). The milky juice of unripe fruits removes freckles and blemishes from the skin. Seeds are used as vermifuge, emmen, used to reduce thirst (Chopra, 1954). An enzyme called Papain is used in the preparation of Cholera medicine, cure of diphtheria, cancer, bleeding piles, ulcers, enlarged spleen and ring worm.

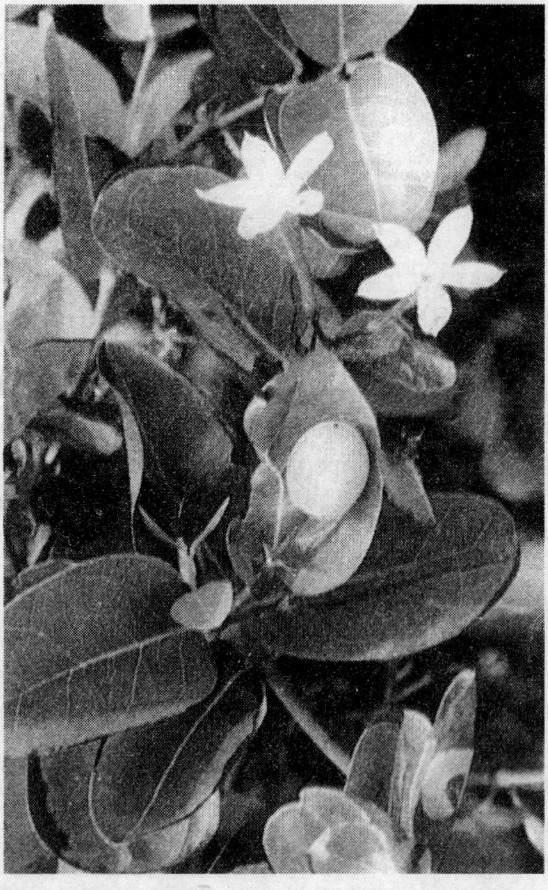

APOCYNACEAE

CARISSA CARANDAS LINN.
KARAUNDA

HINDI.- KARAUNDA, KARUMCHA., **BOMB.**- KARAUNDA., **BENG.**- KARAMCHA., **SANS.**- KANACHUKA, KARAMARDA, AVIGHNA., **TAM.**- KALAKKAY., **TEL.**-VAKA., **MAL.**- KARAKKA., **ENG.**- KARANDA., **MAR.**- KARAVANDA., **GUJ.**-KARAMARDA., **KAN.**- KAREKAYI., **LOCAL NAME.**- KARAUNDA.

An arborescent, glabrous, spiny, densely dichotomously branched large shrub or small tree axis and nodes strong, straight simple or forked thorns in pairs. It is variable evergreen, diffuse, erect, suberrect or scandent. Leaves : Subsessile opposite, small coriaceous, 1- 1/2-3", oblong rounded broadly ovate or obovate shining above, tip rounded or obtuse, nerves numerous. Flowers in terminal and axillary peduncled 3-chotomous cymes. Cymes puberulous. Flowers white or pinkish. Calyx : 5-partite, glandular within or not, segments acute, Corolla tube : 3/4-1" long, cylindrical, throat naked, lobes overlapping to the right. Stamens : at the top of the tube, included; anthers laneeolate, cells round at the base. Disc 0, ovary 2 celled; 4-8 ovuled; style filiform, stigma fusiform or columnar euminately 2-fid. Ovules 1-4 in each cell rarely more. Berry 1/2-1" in ellipsoid or globose 4 or more seeded, 2 (or by abortion-1) celled. Seeds usually 2, peltately attached to the septum, albumen fleshy, cotyledons ovate.

It is present throughout the drier sandy or rocky soils of India, native or cultivated, from the Punjab to Ceylon, Burma and Malaca. Distribution Java, Tianoi.

MEDICINAL USE : Fruits are stomachic, antiscorbutic, referigerant and digestive, root is bitter, stomchic and anthelmintic. Unripe fruits are astringent and antiscorbutic. Decoction of leaves is given at the commencement of remittent fever.

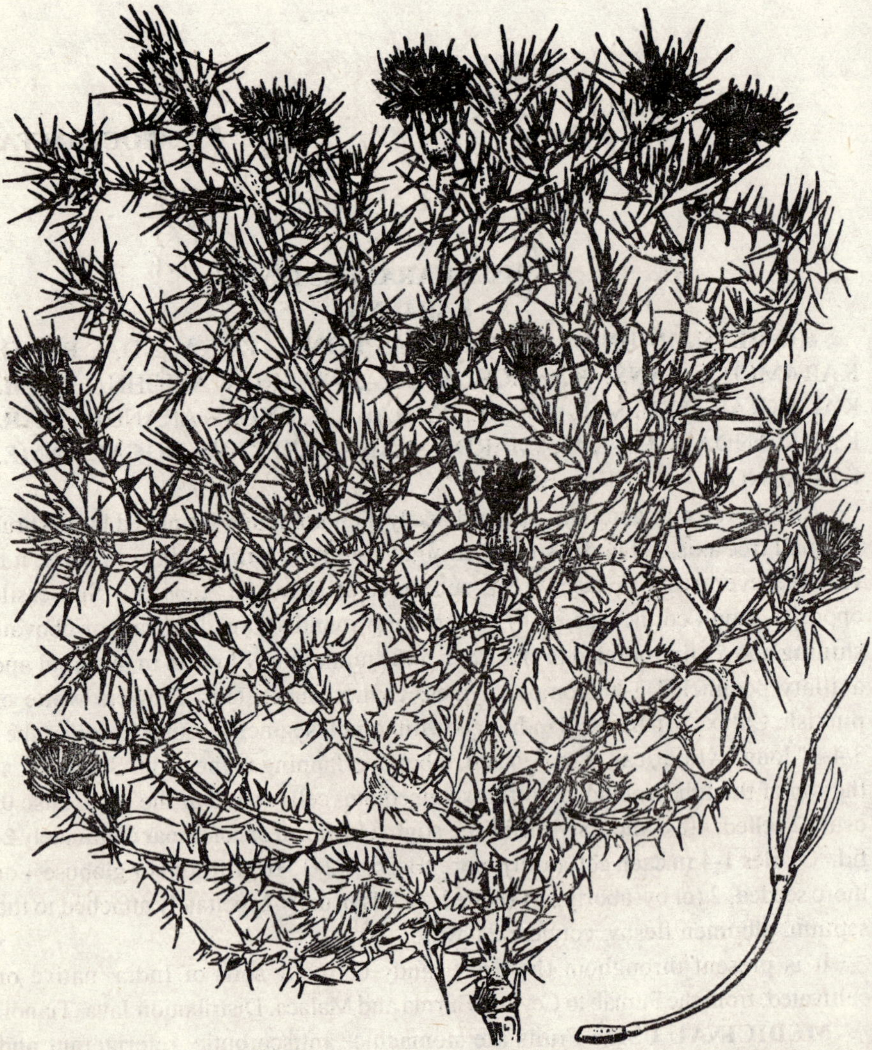

COMPOSITAE

CARTHAMUS TINCTORIUS LINN

BENG.-KAJIRET., **MAL.**- CHENDURAKAM-SINDHI-PAWARI., **ENG.**-SAF-FLOWER., **MAR.**- KARDAI., **ASSAMESE**- FAFRAM., **GUJ.**- KUSUMBI **TAM.**- SENDURAKAM., **HINDI**-KHSUMBAR+KUSUM., **TEL.**- ANGNI SIKNA., **KANN.**- KUSUBI., **LOCAL NAME**-KUSUM.

It is a glabrous shrub a thistle like annual with brownish stems bearing elliptic leaves with bristly-toothed margins. The terminal flowers are in head of orange to red colour after flat topped cluster Flower heads. globular with outer leafing spiny margined involucral bracts spreading beyond the florets. The stem is erect, branched above with leaves glandular hairy, the margins with narrow spiny lobes; Flowers and fruits-March to May. Achenes white and shining.

This plant is cultivated for its flowers and achenes. It is found wild and cultivated and is reported from Parkistan and Kashmir. W. Asia Europe, 1500-1800 m. Wasteland, road side common in Kashmir valley. July to September.

MEDICINAL USE : Seeds are used as purgative while roots are used as diuretic (Nadkkarni, 1954) Seed oil has been reported to lower the level of blood serum cholesterol mainly due to the presence of oleic acid and linolic acid. It has also been considered useful in arteriosclereosis, antherosclerosis and infant eczema (Tiwari et, al) 1970).

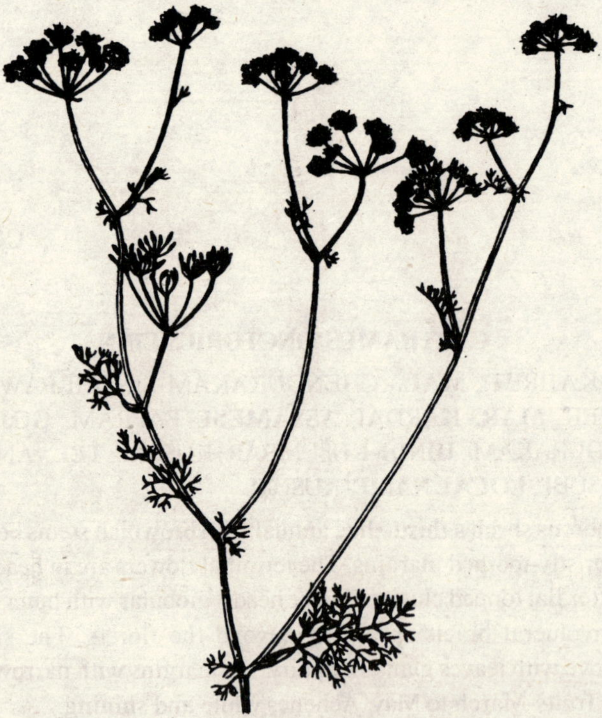

APIACEAE
(UMBELLIFRAE)

CARUM CARVI LINN

BENG.- JIRA., **GAJ.**- SHALAGIRA., **SANS.**- SUSHAVI., **TAM.**- SHIMAISHEMBU., **TEL.**- SHIMAISAPU, URDU-SHAH JIRAH., **BOM.**- VILAYATE ZIRA., **KASH.**- GUNYAN., **LADAKH**- UMBU.

It is an aromatic annual or biennial herb reaching a height of 30-100 cms. Roots thick and fusiform. Stem slender branches hollow and grooved, leaves pinnate, 15-20 cms long, leaflets ovate to lanceolate, linear, entire or dentate lobes, flowers in dense umbels, white, schizocarp oblong oval yellowish brown, mericarps 4-6 mm. long, light to dark brown aromatic with five prominent ribs.

It is found throughout the year in the plains & hills of India. It is considered a native to Europe and west Asia, growing wild in the hills & plains of North India & south India. It is also reported from kinraur, chamba district, Ladakh, Kashmir, chakrata hills.

MEDICINAL USE : Seeds are carminative, stomaehic, aromatic and diuretic. Seed oil is carminative and prescribed in flatulent colie and stomach derangements. Seed vapours give relief in lumbago & rheumatism caraway water finds use in paediatric medicine caraway oil is used for gargle and tooth paste & it is the main ingredient in the scandinavian "Snaps" & German "kummel" It also exhibits neurotropic anti-spasmodie activity & mixed with alcohol and castor oil is used for the treatment of scabies. It also exhibit ante baeterial & antifungal activity.

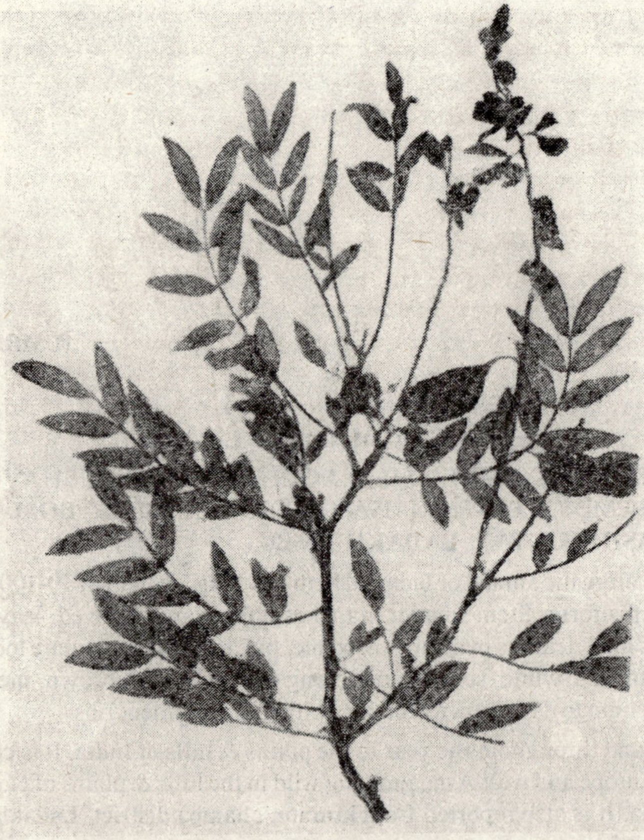

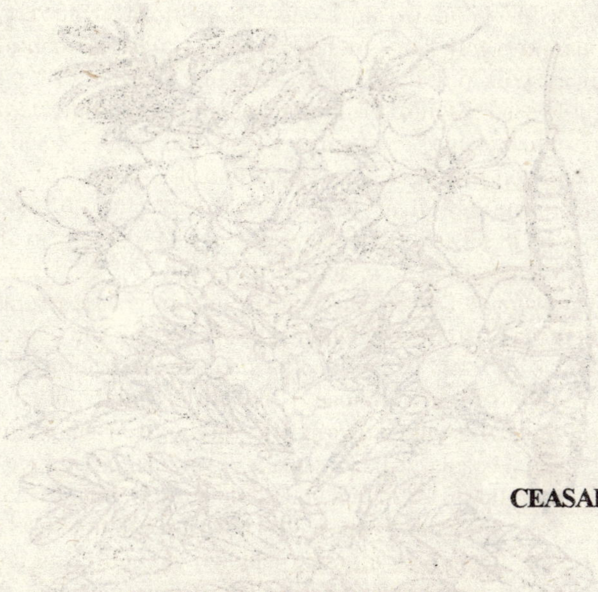

CEASALPINIACEAE

CASSIA. ANGUSTIFOLIA VAHL

Popularly known as Indian Sanai or Teenaveli Seena.

BENGALI- SONAMUKHI., **MARATHI**- SONAMUKHI., **HINDI**- HINDISANA, SENNA, SANAI., **TAMIL**- NALAVAKAI., **MAR.**- SONAMUKHI., **MAL.**- NILAVAKA., **TEL.**- NEHCANGEDU., **B.**- SANNA-MAKKI., **ENG.**- INDIAN SENNA., **SANSKRIT**- BOOMIARI or BOOPADMA., **KAN.**- NILABARIKE.

It is a small shrub, native to Sudan and Arabia and is now cultivated mainly in Tirunelveli and Ramnathpuram districts and to a lesser extent in Madurai, Salem and Tiruchirapali districts or Tamil Nadu. Also grown in a small scale in Cuddaph district of Andhra Pradesh and certain parts of Karnataka. Recently this has been introduced in Mysore.

MEDICINAL USE : Leaves and fruits are used as laxative cathartics, vermifuge and purgative.

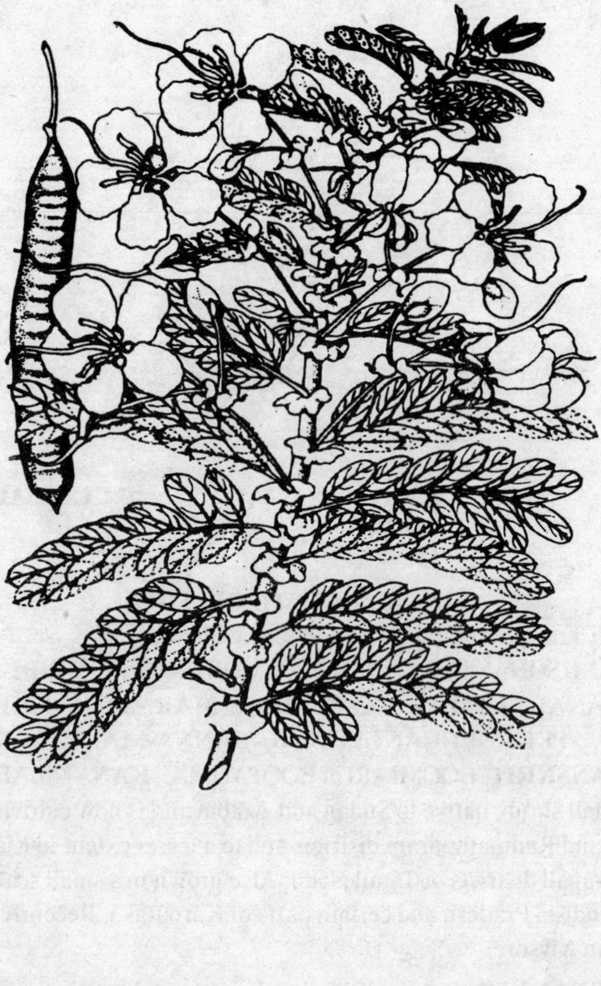

CAESALPINIACEAE

CASSIA AURICULATA LINN.
(Syn. SENNA AURICULATA)
THE TANNER'S CASSIA. AVARAM.

HINDI.- TARWAR., **GUJ.**- AWAL., **MAR.**- TARWAD., **TAM.**- AVARAM., **TEL.**- TANGEDU., **KAN.**- TANGEDU., **BENG.**- TARWAR., **MAL.**- AVARA, AVARAM.

A tall shrub with the virgate branches and large yellow coloured flowers. The underside of the leaves finely grey downy; abruptly pinnate; and nearly sessile, 3-4 inch. long; leaflets 16-24, obovate-oblong, rigidly subcoriaceous; 3/4-1"; obtuse or emarginate with a mucronate stipule large and foliaceous. Flowers : very large and showy, an inch deep, bright yellow, in Copious corymbose racemes. Calyx tube very short; sepals broad or narrow, imbricated. Petals 5, imbricated subequal, usually broad. Stamens normally 10, but rarely all perfect, 3-5 being often reduced to staminodia or all together absent; anthers mostly but not invariably basifixed, dehiscing by terminal pores or with the slit more or less continued longitudinally. Ovary sessile or stalked, many ovuled; style in curved, stigma terminal. Pods 4-5 inch. long by 1/2-5/8 inch; straight, ligulate glabrous, flexible, dark brown, with a distinct space between the liniserrate seeds.

It is found wild in the Central Provinces, the Western Peninsula and Ceylon, often planted elsewhere.

MEDICINAL USE : The bark is astringent and the leaves and fruits are anthelmintic. The root is used in the treatment of skin diseases.

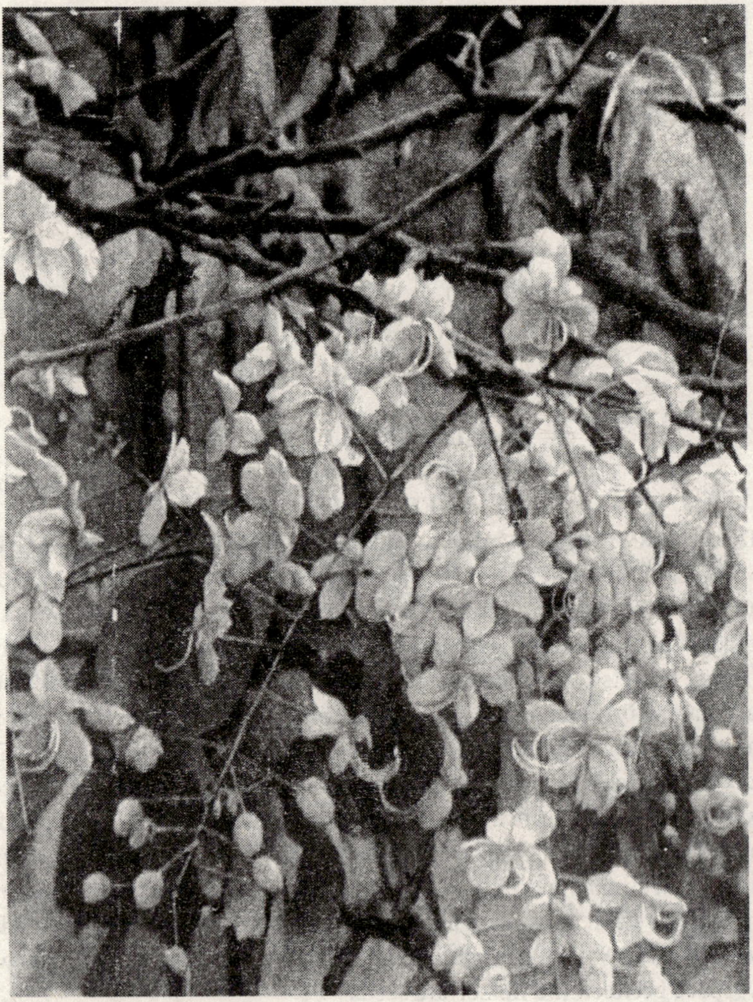

CAESALPINIACEAE

CASSIA FISTULA LINN.
(INDIAN LABURNUM, PURGING FISTULA)

SANS.- SUVARNAKA, RAJATARU., **HINDI**- AMALTAS, GIRIMALAH, SONHALI, AMULTHUS., **BENG.**- SUNDALI, AMULTAS, BUNDARLATI., **MAR.**- BAHAVA., **GUJ.**- GARMALA., **TAM.**- KONNEI, SHARAKKONNAI., **TEL.**- RELA., **KAN.**- KAKKE, KAKKEMARA, KONDRAKYI., **LOCAL NAME**- AMAITAS., **ENG.**- INDIAN LABURNUM, PURGING CASSIA., **KON.**- KAKKAYI., **MAL.**- KONNA.

A middle sized erect deciduous tree, glabrous in all its parts, with a bole 12-15 ft. high and 3-4 ft. in girth. The bark is thick, yellowish or greenish grey. Leaves: A foot or more long; leaflets 8 - 16 large, narrowed to the point. Leaflets 4-8 pairs, 10-15 x 5 cms. long ovate distinctly stalked, usually acute, rigidly subcoriaceous, pale green, strongly veined. Flowers bright yellow in long drooping, lax racemes. Bracts caducous, racemes as long as the leaves; pedicels spreading 1 ½ - 2 inch. Calyx 1-4 - 1/3 rd inch. glabrous; Cadueous. Petals veined bright, obovate, shortly clawed 3-4-1 inch. deep. Stamens: Normally 10- but all are not perfect, 3-5 being often reduced to staminodia or all-together absent; anthers mostly but not invariably basifixed, dehising by terminal pores or with the slit more or less continued logitudinally. Ovary-sessile or stalked, many-ovuled; style incurved, stigma terminal. Pod 1-2 f t, long above an inch. thick. The flowering season is during April - June.

It is reported from Central and Eastern Himalayas to Ceylon and Malacca, ascending to 3000 ft. in Kumaon, wild and often planted. China, Malay isles. It is indigenous to India and naturalised in tropical Africa, South America and West Indies.

MEDICINAL USE : The root, bark, seeds and leaves are used as laxatives. The juice of leaves is applied in skin diseases. The fruit is cathartic and is used in rheumatism and snake bite. Fruit pulp, root bark, seeds and leaves are also used as tonic.

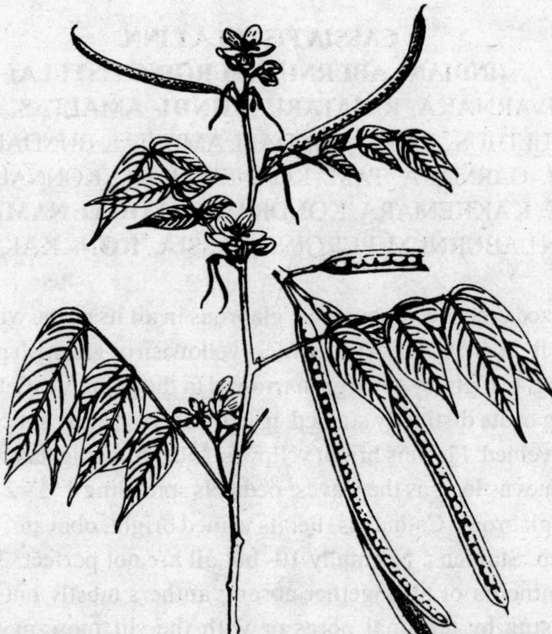

CAESALPINIACEAE

CASSIA OCCIDENTALIS LINN.
(Syn. SENNA OCCIDENTALIS.)

SANS.- KASAMARDA., **HINDI**- KASONDI., **BENG.**- KALKASHUNDA., **TAM.**-NATTAM-TAKARAI, POONAAVARAI., **TEL.**- KASINDA., **MAL.**- NATRAM-TAKARA., **LOCAL NAME**- BAN BHATES, DHADIAL., **GUJ.**- KASUVAYEE., **MAR.**-KASUVAYEE., **KAN.**- DODDATAGACHE., **KON.**-HODU-TAIKILO., **ENG.**- NEGRO COFFEE.

A diffuse subglabrous shrubby herb, a few feet high, usually of annual duration. Leaves 1/2 ft. long; leaf with a single large gland placed just above the base of the common petiole. Leaflets 6-10 ovate oblong or oblanceolate; glaucous, foetid, accuminate, 1-3 inch. long, glabrous or finely pubescent. Flowers yellow in corymbiform, axillary clusters, short peduncled, few-flowered, forming a terminal panicle; bracts thin, ovate-acuminate, caducous; pedicels spreading 1/2-3/4 inch. Sepals 5; obtuse, glabrous, 1/4-1/3 inch; Petals 1/2 in. Pale lilac 5, in no. imbricated, subequal, usually broad; conspicously veined. Fertile stamens 6-7 the anthers subequal or those of the 2-3 lowest larger than the others, three posterior filaments without anthers. Pod. 4-5 inch. by 1/3 inch, transversely partitioned; rather recurved, glabrous, sub-compressed, distinctly torulose, rarely terete. The seeds are 20-30, pale brown usually flattened paralled with the valves. The flowering season is from June to November.

It is scattered from the Himalayas, to Ceylon and Burma probably introduced. Cosmopolitan in tropics.

MEDICINAL USE : The leaves, roots and seeds are used as purgative. The seeds are roasted and used as substitute for coffee in France, Africa and in the North sector of Argentina, seeds are also febrifuge. Roots have been considered diuretic and antiperiodic.

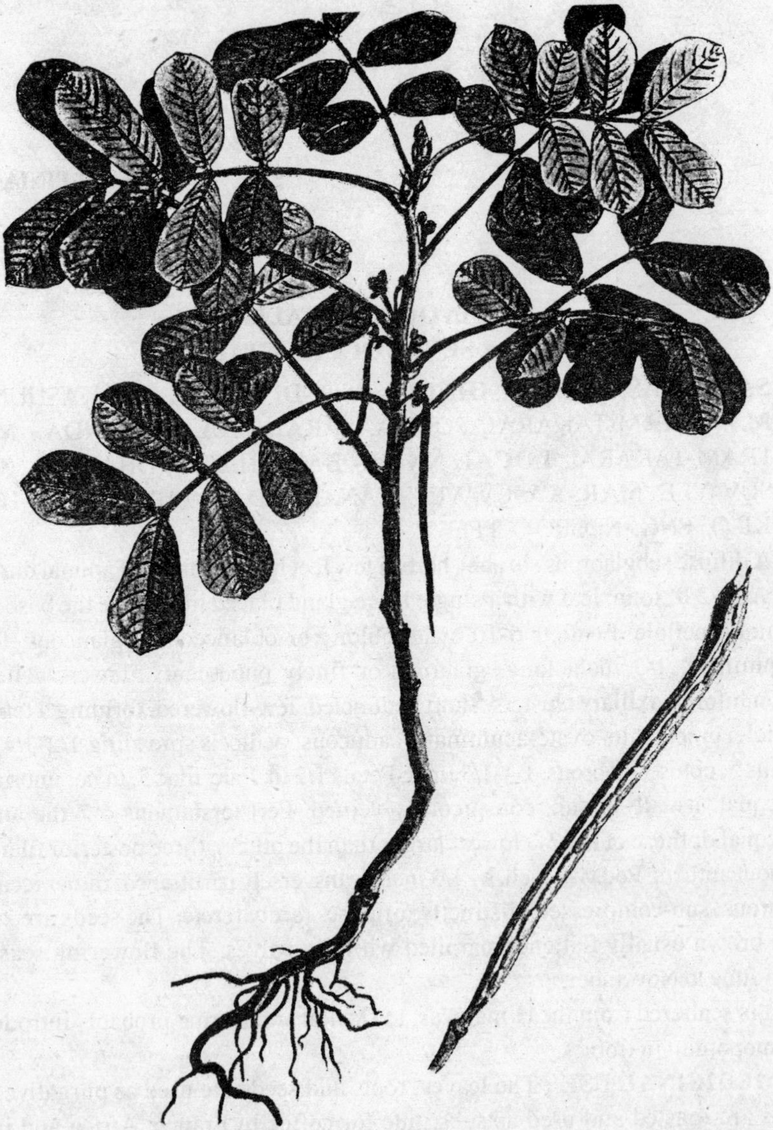

CEASALPINIACEAE

CASSIA TORA LINN
(SYN. C. TOROIDES ROXB)
C.FORETIDA PERS
C.OBTIAFOLIA LINN

ENGLISH- SICKLE, SENNA-FOETID CASSIA., **GUJARAT**- KOYARAYA., **BENG.**- CHAKUNDA, **KON.**- DADDAPAN., **MAL.**- TAKARA., **MARATHI**- TANKALA., **TAMIL**-TAGURAI., **TEL.**- TEGURISA., **HINDI**- PAMAAR, CHAKUNDA., **SANS.**- CHAKRAMARDA, DADAMONI., **LOCAL NAME**- PAWAD, CHAKOWAR.

It is commonly a gregarious foetid annual with usually 3 pairs of ovate leaflets with a gland between the lowest pair and solitary or paired orange-yellow axillary flowers C. 1 cm across borne from the axils of the leaves. Sometimes an under shrub to 120 cm. Petals unequal, obovate, 8-12 mm, stamens 7, Unequal the three upper reducd to staminodes. Leaflets usually 2-4 cm long, hairy or hairless. Pot 10-20 cm. by 2-6 mm. broad, rounded, often curved. Flowers and fruiting August-November.

It is probably native of South America. In the Himalaya to 1500m. wasteland, cultivated areas. August-September. Locally-a common weed along roadsides or in open wastelands often becoming aggressive on unused ground. It occurs throughout India as a weed.

MEDICINAL USE : Decot. of leaves-laxt. leaves and seeds in skin dieseases, for ring worms and itch and in snake bite.

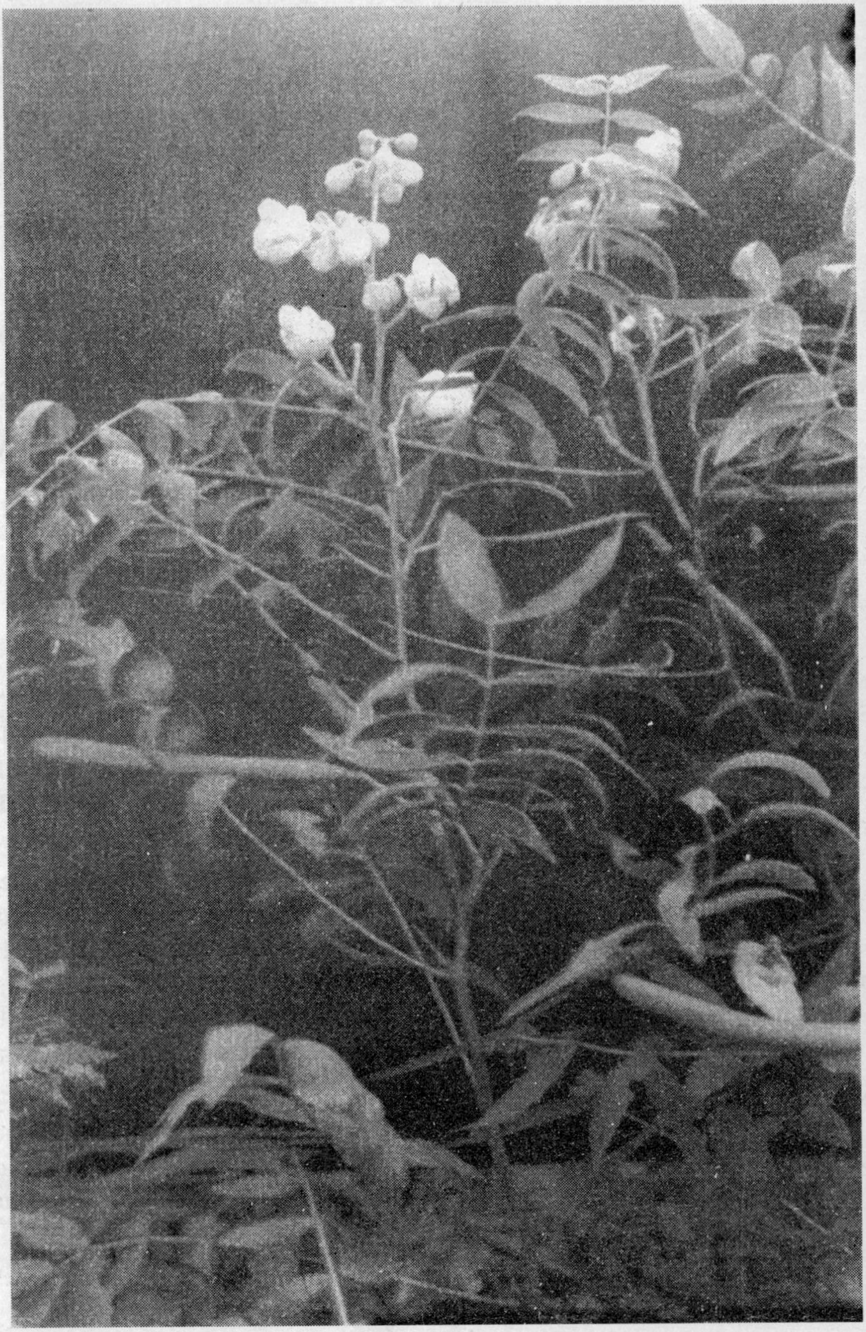

CAESALPINIACEAE

CASSIA SOPHERA LINN
(SYN. C.COROMENDLE LIANA JACQ.)

BENG.- KALAKASUNDA., **ENGLISH**- SENNA SOPHERA., **HINDI**- BAS KI KASUNDA., **MAL.**- PONNANTA, KARA., **MAR.**-RAUTANKALA., **TAM.**- SHUUBIVARAI., **TEL.**- PAIDI-TANGAEDU., **SANS.**- KASAMARDA.

It is a shrubby herb. Leaflets 8-12 pairs, oblong, lanceolate, acute or tapering, rachis with a single gland at base. Flowers yellow, in corymbose racemes. Pods slightly curved, transversly septate. Flowers and fruits July to Feb.

It is found commounly as a hedge around bunglows, It is found through out India.

MEDICINAL USE : Leaves used externally in ring worm. Decoct. of plant used in acute broncht. Plants contains emodin and chrysophanice acid.

CASSIA AURICULATA LINN

H. & B.- TARWAR., **TAM.**- AVARAM., **TEL**-. TANGEDU., **MAL.**- A ARA., **MARATHI**-TARWAD, **ENGLISH**- AVARAM, TANNER'S CASSIA.

It is a shrub occuring wild in M.P. Pannisula, Tamil Nadu and Rajasthan. Cultivatged in other parts of India.

MEDICINAL USE : The bark and roots are astringent. The roots are used in skin diseases while the leaves and fruits are anthelmintic. Seeds are used in opthalmia and conjunctivities as also in diabetes and chylous urine (Chopra et al, 1956, Nadkarni, 1954). Its other species are used in Liv. 52, Bonnisan and Gerriforte.

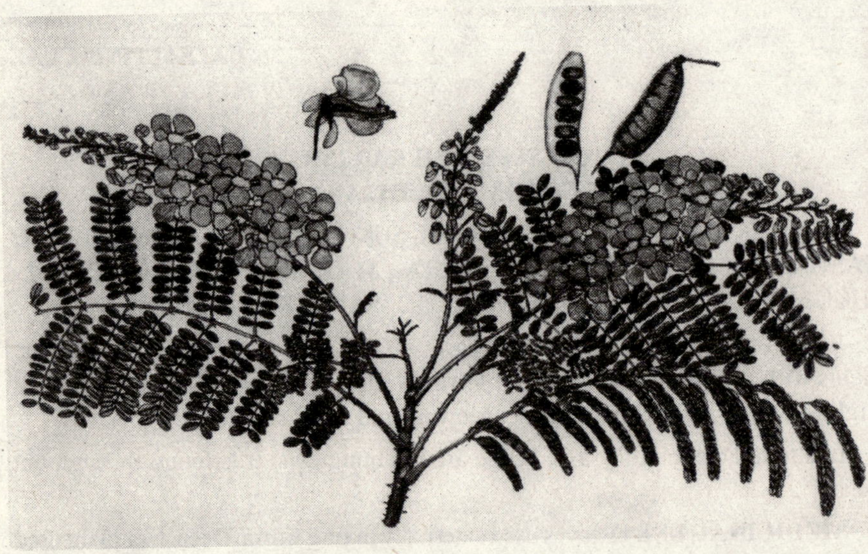

CAESALPINIACEAE

CASSIA SEPIARIA ROXB
(SYN. CAEASALPINIA DECAPELATA (ROTH) ALSTON

A scrawling shrub with twice pinnate leaves, with rachis and branches with prickles, and with large erect spike like clusters of bright yellow flowers. Flower clusters 30-40 cm long; flowers 2-3 cm. across, with rounded unequal petals; Calyx-lobes ovate, 1 cm or more; stamens 10, free, with filaments which are woollyhaired below. Leaves 23-28 cm, with 5-10 pairs of pinnae, each with 8-12 pairs of oblong blunt leaflets 1.5-2 cm long and glaucous beneath. Pod 6-12.5 cm. by 2.5 cm beaked, woody.

It is reported from Pakistan to Bhutan, India, China, Japan, S.E. Asia to 2200 m. Shrubberies, stony open slopes Ravines, March-April.

MEDICINAL USE : Leaves used externally in ringworm. Decoct. of plant-used in acute broncht. Plant contains emodin and chrysophanic acid. (Apothekertg, Ber 1, 1896, 537; wehmer, I, 505).

Properties-similar to C. OCCIDENTALIS.

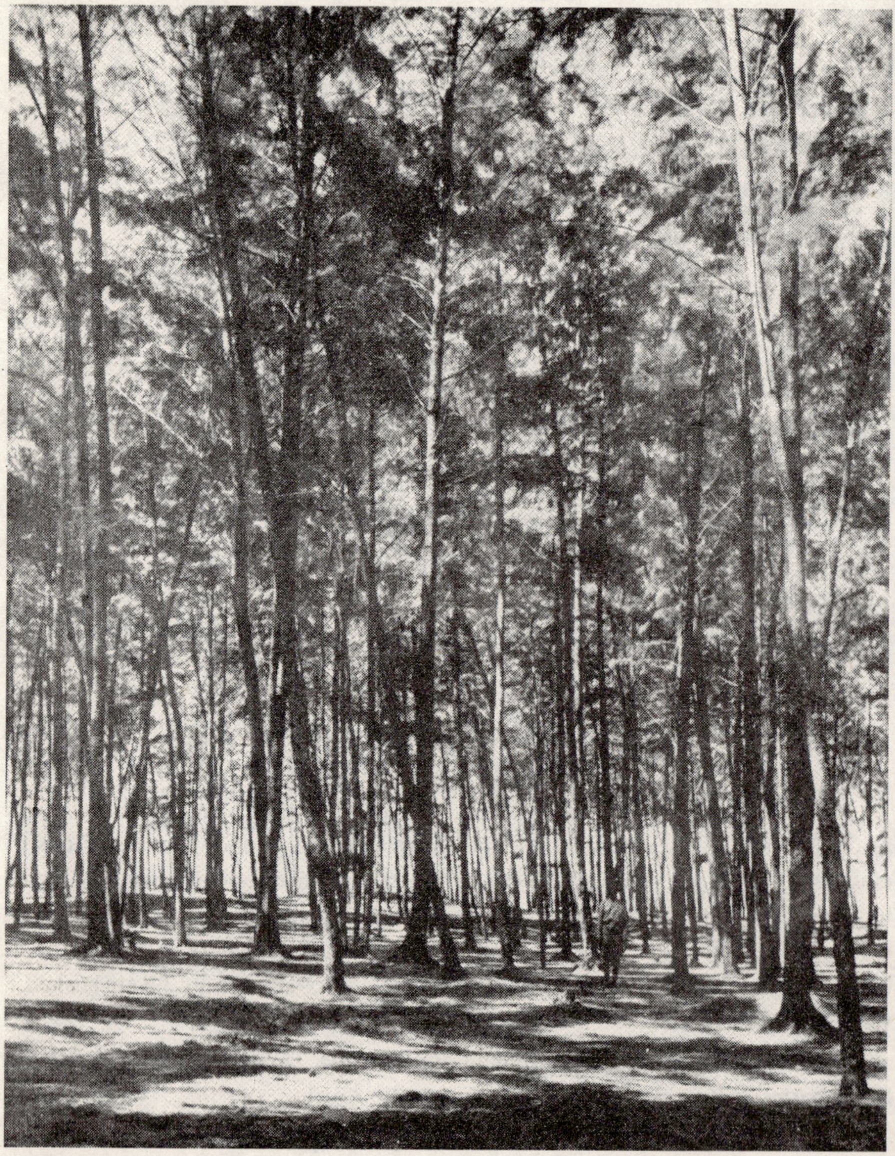

CASURARINACEAE

CASUARINA EQUISETIFOLIA LINN. BEEFWOOD.
(Syn. C. MURICATA ROXB)

HINDI- JANGLI SARU, JANGLI JHAU, JANGLI SARU., **BENG.-** JAU., **MAR.-** SURU., **GUJ.-** VILAYATI SARU., **TEL.-** SARUGUDU, CHAVUKU, SARUKKU., **TAM.-** SAVUKKU., **KAN.-** SARVEMARA, CHABAKU., **MAL.-** CHAVUKKU., **LOCAL NAME-** VILAYATI JHAU., **ENG.-** CASUARINA., SHE-OAK., **BOMB.-** VILAYATI SARO., **BURMA.-** KABWI, TINYU., **CEYLON-** KASA.

Tree or shrub, often of creeping habit with long or short slender green branches, cylindrical and deeply grooved, or sub 6-8 angled; jointed; rush - like, with whorls of 6-8 scales, similar to the twigs of EQISETUM (hence the name EQUISETIFOLIA. The leaves are redueed to minute scales. Internodes terminating in a short sheath of connate subulate scales (leaves). Flowers are female and male. The terminating male are borne in simple or compound spikes about ½inch; usually terminating on green branchlets, but sometimes sessile. The internodes are short and at every node is a cup (formed of the combined bracts) with several stamens hanging out over the edge. Each stamen represents a male flower and has 2 - leaved perianth and 2 bracteoles. The female flowers are borne in peduncled dense shperical or ovoid heads, sessile or terminating. Short usually lateral branchlets, MALE F1. sepals 1 or 2, concave, circumstiss at the base. Stamen 1, 1 inflexed in bud; anthers large, FEM F1. ovary minute, 1-celled; style 2- fid; arms filiform, stigmatose to the base. Ovules 2, collateral, semianatropous. Fruit 3/4 inch in diameter with 12 rows of puperlous achenes, handened braets puberulous, obovate - oblong, mueronate an oblong or cylindrical cone formed of the enlarged hardened bracts and bracteoles, together forming 2-valved cavities enclosing the compressed winged achenes; wing terminal, tipped by the style. The seed is single seeded, flattened, terminally winged out of seed like appearance enclosed in the woody bracteoles, which separate at maturity. The flowering season's March to May and fruiting season is June - July every year.

It is found on the east side of the Bay of Bengal, from chittagong Southward, cultivated elsewhere in India.

Distributed, Malay Islands, Australia, Pacific.

MEDICINAL USE : Bark astringent, useful in diarroea and dysentry. Decoetion of leaves used in colic. Its fruits known as gokhru, when boiled with water forms a deecoction. This deccoction serves as a tonic in kidney disorders.

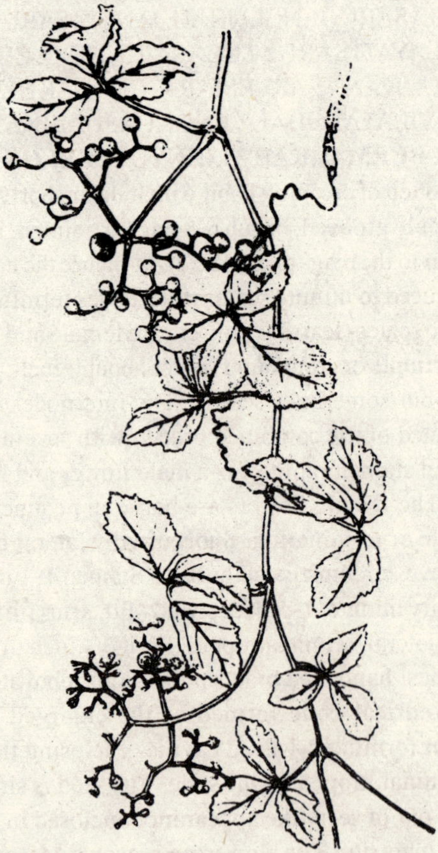

VITACEAE

CAYRATIA CARNOSA (WALL) GAGNEP.
(SYN. VITIS TRIFOLIA LINN.)
(SYN. VITIS CARNOSA) WALL.

HINDI- AMALBEL., **BENG**.- AMALLATA., **MARATHI**- AMBATBEL., **TEL**.- KURUDINNE., **TAM**.- TUMANS., **MAL**.- SORIVALII.

A creeping or twining shrub. Leaves trifoliate. Leaflets variable, crenate-serrate. Tendrils branched. Flowers greenish white, hermaphrodite, petals four, in umbellate cymes. Fruit a berry, globose, black two to four seeded. Flowers-rainy season, fruits- rainy and winter season.

It is considered as a Weed occurring commonly in waste and open lands with little bit of moisture. It is also reported from Tropical Himalayas and throughout the hotter parts of India.

MEDICINAL USE : Root astringent, ground with black pepper applied to boils. Leaves made into poultice employed in the treatment of yolksores stem, leaves and roots contain hydrocynic acid (Burkill, 11-2248), philipp. Agricul, 1928,335).

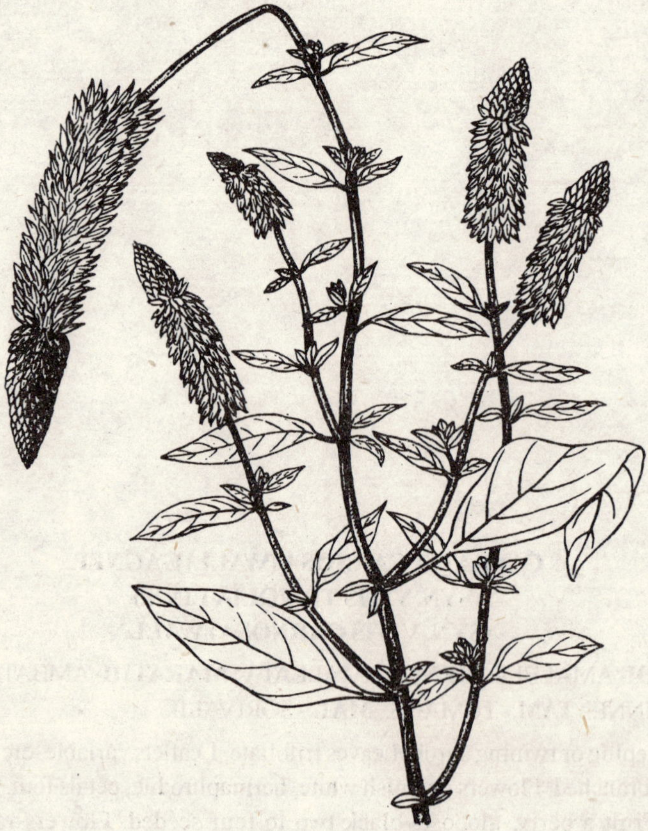

AMARANTHACEAE

CELOSIA ARGENTEA LINN

H.- SAFAID MURGHA., **B**.- SWET - MURGA., **BO.**- KURDU., **P**.- SARWALI., S.- VITUNNA., **TEL.**- GURUGU., **LOCAL NAME**- CHILMIL, SARWAN, SARAI.

It is an erect, glabrous, tall herb approximately 40 cm. height, stems are angular and branched. Leaves are linear, ovate, lanceolate tapering at ends size is approx. 7.5- 14 x 2.8-5 cm spikes terminal, dense, conical to long oblong being an aggregate of both central basal side lateral; pinkish white, Flowers pale-pink closely imbricate. Capsule ellipsoid. Seeds brown or black polished.

It is found as a common weed in cultivated and fellow fields. Flowers and fruits are avilable from August to October.

Grown in gardens for ornamental purposes or found as an escape in the plains and upto a height of 5,000 ft. on the Himalayas.

MEDICINAL USE : Seeds in diarroea aphrodis; useful in blood diseases and mouth sores, for clearing the vision and for diseases of the eye. It is also used as a haemostyptic and in opthalmic treatment in Himalaya Drugs.

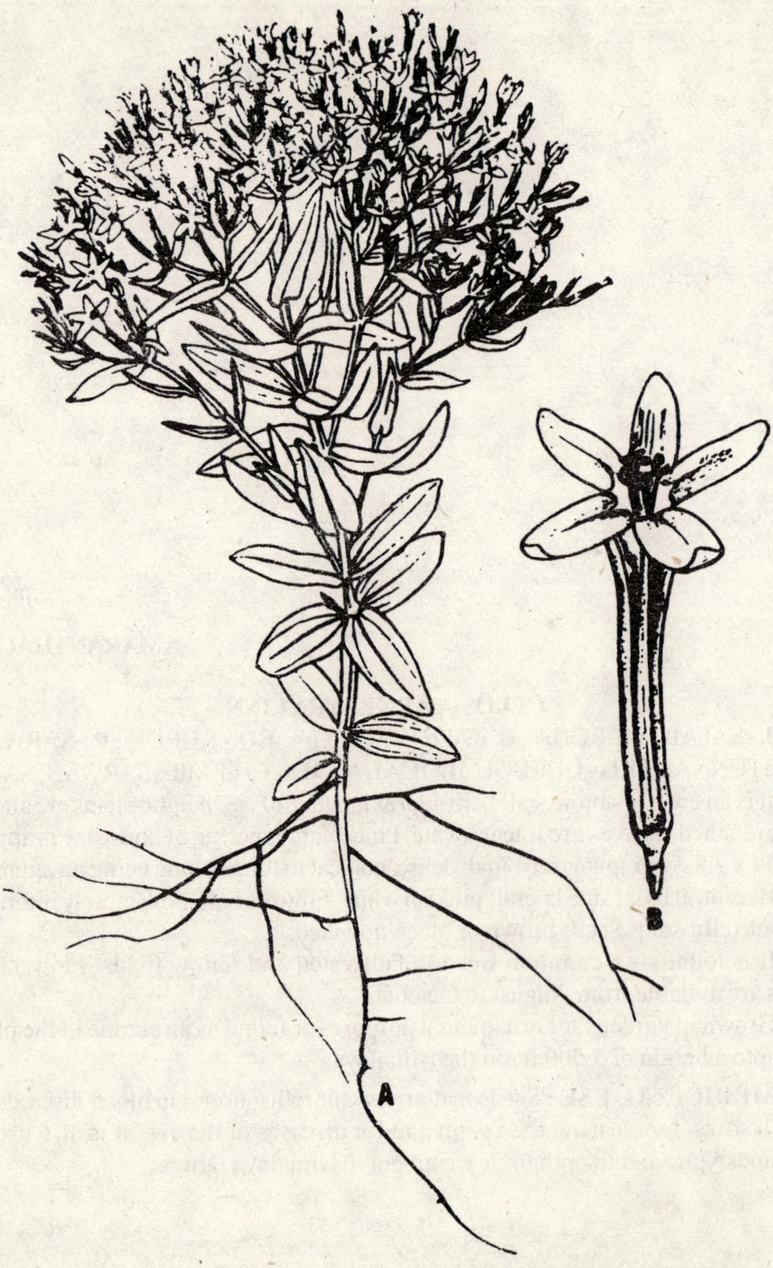
B
A

GENTIANACEAE

CENTAURIUM ROXBURGHII (G. DON) DRUCE
(Syn. ERTHRAEA ROXBURGHII G. DON.

HINDI- BARIK, CHARAYATAH., **BENG.-** GIRMI., **BOM.-** KURUNAI, LUNTAK., **MAL.-** THUPORAPPENPULLU.

An erect, glabrous, elegant herb, 5-10 cm. tall. Leaves decussate, asending, crowded - leafy, variable in shape. Flowers rosy or scarlet sometimes dull white, conspicuously bracteate, axillary and terminal, dichotmous cymes forming a lax head.

Calyx spathe like and split to the base (bell shaped) stand end oblong - lanceolate, 4-5 mm. twice as long as keel. Capsules as long as or longer than the calyx, many seeded seeds minute, ovoid, black, reticulate. Abundant in April and May.

It grows in moist, sandy and silky soil as an escape on waste lands gardens and lawns.

It is found throughout India, ascending upto 2,000 ft. and common in cultivated ground.

MEDICINAL USE : Plant bitter, stomach, substitute for chiretta in fever.

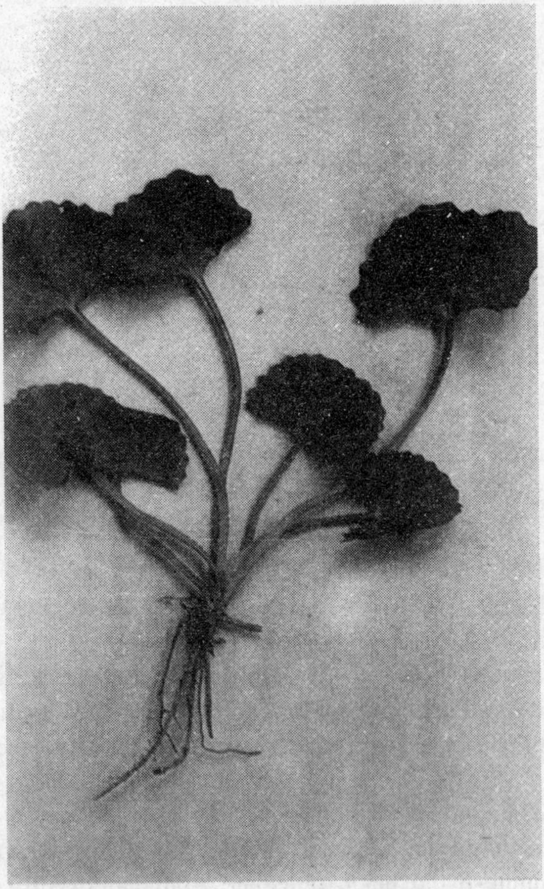

UMBELLIFRAE
(HYDROCOTYIACEAE)

CENTELLA ASIATICA(L) URBAN
(SYN. HYDROCOTYLEASIATICA LINN.)
INDIAN PENNYWORT

BENG.- THOLKHURI., **HINDI**- BRAHMA-MANDUKI, KHULAKHUDI., **MAR**- KARIVANA, KARINGA., **TAM.**- VALLARAI., **TEL.**- BRAHMI, SARASWATAKU., **BOMB.**- KARIVANA., **SANS.**- MANDUKAPARNI., **ENG.**- ASIATIC PENNYWORT., **ARAB.**- ARTAYNIYA-E-HINDI., **SINH.**- GOTUKOLA., **LOCAL NAME.**- BRAMI.

A prostrate perennial taintly aromatic herb, rooting at the nodes. Leaves: several at each node, ½ - 2½ inch. diam; usually glabrous or nearly so; orbicular, reiniform entire crenate or lobulate; petiole long pubescent or glabrous. Peduncle short, about 1/4"; often 2-3 nate, laxly pubescent or glabrous; bracts small ovate being 1/8 -1/6 inch embracing the flowers not scattered among the pedicels. Pedicels O,umbel 3-6-flowered, flowers pink sometimes unisexual; Calyx-teeth O or minute. Petals entire obtuse, imbricate, subpersistent; secondary ridges as distinct as the primary. Carpels oblong subcylindrical, curved, slighhtly compressed, much longer than broad reticulate-rugose, often crowned by the subpersistent petals, each with 9 curvilinear subsimilar ridges, and 2 within the commissure. Pericarp thick and woody white. Fruit : 1/8-1/6 inch; 2 seeded, indehicent, laterally compressed. Seed: Compressed laterally; pericarp much thickened; endocarp is greatly thickened and that is adnate to the exocarp; brown, dull and oblong. Flowering season is from April-July.

Throughout India, alt. 0.2000ft. from the Himalaya to Ceylon and Malacca; frequent. Tropical and sub-tropical regions.

Locally it is common and abundant along the irrgation channnels crossing the fruit orchards as well as suburbs forming a mat-like growth.

MEDICINAL USE : Used as an antidote to cholera and heat effects and also to cure, madness. It may cuse influenza if taken in winter. Plant as a whole useful alterative and tonic in diseases of skin, leprosy, nerve and blood. Leaves are taken as tonic and for improving memory, useful in syphilitic skin diseases both internally and externally.

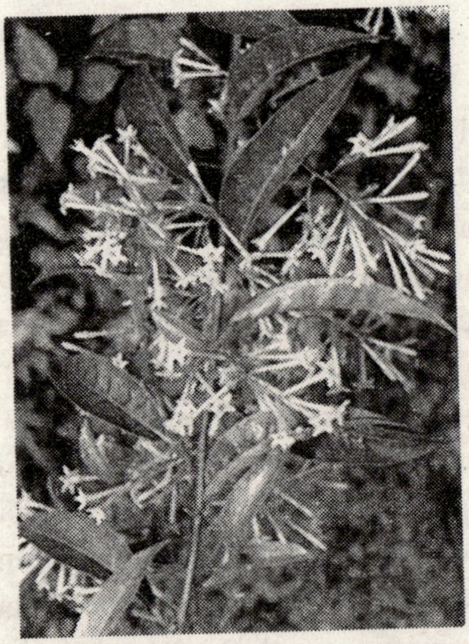

SOLANACEAE

CESTRUM NOCTURNUM LINN.
(NIGHT BLOOMING JESSAMINE)

ENG.- LADY OF NIGHT., **HINDI**- RAAT KI RANI., **LOCAL NAME**- RATKI RANI., **TEL.**- BAGADA CHETTU., **PUN.**- RAATKI RANI.

An evergreen foeted and diffused shrub with ovate lanceolate long-pointed shining leaves. Stem upto 4 cm.; branches green, slender, Leaves entire, 8-12 cm.; alternate and in unequal pairs, thin, oblong-ovate to elliptic, shining, tapering at the ends. Inflorescence Cymose : dichotomous or racemose, lateral or terminal. Flowers greenish yellow, in axillary and terminal, umbelliform racemes. Calyx : 5 or 10 lobes, rarely 4-lobed or subentire, unaltered or enlarged in fruit. Corolla tube : short, rotate, in duplicate-valvate limb 5-(rarely 4-6) lobed, plaited in bud. Stamens 5 (rarely 4-6) filaments short in the corolla tube; anthers oblong, narrowed upwards connivent into a cone, opening by terminal pores or short slits. Ovary 2-celled, (rarely in cultivated forms) 3-4 celled, style columnar stigma small. Berry small or large, capsular; seeds very many, discoid; scarcely compressed; embryo straight. Flowering season is July-September.

Native of tropical America, commonly cultivated in India and the Himalaya to 1500 m. Semi-naturalized in cultivated areas, hedges; common August-October.

MEDICINAL USE : The whole plant extract possess a saponin which exhibits cardiotonic and cardiotoxic activity.

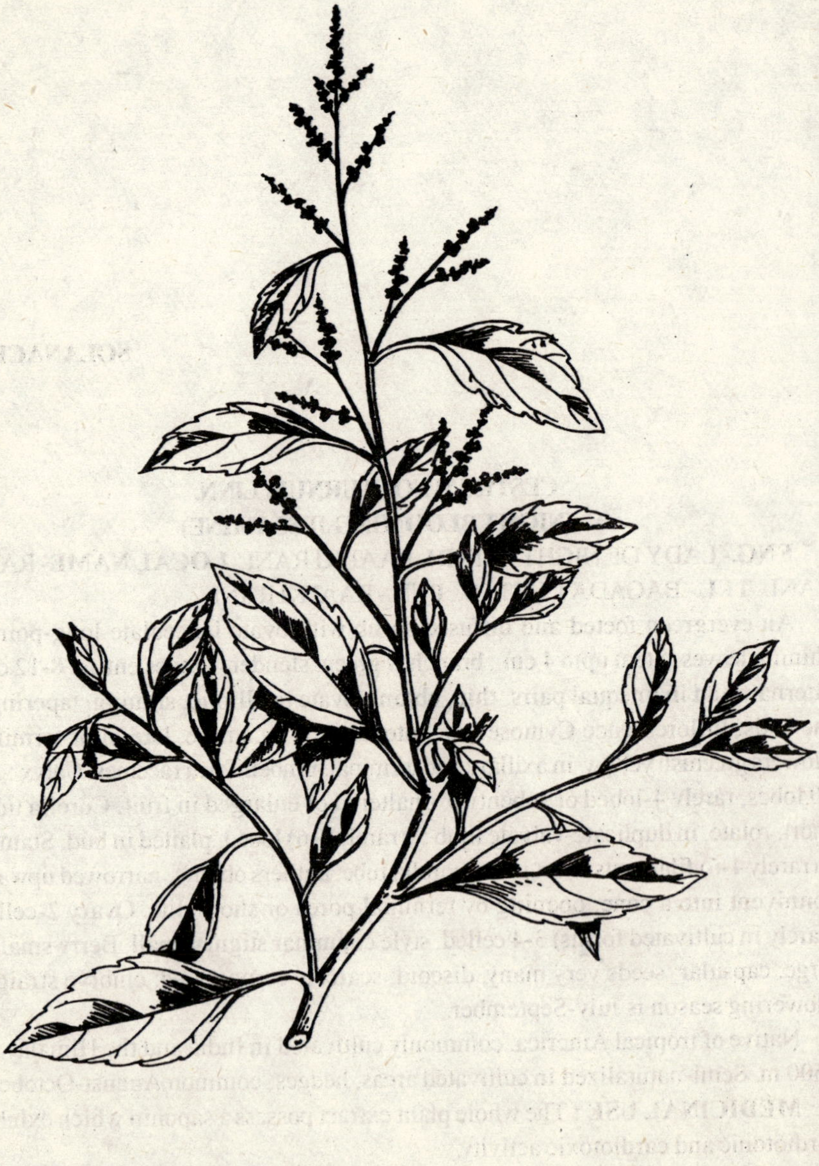

CHENOPODIACEAE)

CHENOPODIUM ALBA LINN

SANS.- VSTUK., **ENG.**- PIGWEED, LAMBS QUARTERS., **BENG.**- CHANDAN, BETU, BETHU, SAG., **BOMB.**- CHAKWIT., **PUNJ.**- BATHU., **HINDI**- BETHU SAG, BATHUA., **TAM.**- PARUPUKKI-RAI., **TEL.**- PAPPUKURA., **LOCAL NAME**- BATHUA, CHANDAN BATHUA, BATHU.

An erect or prostrate herb, green or coated with white scentless or foetid herbs mealy granular pubescence. Stem angular; woody in tall plants; 1-10 ft. rarely slender or decumbent, often striped green, red or purple. Leaves:- variable in size alternate, entire lobed or toothed; rhombic deltoid or lanceolate acute or obtuse; irregularly lobulate, upper narrower more entire; in cultivated forms leaves are extermely variable, 4-6 inch long, with the petiole sometimes as long or longer. Flowers in terminal and axillary clusters, forming compact, panicled spikes, the terminal spikes becoming thyroid. Sepals 3-5, keel covering the utricle, herbaceous (not succulent in fruit). Stamens 1-5; disc., ovary free, depressed or compressed styles 2-3; utricle membranous, included in the perianth. Embryo is perfectly annular. Seed horizontal or rarely vertical testa crustaceous, albumen floury; the cultivated forms a vary from green to red. The flowering period is from August - December every year.

Tropical and Temperate Himalaya from Kashmir ro Sikkim, ascending to 12,000 ft. (Wild or cultivated), and in Western Tibet to 14,000 ft. Plains of Bengal the gangetic valley and Punjab, KHASIA Mts. cultivation.

Deccan Peninsula.- Distribution Umbiquitous.

Locally it is a common winter and summer weed in waste places and dry, gravelly soils of ancient buildings and cultivated grounds. It is also cultivated as pot herb.

MEDICINAL USE : The plant is considered as a whole laxative and anthelmintic. The essential oil contains carotene and vitamin C. It also helps in curing. Piles, gallstones. In summer its inelusion in food is cooling and refreshing.

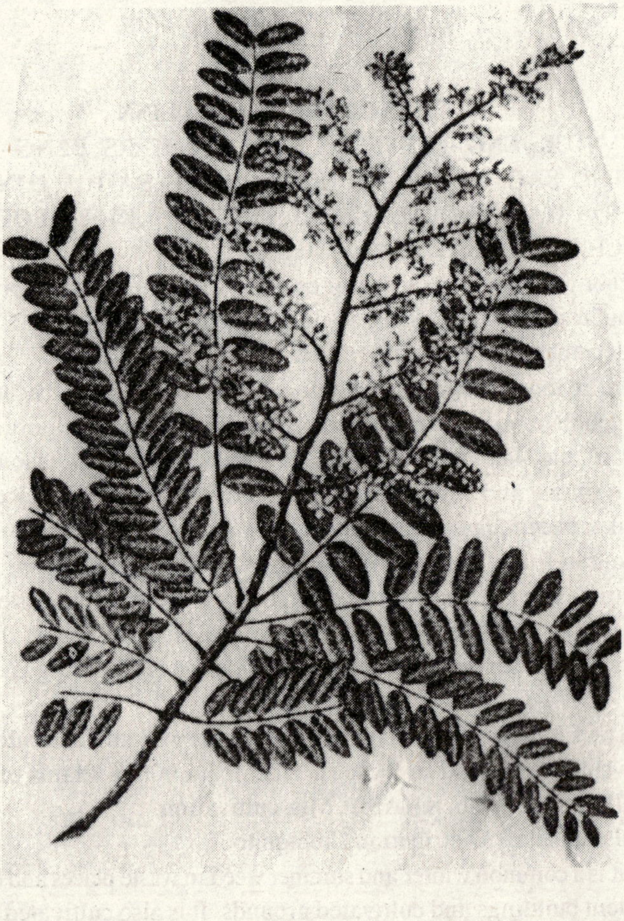

RUTACEAE

CHLOROXYLON SWEETENIA DC.

ENGLISH- EAST INDIAN SATINWOOD TREE., **HINDI**- BHIRRA, GIRIYA, DHAUR., **BO.**- BHERIA., **TAM.**- PORASU, KARAMBORYA and MODIRAI., **TELGU**- BILLU, BILLIDU, K. HURAGALUMORA, MASSI., **MARATHI & GUJ.**- HALDA, BHARIYA BILLY, HARDI., **MYSORE**- HURAGALU., **BOMBAY**- BITTU, MAYRIA, HARDI, HULDA., **M.P.**- BHEYRA, GIRIYA, BHEYRU, MIRR., **SRI LANKA**- BARUTA, MUTIRAI.

It is a tree with a short stem and diffused top. In Sri Lanka this tree acquires a larger size. It is a very stout plant and can withstand any adverse environmental conditions. Its wood is variously coloured and shining like satin. The bark is rough and canvas coloured. The leaves are bipinately compound. The pinnatefid pairs vary from 10-16 arranged in an opposite manner. The flowers are found in terminal clusters and are greenish in colour, while small flowers are somewhat longer and olive coloured and sometimes black in colour. The seeds are brown in colour.

It is reported from dry deciduous forests in the indian Peninsula, extending in the north to the Satpuras and Chhota Nagpur.

MEDICINAL USE : Bark - Astringent.

Leaves- applied to wounds and prescribed in rheumatism. Plant as a whole is irritant. It contains an alkaloid chloroxylonine which is a powerful irritant.

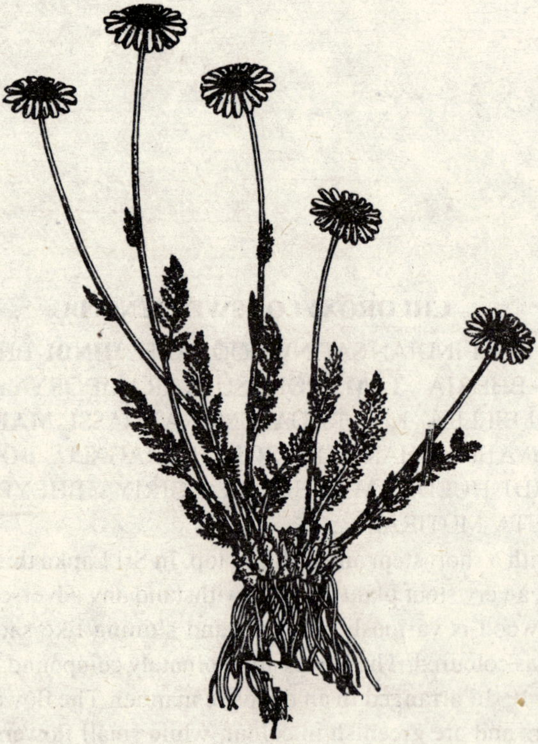

COMPOSITAE

CHRYSANTHEMUM CINAERIFOLIUM (TRE-V) VIS
(Syn. PYRETHRUM CINERAIFOLIUM TREV)

ENG.- DALMATIAN, PYRETHRUM, DALMATIAN, INSECT FLOWER.

A glaucous pernnial herb, 18-24 inch high with finely cut leaves and numerous flower heads, 6-9 mm. diam. when closed and 9-12 mm. diam when open. Rarely shrubs. Leaves alternate, entire toothed lobed or pinnatifid. Head large, terminal, long peduncled, or smaller and corymbose, heterogamous, rayed (very rarely disciform); ray-floret. female 1-seriate, fertile, liqule spreading white-yellow or rosy; disk - flaret, hermaphrodite fertile, tube terete or 2-winged, limb 4 - 5 fid. Involuere hemispherie or broader; bracts infinite-seriate, broad, appressed, inner with scarious tips, outer shorter often with scarious coloured margins; receptacle various, naked. Anther bases obtuse, entire. Style arms of hermaphrocdite with truncate penicillate tips. Achenes substerete or angled, variously ripped or winged, pappus O or short, or a cup of auricle.

As far as eighty species are reported from North temperate regions.

C. CINERATIAEFOLIUM is a native of Dalmatia, Herzegorina and Montenegro, and is cultivated on a commercal scale in Algeria, Dalmatia, Austrailia, Brazil, Bulgria, California, China, Japan, France, Italy, Kenya, Persia, Kussia, Spain and Switzerland. Cultivation has also been under taken in England and India.

MEDICINAL USE : Dried and powdered flower heads are acrid and bitter and cause a numbing sensation to the tongue and tips.

Pyrethrum is a contact poison and it takes part in the formation of important insecticides. It also occupies an important place in anti-malerial measures. It is also used as a live stock spray against parasites.

Preparations of flower heads are effective in pediculosis, scabies and against intestinal parasites of animals. (Bhagat et. al., 1968).

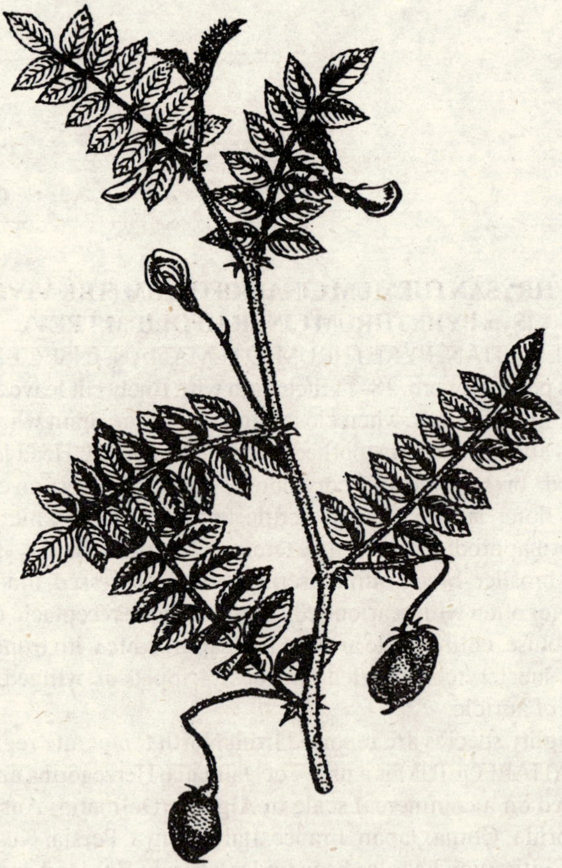

PAPILIONACEAE

CICERARIETINUM LINN.

BENG.- CHOT-ABUT, CHOLA., **ENG.**- CHICKEN-PEA, BENGAL GRAM., **HINDI**- CHANA., **GUJ.**- CHANA., **KAN.**- KADALE., **KON.**- CHANO., **MAL.**- KATALA., **MAR.**- HARBARA., **PUNJ.**- NAKHUD, CHOLA., **TAM.**- KONDAKKADALAI, KADALAI., **TEL.**- SANAGALU., **BOMB.**- CHANA., **SANS.**- CHANAKA.

Gram or chick peas are also called garbanzos or garbarzo beans. Gram is extensively consumed by both animals and human beings. It is a much branched viscous-pubescent annual herb reaching to a height of 1-2 ft. All the parts of the plant are covered with glandular hairs. Leaves : are pinnately compound; 1-2", with usually a terminal leaflet; stipules small with a few long teeth; leaflets close; oblanceolate or oblong; rigid leaflets and stipules strongly veined, deeply toothed. 1-1.5 x 0.5-0.7 cm. Peduncle 1/2 - 3/4 inch. Flowers :-Pink, blue or white, solitary in the axils of leaves. Calyx : 1/4-1/3 inch; calyx tube oblique; teeth laneeolate subequal; 2-3 times the tube. Corolla:-exserted; standard broad, exceeding the wings and keel; scarcely half as long as the calyx; stamens : diodelphous; anthers uniform. Ovary : sessile, 2 or many ovuled; style incurved beardless, stigma capitate. Pod : sessile, oblong, turgid, narrowed into the persistant style; pubescence of pod short and fine, oblong 3/4-1".

Commonly cultivated in the Northern provinces and Nilghiris, cultivated in various temperate and tropical countries. It is a cold season crop. the flowering and fruiting season is winter. It is believed that Indians introduced it in East and South Africa and the West Indies. India accounts for 90% of the total world Production of Gram. The other gram producing regions are the Meditranean (Iran, Iraq, Morocco, Algeria, Greece, Italy, Portugal, Spain), Ethiopia and Mexico. In India it is chiefly grown in Punjab; Uttar Pradesh, Bihar, Madhya Pradesh and Andhra Pradesh. Northern India accounts for nearly 90% of the total covered area and about 95% of the total annual production; which are 24 million acres and over 6 million tones respectively.

MEDICINAL USE : 1. Gram flour is used as a substitute for wheat flour for diabetic patients.

2. If forms an important ingredient in all types of face packs.

3. The plant is refrigerant. Seeds are astringent and antibilious. When roasted, the pulse is considered to be aphrodisiac. Fried seeds are diuretic. The leaf juice is stomachic and laxative.

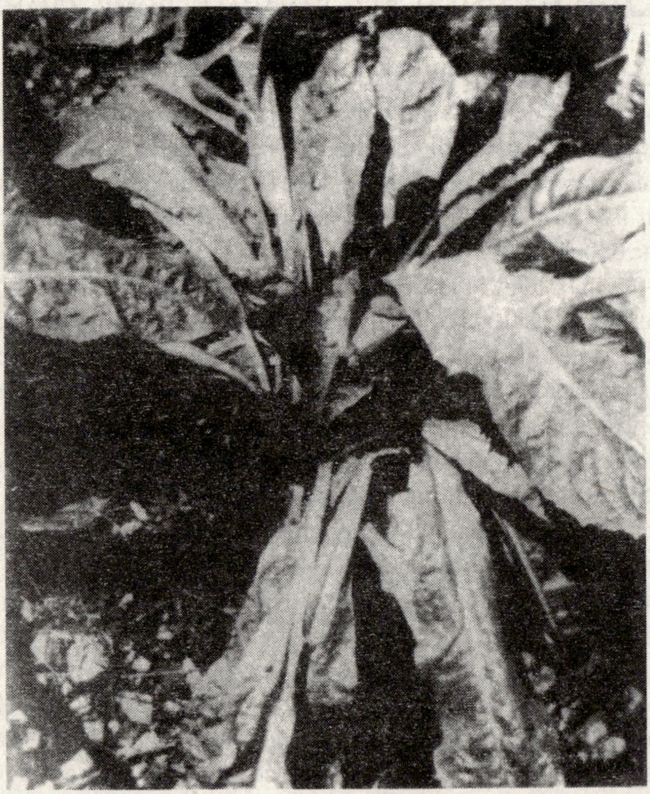

COMPOSITAE

CICHORIUM INTYBUS LINN.
(Syn.CHICORY, WILD ENDIVE.)
INDIAN NAME- KASANI, KASHINI, KASNI.

ARAB.- HINDUBAR, INPYBA., **HINDI**- KASNI., **BENG.**- KASNI., **BOMB.**- KASNI., **TAM.**- KASHNI., **TEL.**- KASHNI., **LOCAL NAME**- KASNI.

An errect or prostrate, glabrous perennial hispid herb with fleshy tapering root. Stem is 1/3 ft; angled and grooved; branches rigid and spreading; divaricate and sometimes spiny. Latex white; Leaves: upper subentire, lower pinnatifid, oblong-lanceolate, upper chordate-amplexicaul, Stem and leaf nerves beneath hispid. Heads: sessile on the branches or on thickened peduncles, homogamous blue; flowers all liqulate solitary and terminal and axillary clustered, invol. bracts glandular-hispid much shorter than the corolla. flower-heads blue, with ray florets only present; involucral bracts green in two ranks, the outer shorter lanceolate spreading, the inner longer errect. Pappus pale obtuse very short 1 - 1½" diam; invol, bracts herbaceous; ligules bright blue rarely white or pink, truncate, 5 toothed. Achenes angled, pale, mottled, glabrous, sub 5-angled, the outer sub comprecssed and infinite - ribbed or stariate, or base contracted, tip truncate or the margin slightly produced; pappus pales short, 2-3 serriate. The flowering season is April - May.

Reported from North Western India; Kumaon (cultivated or an escape?) Westward to the Altantic Pakistan and Kashmir, West Asia, Europe. 1500 - 2400 mts. cultivated areas; quite common in the Kashmir Valley. July - September wild in Punjab N. W Frontier Province and Hyderabad (DN) cultivated in Nadiad, Broach and Amalsad in Bombay.

MEDICINAL USE : It is used as tonic in fevers, vomiting, diarroea and enlargement of the spleen and its root as a stomachiac and diuretic.

Wild form of the plant considered tonic, emmengouge and alexiterie (Kirt & Basu, loc. cit.)

Roots when dried, roasted and ground, are mixed with coffee.

Comnercially it forms an essential ingredient of Liv 52 Bonnisan, Geriforte and Herbolex.

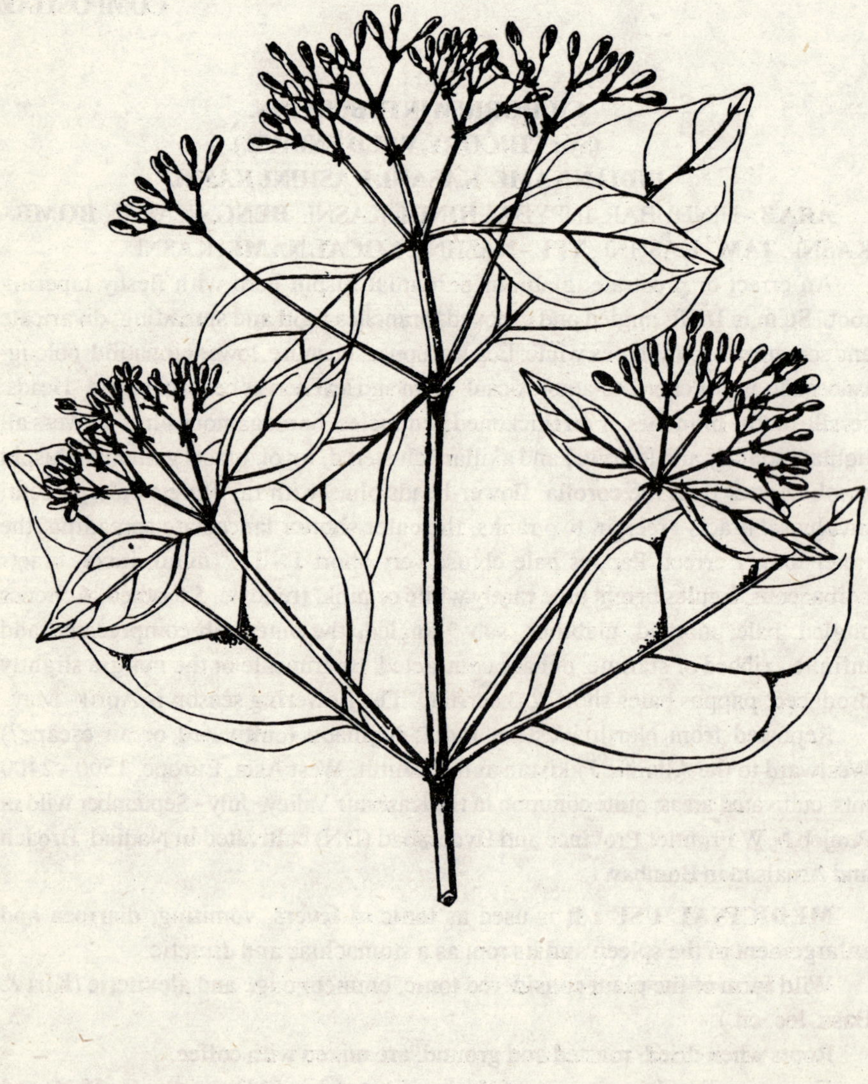

RUBIACEAE

CINCHONA LEDGERINA MOENSEX TRIMEN (SYN. C.CALISAYA WEDD.)

ENG.- CINCHONA BARK, PERUVAN BARK, QUININE, JESUITS BARK., **TAM.**- KWAINAAMARAM., **HINDI**- CINCHONA.

Cinchona is the bark of the tree yields the drug Quinine attaining a height of 50 ft. or more it is a large tree with a stout straight bare trunk, the bark is thick which may blight coloured, pale, brown or dark brown or whitish, on the species fissured and smooth depending on the species. The leaves are entire, opposite, leathery, elliptical or elliptical-lanceolate, petiolate, with interpetiolar stipules. The flowers are yellow or pink coloured which are borned in terminal painicles. They are produced from the third or fourth year of growth. Calyx-Tube adnate to the ovary; limb various. Corolla regular, usually 4-5 lobed; lobes valvate, imbricate or contorted to the left; stamens as many as the lobes, inserted on the mouth or tube of the corolla, filaments short or long; anthers 2-celled, usually dorsifixed and dehiscing laterally or in front. Ovary 2-10 celled. Style simple or cleft, stigmas various; ovules one or more in each cell. Fruit, capsular, drupaceous or of dhicent or indhiscent cocci, 2-10 celled. Seed various, cotyledons flat or semiterete.

The plants are limited in distribution. They grow in the tropics between 10 North and 20 South of the Equator at altitudes more than 1,000 ft. They grow in regions of very high temperature and high rainfall (60" or more). Cinchona is thoroughly naturalized in India. C. CALISAYA (yellow cinchona bark, grows best at the Himalayan plantations and Sikkim. C. LEDGERIANA being in abundance in Madras and Bengal plantations.

MEDICINAL USE : The barks and all preparations of Cinchona are specially valuable in intermittent fevers. In small doses they act as tonics in dypepsia, gastric catarrh, adynamier and Convalescence from fevers. The alkloids quinine guinidine, cinchonidine, cinchonine are valuable as antipyretics. They have been used in the prophylaxis treatment of malaria, whooping cough, hay-fever, enlargement of spleen, hemierania and other neuralgic affeetions. It is also used in small pox, septic fevers, pneumonia, acute rheumatism, acute tonsillitis, acute nasal catarrh , pyaemia etc., For abscesses cavities and ulcers, it is used as an antiseptic. In sore throat it is used for wash and gargle. The indiscriminate use of quinine in continuous and large doses for a long time weakens the heart, produces restlessness and cachexia.

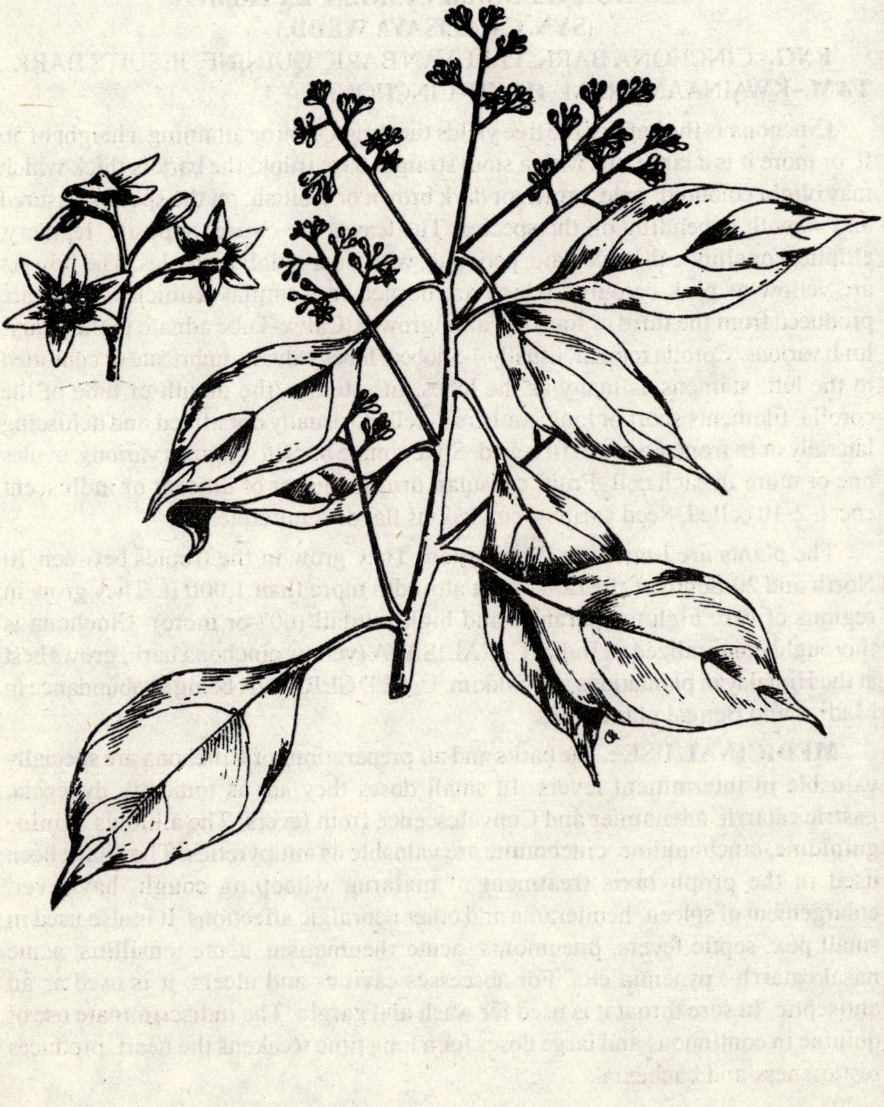

LAURACEAE

CINNAMOMUM CAMPHORA (L) T. XIEES & EBERM

ENG.- CAMPHOR, CINNAMON., **HINDI**- MUSHKAPUR., **KANNADA**- CHANCHE, KARPURA, KUMUDA, PACHKARPURA, TUHINA., **SANS.**- KANPURA., **TAMIL.**- KARUPPURAM, PUGALNISUVANDIRAM., **TELGU**- KARPURAMU, SITABHRAMU.

It is a medium sized ever green tree. Mainly it is considered as an ornamental plant. The leaves are dark green above and pale glaucous beneath arranged alternately, coriceous, leaves are 5-9 cm. with a short slender leaf stalk about a third as long as the blade. Leaf is elliptic long pointed 3 veined. Panicles axillary with tiny greenish yellow flowers in small spreading branched clusters, each to 5 cm. across. Flower C. 3 mm. across with 6 lobes hairy within; fruit globular C. 9 mm. across with a thickened club shaped base. It is grown for a white crystalline substance knowns as Japan camphor which is obtained from the leaves & twigs used in medicine.

It is a native of China & Japan. Cultivated in HImalaya to 1500 m & some time naturalized; common in kathmandu. April-May.

MEDICINAL USE : Externally it is utilized in cases of inflamations bruises & sprains. It is also used for rheumatic pains. Internally it is used in diarrhoea & as cardiac stimulant. Mixed with any oil it is a good remendy for skin itch, exzema & skin infections.

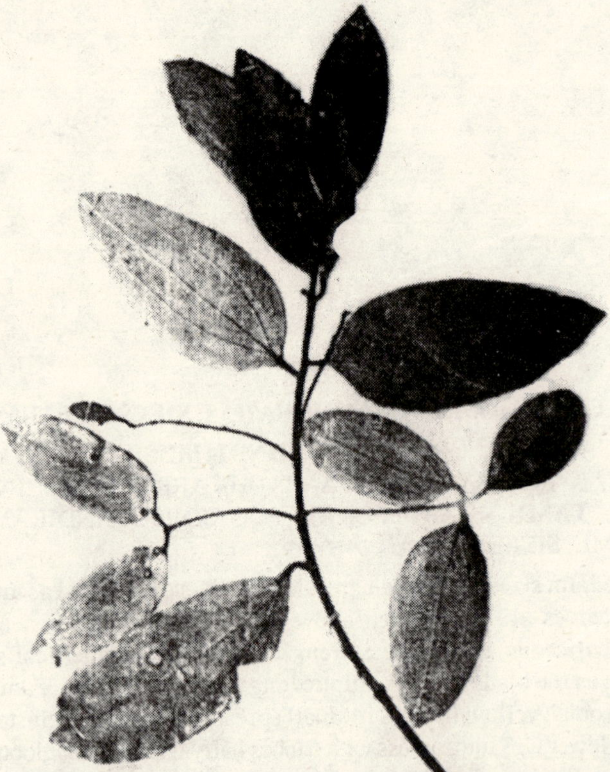

LAURACEAE

CINNAMOMUM ZEYLANICUM BREYN.

ENG.- CHINESE CASSIA, CINNAMON., **HINDI**- DALCHINI., **PUNJ.**- DALCHINI., **KASHMIRI.**- DALCHINI., **BENGALI**- DALCHINI., **KAN.**- DALCHINI., **MAL.**- KULIT-MANIS., **SANS.**- TAMALA PATRA., **SANS.**- KURUNDU., **TAM.**- LOWANGA PATTAI, IIAYANGAM, CANNA LAVANGA PATTAI., **TEL.**- DASMCHAKKALU, LAVANGAMU.

CINNAMON of COMMERCE is dried inner bark which is available in the form of long sticks termed quills', and has a delicate fregrance and warm sweet taste.

It is a small evergreen tree attaining a height of 20-25 ft. and sometimes reaching a height of 60 ft. as in Ceylon. Leaves :-Opposite or alternate, usually triple-nerved; 4-7 inch; glabrous, very coriaceous ovate or ovate-laneeolate; sometimes five nerved; obtuse of subacute, reticulate beneathe. The flowers are borned in branched large axillary stalked clusters. Panicles often larger than the leaves sub silkly pubescent, perianth 1/4 inch. long, fruiting peduncle campanulate 1/3 inch; diam. crowned with the rounded perianth-lobes, fruits oblong 2/3 inch. long apiculate dry.

It occurs wild in the Southern Coastal regions of Western India up to an altitude of 6,000 ft., and in Ceylon. It is abundant in the regions 100-700 ft. above sea level, and is fairly common up to 3,500 ft. It is also reported from Tenasserin, Burma and the MALAY Peninsula; Deccan Peninsula and Ceylon, indigenous or cultivated.

Distribution cultivated in the Malay Islands, and elsewhere in the tropic.

MEDICINAL USE : Ceylon bark oil is used in liqueurs etc. It is also a fungicide. It has the cordial and carminative proeprties of cinnamonmum without its astringency and is employed as adjuvant in stomachic and carminative medicines. As a powerful local stimulent it is sometimes prescribed in gastrodynia flatulent, colie and gastric debility. The dosage is 1-3 minims (U.S.D., 295, BP., 373).

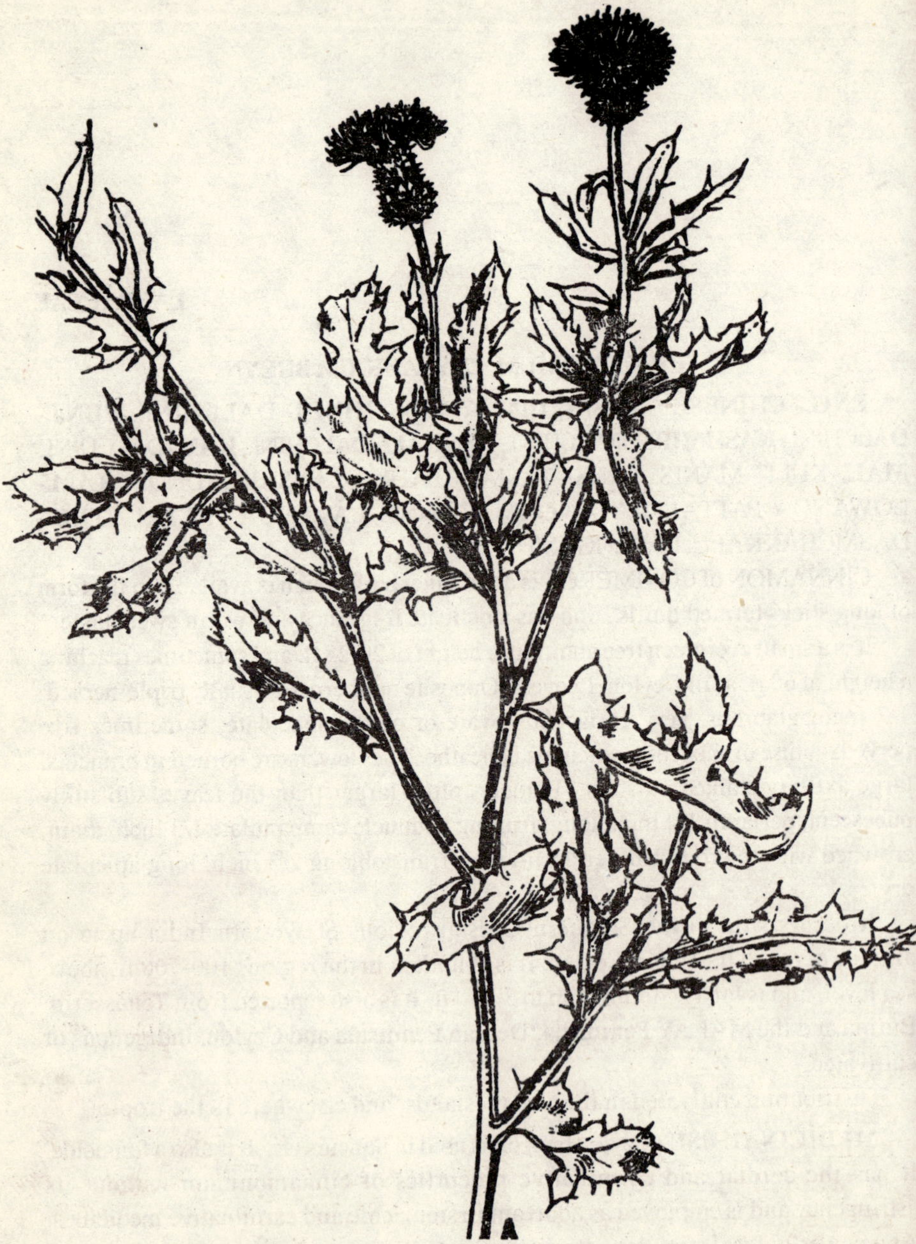

A

COMPOSITEAE

CIRSIUM ARVENSE (LINN) SCOP
(Syn. CNICUS ARVENSIS HOFFM.)
(Syn. SERRATULA ARVENSIS LINN).

LOCAL NAME- KATELI, KATALA, RISSA.

It is an erect herb very variable 0.6 - 1 m. tall. Underground roots are for-creeping and producing many erect stems. Stems much branched, leaf, mostly 50 - 100 cm. Leaves lanceolate to oblong in outline, entire or pinnately lobed, with triangular lobes with weak to stout marginal spines, hairless or scaresely cobe-web-hairy. Flower heads pale purple, 1 to 5 shortly stallked and borne at the ends of the branches. Involucre mostly 1.2 - 1.7 cm. long with adpressed braets with short terminal spines, the outer braets blunt, the inner longer with recurved tips, florets unisexual, 1.3 - 1.8 cm. Achenes small. Pappus pale brown. Flowers and fruits - February - April.

It is commonly found in waste places, cultivated areas and a long field edges. Common in Kashmir - March - August. It is also reported from Bengal and Gangetic Plains, from the Sunderbans North-Westwards to Punjab, Western Himalayas from Kashmir to Kumaon.

MEDICINAL USE : Plant emetic, tonic, diphor. The plant contains a volatile alkaloid and cnicin, a crystaline bitter glycoside, possessing emetic and emmen properties. Its' another species CIRSIUM VULGARE (U. S. D. 1629) is also used medicinally. Some thistles have medicinal properties.

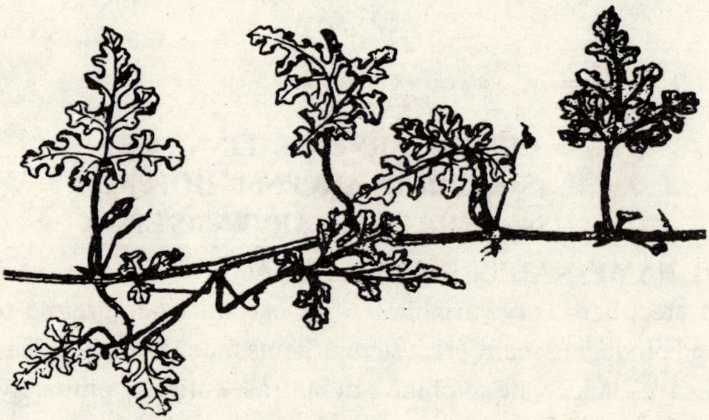

CUCURBITACEAE

CITRULLUS COLOCYNTHIS SCHRAD
(Syn. CUCUMIS COLOCYNTHIS L.)
(Syn. COLOCYNTHIS VULGARIS SCHRAD).

ENG.- COLOCYNTH, BITTER APPLE, INDIAN WILD GOURD., **HINDI**- INDRAYAN., **LOCAL NAME**- GADUMBA KI BEL, INDRAYAN., **KAUR**- TUMBA, HARPENDUA., **SANS.**- MAHENDRA - VARUNI., **H & B &B.O.**- INDRAYAN., **B.** MAKHAL., **TAMIL**- PEYTTUMMATTI, PEIKKUMMATTI., **TEL.**- ETIPUCHEHHA., **MAL.**- PEYKOMMUTHI., **GUJ. & BENG**.- INDRAYAN, MAKHAL., **KAN.**- HAAVUMEKKAL., **KON.**- KAVANDALI., **MAR.**- KADU - INCHAVANI., **PUN.**- GHUMBA.

It is a perennial, trailing, scabrid herb, leaves ovate or triangular in outline, deeply - 3 lobed; lobes sinuately pinnatifid; Flowers, axillary and short stalked. The tendrils are long curved and branched. Fruits globose, striped with dark green and white; pulp spongy, very bitter flowers-May to July; fruits August-October.

It grows commonly in the sandy tracts near Najafgarh, Khera Nangloi and Narela. It is known native to Asia and Africa but found in N. Indian, M.P., Gujarat and South India.

MEDICINAL USE : Fruit and seed-purg.

Roots-purg; used in ascites, jaundice, urinary diseases and rheumatism. Fruit and root-antid, to snake poison extract from fruit pulp is highly effective against bacteria.

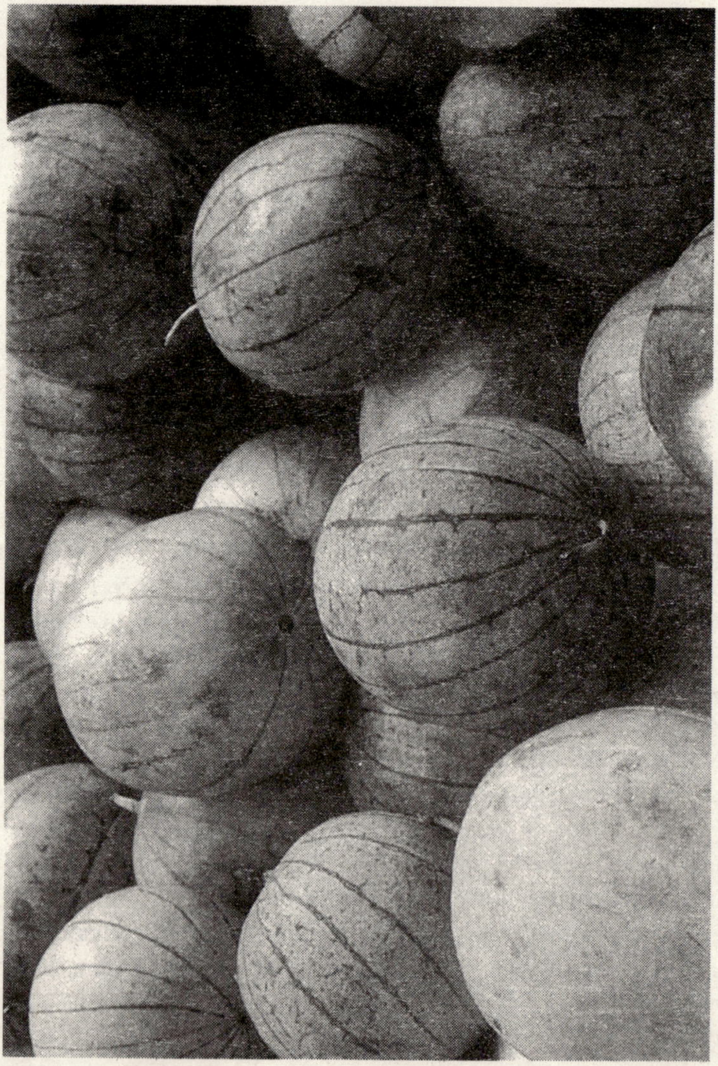

CUCURBITACEAE

CITRULLUS VULGARIS SCHRAD (V.CUCURBITA CITRULLUS LINN)

ENG.-WATER MELON., **ASSAMESE**- TARMUJ., **BENG.**- TERMUJ., **ORIYA**-TARBHUJA., **TELGU**- PUTCHA., **TAMIL**- TURBUZA, PALAM, PANNA, **MALAYALAM**- THANNIRMATHAN, **KANNADA**- KALLANGADI., **MARATHI**-KALINGAD., **GUJARATI**- TARBAR, TERBOOJ., **PUNJABI**- TARBOOZ., **LOCAL+ HINDI NAME**- TARBOOZ, TARBUJZA.

It is a climbing hispid annual. Leaves are lobed, Flowers large in size yellowish white. Fruits large sub globose ellipsoid, yellow, dark green or mottled; striped etc. Pulp of the fruits is white, yellow or red. Fruits are found in June-July. It is also most exclusively grown in barren sandy soils, though cultivated all over India.

MEDICINAL USE : The juicy flesh of the fruit is very sweet, water melon juice to which salt and pepper is added from a popular drink in the summer. Small unripefruits are also used as vegetable. It has got traces of vitamin A and has cooling effect. Fruit is cooling, diuretic, seeds cooling aphrodisease, tonic, diuretic seed oil substitute for almond oil; seeds rich source of an enzyme, urease, juice contains citrulline.

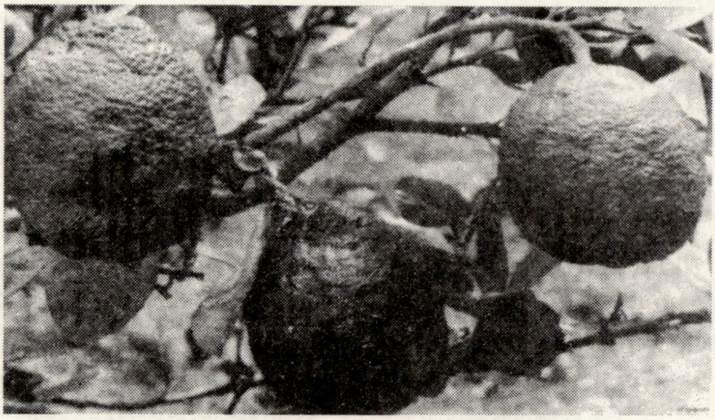

RUTACEAE

CITRUS AURANTIFOLIA (CHRISTM) SWINGLE.
(SYN. C. MEDICA VAR. L. ACIDA OF WATT. (LIME).
(SYN. LIMON AURANTI FOLIA CHRISTM)

HINDI- KHATTA, NIMBU, KAGHZI-NIMIBU, NARANG, SANTRA., **LOCAL NAME**- NIMBU, KAGHZI NIMBU., **TAM.**- NARANGAM, NARATTAL, ELUMICHAI, KAMALA, APZAM., **TEL. & ENG.**- LIME, SWEET or CHNESEORANGE, ORANGE., **KAN.**- HERALAY, NIMMA, KITTALAY., **MAL**- KARNA, ERUMICHINARAKAM., **MAD.**- HURANA RAKAM., **BENG.**- KAGHZI NIMBU., KAMLA-NEBOO., **GUJ.**- SUNTRA, NARANGI., **MAR.**- SUNTRA, NARANGI., **KON.**- SONNA-RINGA., **PUN.**- SANTRA.

An arboreous tree, usually spinous. Young shoots are glabrous greenish and white. Leaves: alternate, 1-foliolate, coriaceous, persistant; petiole often broadly winged. Leaves contain translucent oil glands in the leaves, which give a strong aerid aroma when crushed. The leaves are usually trifoliate or compound. Inflorescence terminal, branched, often flat-topped. Flowers bisexual, usually regular, axillary, solitary fascicled or in small cymes, pure white sweet-scented. Calyx: Cupular or urceolate 3-5 fid.,Petals 4-8, linear-oblong, thick, imbricate; stamens 20-60, inserted round a large cypular or annular disk; filaments variously connate, compressed at the base; anthers oblong and with a thick glandular basal disk. Ovary infinite celled, superior, with 4-5 fused carpels. Styles stout decidous, stigma capitate; ovules 4-8, 2-serrate in each cell. Berry-large; oblong or globose, fleshy, many celled; septa membranous, cells few seeded and filled with horizontal fusiform cells distended with juice. Seeds horizontal or pendulous, testa coriaceous or membranous; embryo sometimes 2 or more in one seed catyledons plano-convex, often unequal, radicle small, superior.

Distribution about five tropical Asiatic species, and 2 Australian. It is also reported from hot valleys along the foot of the Himalaya, from Garwal Last Wards to Sikkim and in the Khasia Mts. It is cultivated in the plains and up to 4,000 ft. Madras tops in the productionof this fruit. Other producing areas are Bombay, Bengal, Punjab, Madya Pradesh, Hyderabad, Delhi, Patiala, U.P. and Baroda.

MEDICINAL USE : Lime is an excellant source of vitamin "C". Which is very essential keeping digestion good; in a healthy skin, gums and teeth and for restoring and maintaining general resistance of the body. Lime is an appetizer, stomachic, antiscorbutic and anthelmintic (Kirt. and basu, I, 489, 1935). It checks biliousness. Salted lime peel is recommended for indigestion. It prevents blood from clotting and keeps blood vessels elastic.

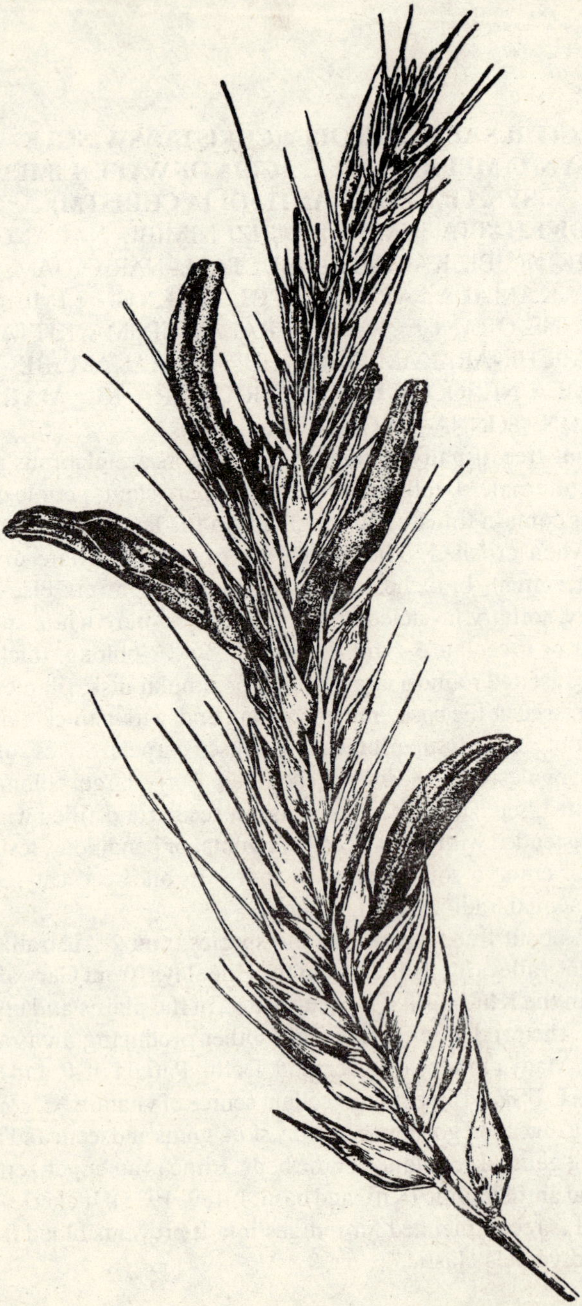

CLAVICIPITACEAE

CLAVICEPS PURPUREA (FR.) TUL.
ENGLISH-ERGOT.

It is a small herbaceous plant ½ to 1" tall. It is triangular and rust coloured and is known as a fungous parasite. It is found on a number of grasses particularly rye; it is poisonous but not fatel.

It is mainly cultivated in the Nilgiris and at Chakrohi farm in Jammu.

MEDICINAL USE : Dried sclerotium, known as ergot is used in medicine in contraction of uterus and bladder. It also controls bleeding. Ergotamine is also used as a remedy for migraine. Ergotamine tartrate and ergometring maleate are two important ergot alkaloids used in medicine in form of tablets, and ampoules. Strains of ergot have been commercially produced in drug forms of the CIMPO, and the PRL Jammu and pure alkaloids are reported to have been prepared on large scale.

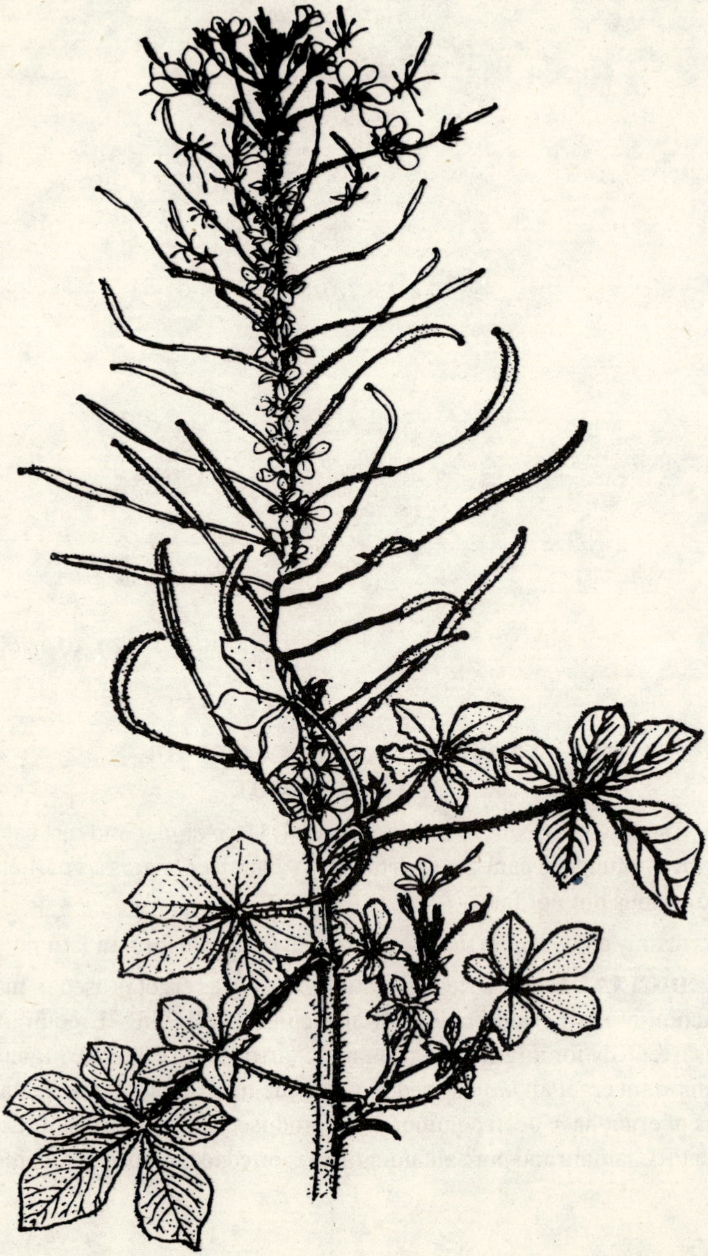

CLEOMACEAE
(CAPPARIDACEAE)

CLEOME VISCOSA LINN.
(Syn. POLA-NISIA ISOCANDRA LINN. W & A.)
(Syn. CLEOME ISCANDRALINN)
Popularly known as wild or Dog Mustard.

ENG.- STICKY CLEOME., **HINDI**- HUR HUR, HUL HUL., **LOCAL NAME**- HULHUL., **BENG.**- TILPARNI, HUKHURIA., **GUJ.**- TILYANT., **KAN.**- KAADUSAASIVE, NAYIRELA., **KON.**- SIRIKALA., **MAR.**- ARYAVAL, KANPHUTI., **PUNJ.**- BOGRA., **TAM.**- NAYI-VELAI, KEERAI, NAYIKKADUGU., **TEL.**- NAELANAMINTA, KUKHAVOMINTA.

An erect, branching-glandular-pubescent herb 10-60 cm. high. The whole plant is covered over by mixed simple and glandular hairs. Leaves : softly pubescent, 3-5 foliate; leaflets ovate or obovate; unequal in size; leaflets equalling or shorter than the petiole upper usually subsessile. Flowers yellow, solitary, axillary or in leaf-bearing terminal racemes. Racemes are long pedicelled flowers 1/2"- 2" long. Sepels-4, spreading petals 4, regular or ascending; reflexed. Stamens : 12-20, sessile on the disk, ovary sessile or with a short gynophore style short or 0; ovules many, on 2 parietal placentae. Capsule 2 - 3 1/2", striate, narrowed to the tip; glandular pubescent oblong or linear; valves 2 seperating from the seed-bearing placenta. Seeds reniform, small and granular.

It is abundantly present throughout the tropical and Warm India and the rest of the World. Locally it comes up after the first monsoon shower in the waste and dry sandy soils.

MEDICINAL USE : The leaves are rubefacient, vesicant and sudorific. The juice of the leaves mixed with ghee is used in the treatment of inflammations of the middle ear. The leaves are used also in external applications for wounds and ulcers. The seeds also possess rubefacient vesicant and anthelmintic properties. Leaves have a pungent flavour and bark is irritant and acrid; externally it is rubefacient and vesicant.

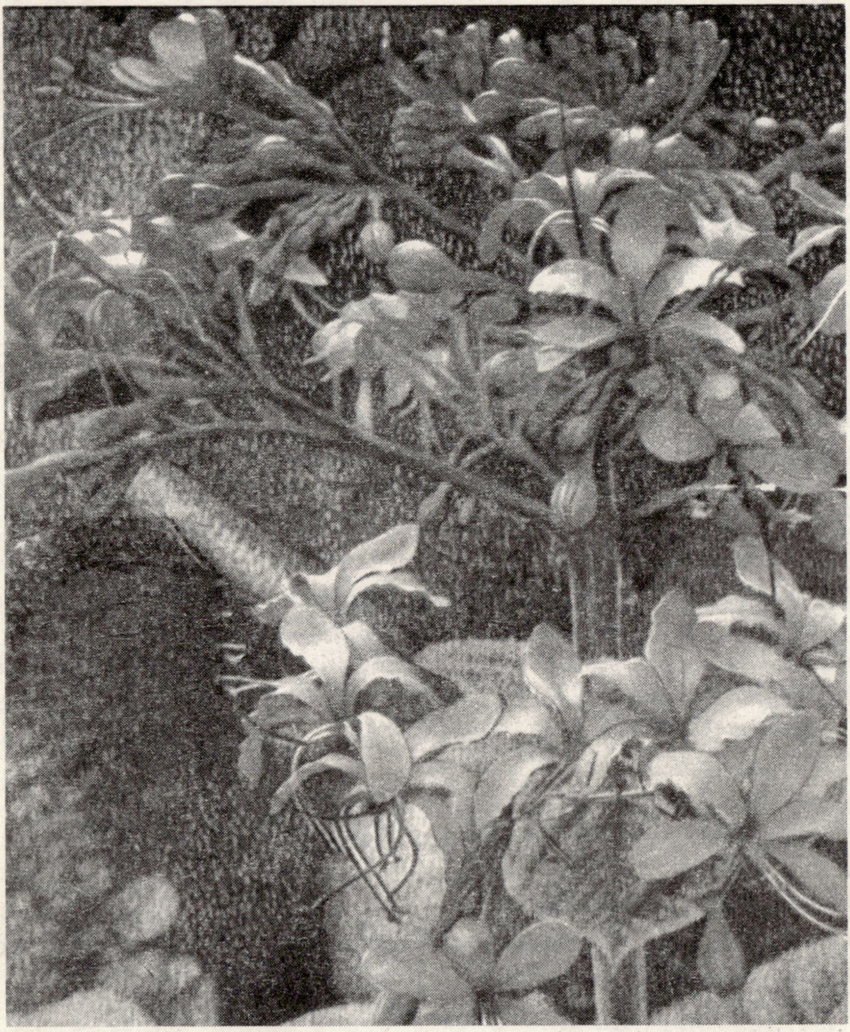

VERBENACEAE

CLERODENDRON INERME (LINN.) GAERTN
(Syn. VOLKAMERIA INERMISL.)

SANS.- KUNDALI, VANAJAI., **HINDI**- LANJAI, SANGKUPI., **BENG.**- BONJOI, BATRAJ., **BOMB.**- VANAJAI., **MAL.**- NIRNOCHI., **TAM.**- PINARICHANGANGUPPI, ANJALI., **TEL.**- TAKKOLAKAMU., ETIPISINIKA., **KAN.**- KUNDALI, NAYITAKKALI.

A densely hairy, straggling trailing shrub with hairy twigs. Stem with very large corky lenticels C. 1-2 inch. Leaves 6 mucilaginous, bitter and fragrant, variable, ovate, elliptic, elliptic-oblong to obovate, glabrous and subfleshy; opposite 3-4 nate long stalked with a rounded or slightly heart shaped base, densely rough-hairy on both sides, simple occasionally lobed. Flowers white sweet-scented with pink centres and long exerted stamens in large lax terminal branched clusters. Each cluster is 3-flowered eyme from uppermost leaves. Calyx : Campanulate truncate or 5-toothed, or sub-5-partite, persistent often accrescent or coloured. Corolla tube slender, cylindrical, usually long filiform; limb 5-fid; spreading, more or less oblique; silky-haired much enlarged in fruit. Stamens : about three times as long as corolla; 4; overy : imperfectly 4-celled, 4-ovuled; style filiform, shortly bifid. Fruit a spongy drupe, black when ripe seated in the enlarged red Calyx, globose, sacculent, more rarely nearly dry 4-grooved, seperating into 4 pyrenes of which 1-3 are often supressed. Seeds oblong. Flowering season from July to November.

Reported from India and Ceylon near the sea from Bombay to Tenosserin. Uttar Pradesh to Sikkim. India S.E. Asia to 1,500 meters.

MEDICINAL USE : Fresh and dry leaves possess alterative and febrifugal properties. A poultice of the leaves is used to resolve buboes. A liniment useful in rheumatism is obtained by boiling the root in oil.

Leaves contain amorphous bitter principal, resin, gum (Dymock, Warden and Hooper 111, 76).

Medicinal properties of this plant resemble those of SWERTIA CHIRAYITA.

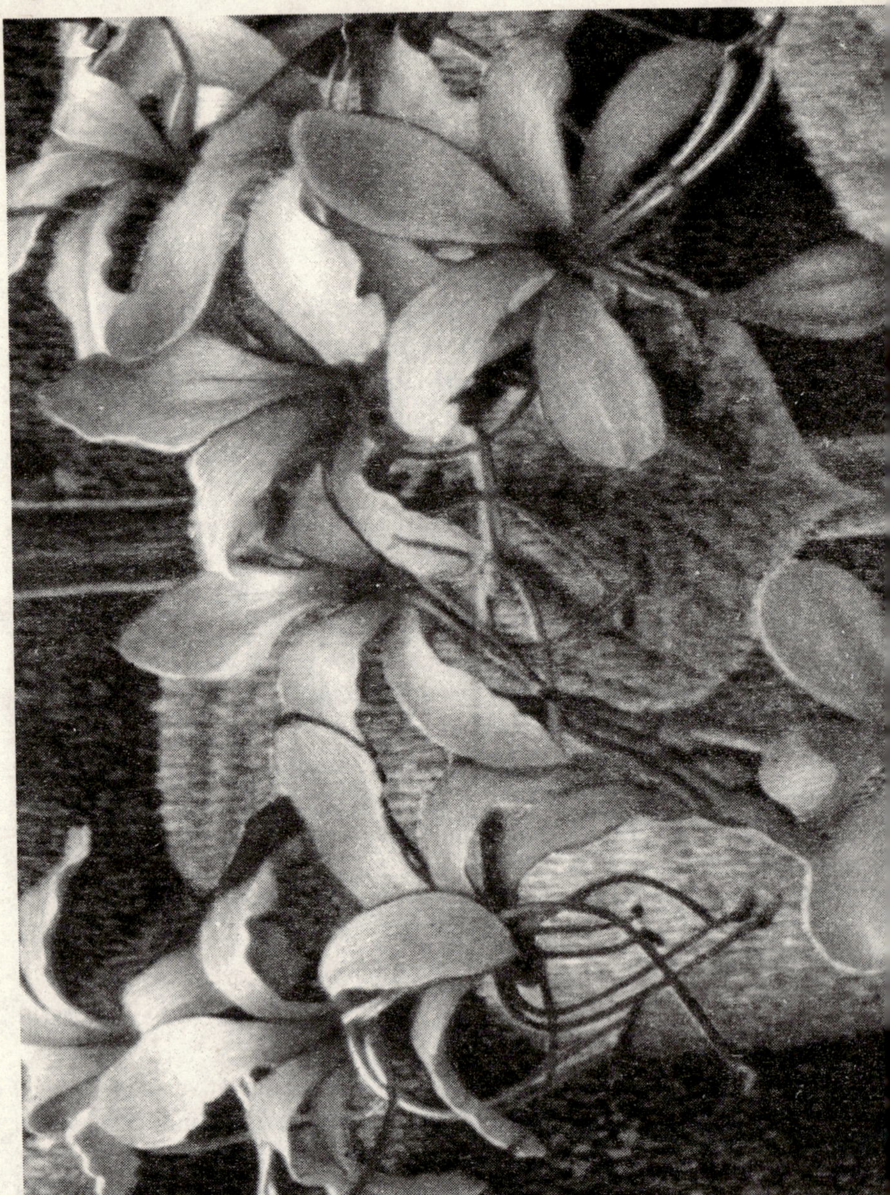

VERBENACEAE

CLERODENDRON INFORTUNATUM (AUCT-NON) LINN (SYN. C. VISCOSUM VENT)

HINDI- BHANT., **BENG.-** BHANT, **BOMB**.-BHAT., **SANS.-** BHANTAKA, ARHICHUDA., **TAM.-** PERUGILAI, ANGAARA, KARUKANNL., **MAL.-** PERUKU, PERUVELLAM., **KAN.-** NAYI-BELA, BASAVANAPADA, IBBANE., **MAR.-** KARI, BHANDIRA., **PUNJ**.- KALIBASUT., **SANS.-** BHANDIRA., **TEL**.- GURRAPUKATTIYAKU, BAKAOA

It differs from C. INERME in having leaves ovate acuminate entire or serrulate mature, panicle open villous, corolla-tube exceeding the glandular Calyx-lobes ½ inch.

It is shrub, 4 ft. often gregarious, yellow or white-villous upwards, sometimes a small tree according to a note in Herb Wallich. Leaves are 4.8 inch, base chordate or obtuse, carrying from round-ovate to broad-oblong in the Decean example usually entire in the North Indian denticulate, some what roughly hairy above, beneath densely villous or thinly hairy often with small obscure round glands; petiole 1-4". Panicle 6-12 by 4-8"; erect, branchiate, sometimes leafy on the main rachis, upper branches and Calyces more or less reddening; bracts of the cymes usually caducous. Calyx, in flower, 1/3rd inch divided nearly to the base, segments broadly lanceolate very acute, suberect. Corolla pubescent without white pink tinge; tube 2/3 inch. Drupe 1/3rd inch diameter; black; Calyx in fruit enlarged sometime 1-1/2 inch diameter.

Found Throughout India from Gurwhal and Assam to Ceylon and Singapore, in the warm region, very common in Malaya.

MEDICINAL USE : The leaves are used as bitter tonic, antiperiodic in malaria vermifuge, laxative and cholagoque. The leaves and roots are used externally for tumours and certain skin diseases. Fresh leaf juice is used as an injection into the blood for return of ascarids. Root rubbed down with buter milk is given in Colie. The drug is also used in Scorpion-sting and snake-bite. CLERODENDRUM sp. is a very useful product of Capyna compound of Himalaya Drugs.

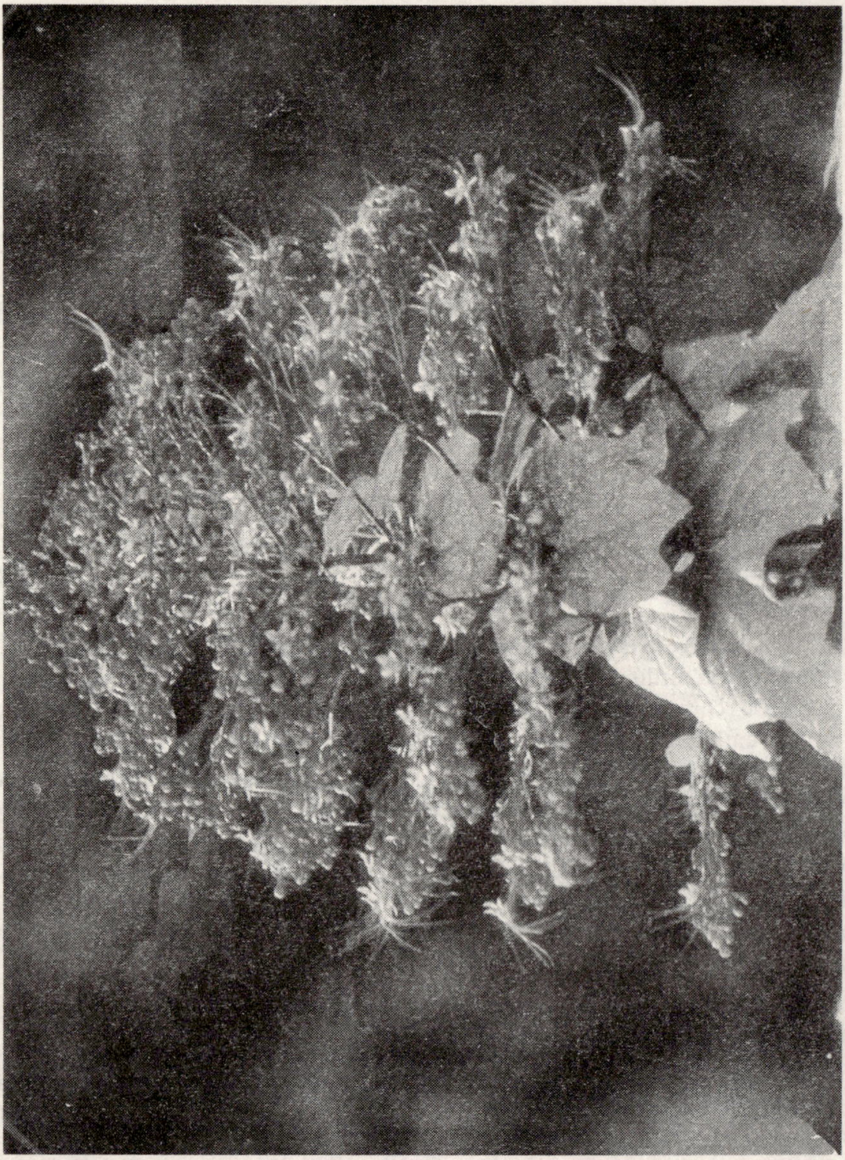

VERBENACEAE

CLERODENDRON JAPONICUM (THUNB.) SWEET.
(Syn. C. FRAGRANS. (VENT); C. BRACTEATUM (Wall).

ENG.- GLORY TREE., **HINDI**- ATTARDANA, MADANMOHAN.

It is a sweet smelling shrub or undershrub, native to China and Japan; grown as an ornamental for its very fragrant flowers. Leaves are large and heart-shaped; ovate, acuminate, entire, mature, villous, opposite, 6 by 3-4', base from cordate to cuneate, softly hairy above, villous or almost woolly beneath leaf blade serrate; leaves beneath glabrate, with many round glands. Bracts are numberous, ovate or oblong. Petiole 1-3' long connected by a dense ring of hairs. Inflorescence fulvous-villous with conspicuous terminal branched clusters of scarlet flowers. Calyx ½' divided more than half-way down; segments ovate lanceolate, suberect. It is red in colour, ovoid, nearly half as long as corolla-tube. Corolla pubescent, white; tube 1; lobes ¼'; elliptic. Corolla lobes are oblong and spreading. Drupe 1/3'; purple.

Originally it was native of tropical Asia; naturalized in cultivated areas and also in gardens in Nepal. To 1800 M. in July to October. It is reported from Sikkim and Bhutan, about 2-5000 ft.; Cachar and Khasi Mts up to 4,000 ft.; It is found in plains of India as wild plant.

MEDICINAL USES: Leaves with black Pepper are used in Colic Pain.

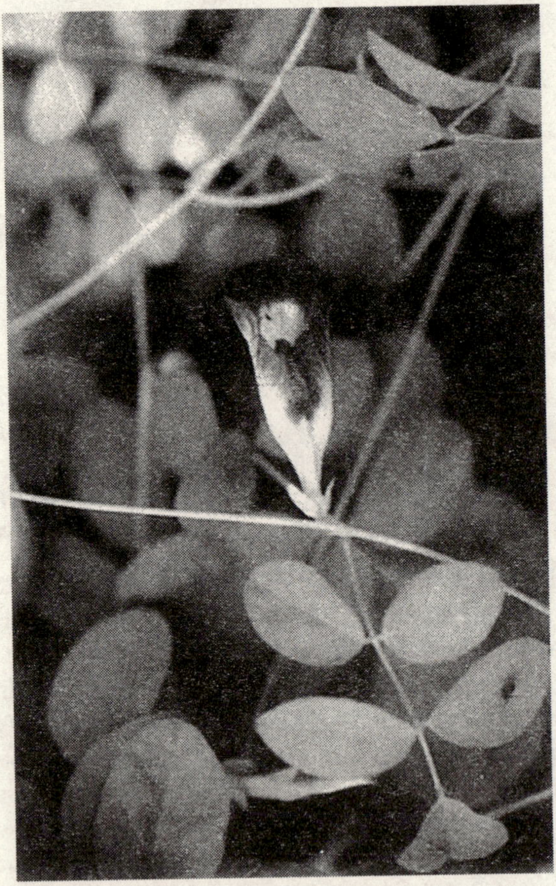

PAPILIO NACEAE.

CLITORIA TERNATEA LINN

S.- APARAJITA., **H. & B.-** APARAJIT, (THUNB.) SWEET. **M.-** KAKKANAN., **BEN.-** NILA APRAJITA., **KAN.-** SHANKAPASHPA., **ENG.-** BUTTERFLYPEA., **KAN.-** SHANKASPUSHIPI., **GUJ.-** GARANI., **MAL.-** ANAL, SHANKAPU SPARMA., **HINDI-** APARAJITA., **MARATHI-** GOLKURNA MULA., **LOCAL NAME :** GOKAREN., **TAM.-** KODI, KAKKA NAIV SHANENPUSHPAM., **TEL.-** DINTANA.

A rambling beautiful climber Leaflets 5-9 oval or oblong. Flowers more or less uniformly white or blue in the standard with white centre. The rest blue or white, solitary, axillary, pods stipitate, flet, flowers and fruits November- Feb.

A Common garden plant occuring among hedges, all varieties tropical region from the Himalaya to Ceylon abundant in South India also found as an escape.

MEDICINAL USE : Seeds purg apert. leaves powerful, cathartic action, root bitter, Cath, perg. diur., root bark diur, laxt. plants used in snake poison (Nadkarni 1954). Commercially it is known as a diuretic and laxative.

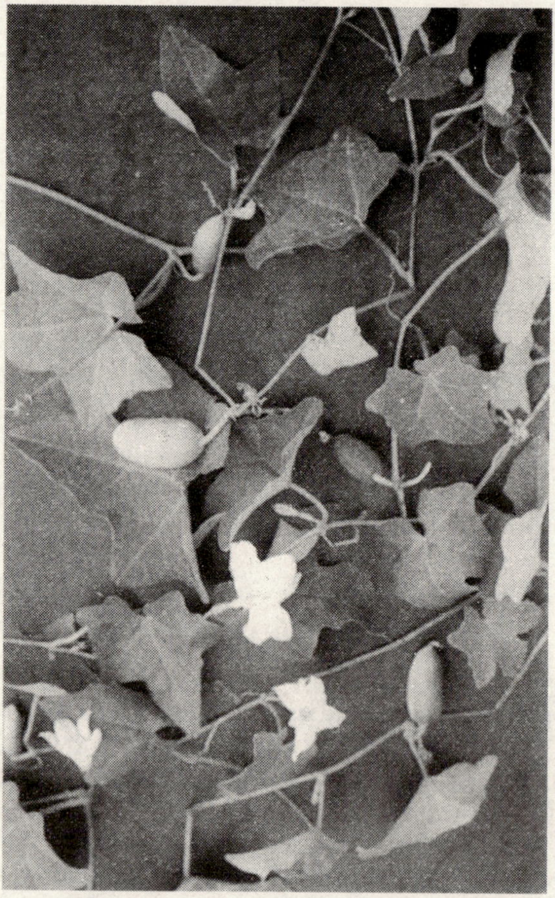

CUCURBITACEAE

COCCINIA CORDIFOLIA SENSU AUCT NON (L) COGN.
SYN. C. INDICA WANDA
SYN. CEPHALANDRA INDICA NAUD. IVYGOURD
SYN. C. INDICA WEIGHT AND ARN
SYN. BRYONIA CORDIFOLIA L.
SYN. C. GRANDIS (LINN) VOIGT

SANS.- BIMBA., **HINDI-** KANDURI, KUNDRU., **KANDURIK-** BEL., **ENG.-** KOVAI FRUIT, IVY GOURD., **PUNJ.-** KANDURI., **BENG.-** TELAKUCHA., **BOMB.-** BHIMB., **TAM.-** KOVAIKAI, KOVAI, KOVAKKKODI., **TEL.-** KONDAKAYA, KONDATIGA., **MAR.-** BIMBI, TENDLI., **RAN.-** TONDALA., **GUJ.-** GHOBE, GLURU, GHOLI., **KAN.-** TONDEKAI., **MAL.-** KOVA., **LOCAL NAME-** KUNDRU KANDURI, KATRU, RAM KACHRIYA.

A climbing or prostrate perennial herb growing wild throughout India with long tuberous roots and ovoid or elliptic fruits. The tendriles simple and straight or bifid scarecely hairy. Leaves: petioled, 5-angular or 5-lobed, toothed. 2-4" in diameter; 'papillose; scabrid, Chordate, shining; margin distantly glandular-tipped. Flowers dioecious moderately large, all solitary and white in the Indian species, ebracteate. Male:- calyx-tube companulate short, limb 5 lobed; peduncle 1"; jointed below the flower; calyx-lobes linear-oblong; corolla nearly 1"; lobes long triangular, corolla companulate 5 lobed about 1/2 way down; stamens 3; anthers exsert, connate, one 1-celled, two 2-celled, cells conduplicate. Female:-calyx and corolla as in the male; ovary oblong smooth style long with 3 bifid stigmas; ovules many, horinzontal; placenta 3, vertical. Female peduncle about 1/4 inch. Fruit:- Bright scarlet 1-2 by 1/2-1" fleshy indehiscent, cylindrical, smooth, ovoid or oblong when ripe. It is present in the axil of the leaf opposite the tendril. Seeds:-Many, ovoid, compressed, margined and embedded in red pulp. The flowering season is March-October and fruiting season is October to December.

It is commonly distributed throughout India and is reported from Malaya and Africa.

MEDICINAL USE: The dried bark is a good cathartic. Leaves and stem are antispasmodic and expectorant. Nadkarni, 1954 reportes that the plant is responsible for reducing sugar in blood in diabetes and is declared by some as Indian substitute for Insulin. However, Koman (1920) reports that none of these properties could be verified.

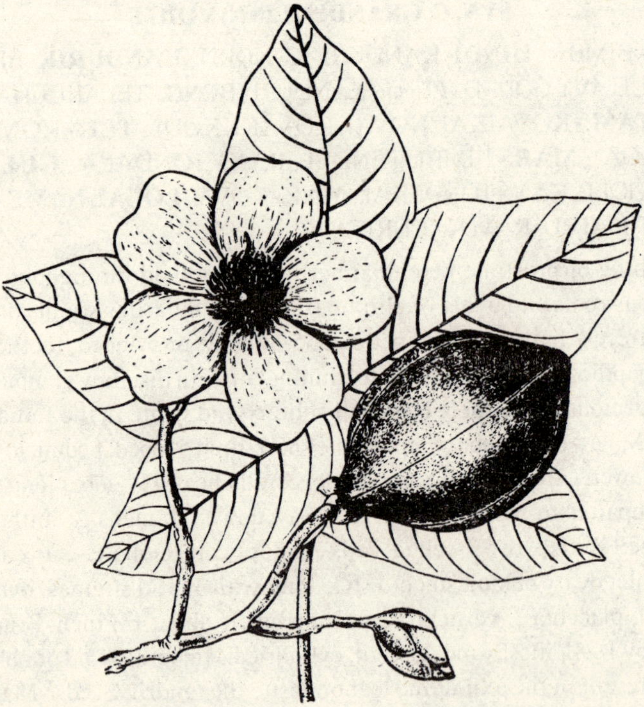

COCHLOSPERMACEAE

COCHLOSPERMUM RELIGIOSUM (LINN) ALSTON (SYN. C. GOSYPIUM D.C.)

ARAB.- KATIRA., **H.**- KUMBI., **MAL.**- APPA KUTAKKA., **MARATHI**-GANGLAY., **TAM.**- TANAKKU., **TEL.**- KONDAGOGN., **ENG.**- WHITE SILK-COTTON., **HINDI**- PILIKAPAS, KUMBI.

It is also known as silk cotton tree. It is a medium size soft wooded plant. It is 2.4-5.4 m. tall and 30 mm across. Leaflets 5 lanceolate glabrous- Flowers large bright yellow in big clusters found terminally on branches. From December- April, the leaves continue to drop but flowers keep on blooming. The fruit is a capsule in shape. They very from 5 to 7.5 cm. They ripe in from June to July.

It is reported from Garhwal, Bundelkhand, Bihar, Orissa, Bengal, Madhya Bharat, Deccan, and Western Pennisula and Madras State in dry forests, especially in stray hills, in all districts but less on the W. Coast.

MEDICINAL USE : Tree yields a gum which is sweetish, cooling, sedative, used in cough and ghonnorea, Dried leaves and flowers are stimulant.

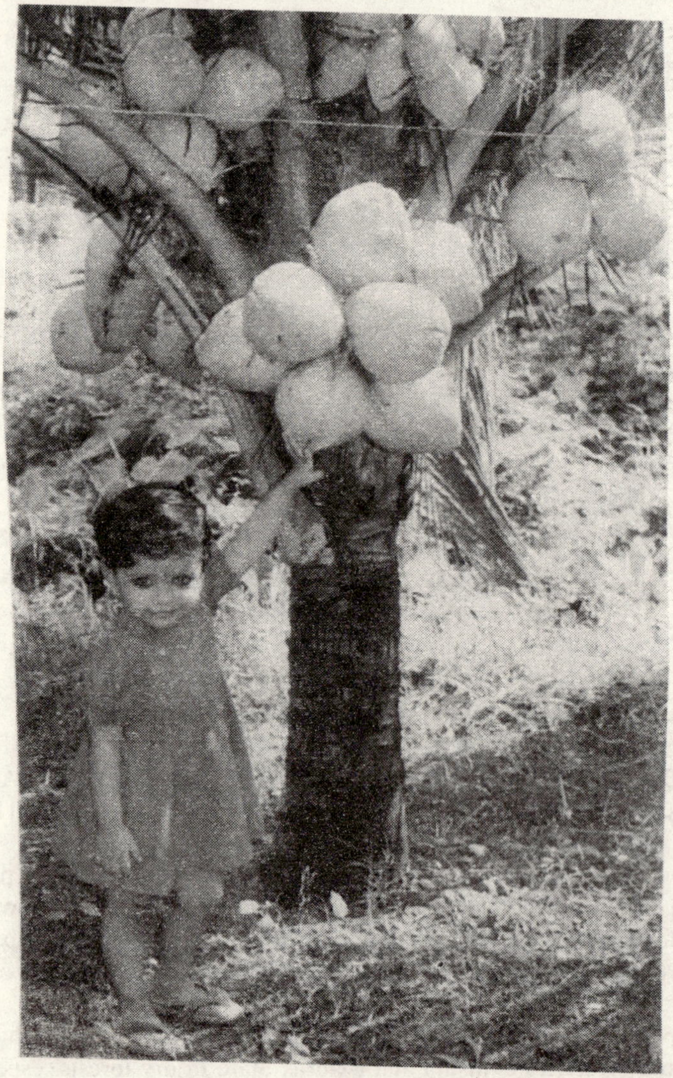

PALMAE

COCOS NUCIFERA LINN.

BENG.- NARIKEL, DAB., **ENG.**- COCONUT PALM., **GUJ.**- NARIYAL, NALIAR., **KAN.**- TENGU., **KON.**- NARLA-MADDO., **MAL.**- TENGU, NARIKELAM., **MAR.**- NARAL., **TAM.**- TENGU, TENNAIMARAM TEMALA., **TEL.**- TENKAYICETTU, NARIKELAM., **SANS.**- NARIKELA., **BOMB.**- MARIKEL., **HINDI**- NARIYAL.

Unarmed, monoecious palms; tall and stately growing to a height of 40-80 ft, stem flexuous, annulate rarely branched, it is marked by ring like leaf scars which are not prominent, bearing a crown of large, pinnate leaves. The trunk is short (1 - 1½ ft. in diam.) straight or gently curved rising from a swollen base surounded by a mass of roots. The leaves are 6-18 ft. long, pinnatisect; leaflets 2-3 ft. long, narrow and tapering coriaceous and flaccid; Petiole 3-5 ft. stout. In the axil of each leaf is a spathe enclosing a spadix, 4-6 ft; stout, straw or orange - coloured; branches flexuous; spathes 2 or more, lower short, upper fusiform or clavate; lower spathe 2-3 ft; oblong, hard, splitting lengthwise. The female flowers are relatively few, borne at the base of the panicle; usually one inch long, 2 bracteolate, disk annular perianth greatly accrescent; sepals imbricate; petals shorter, convolute with imbricate tips; disk annular or O; ovary 3-celled, usually 1-ovuled; style short, stigmas recurved; ovules subbasilar. The male flowers are numerous, small and sweet-scented, borne towards the top of the panicle. Unsymmetric; sepals small, valvate; petals oblong, acute, valvate; stamens 6, filaments subulate, anthers linear, erect pistillade minute or O. Fruit:- is large and ovoid, terete or trigonous, 1 seeded, style terminal; pericarp thick, fibrous; endocarp bony or stony, with 3 basal pores, the remains of the 3 cells. It is known as drupe. The drupe is green or yellowish. The exocarp (outer husk) is thick and fibrous and encloses a hard and bony endocarp (shell). Adhering inside the endocarp is the testa with a thick albuminous endosperm (pulp). At one end of the shell are three pores below one of which and embaded in the pulp is the small embryo. The cavity of the endosperm is large and is filled in the unripe fruit with a watery fluid (coconut water); it is only partly filled in the ripe fruit. Seed:- choring with the endocarp; albumen solid or hollow, or merely lining the encocarp with a thick hard coat; embryo opposite one pore.

The Plant is cultivated in the hot damp regions of India, Burma and Ceylon, especially near the sea (indigenous in the Cocos Island and N. Andaman, Kurz). All tropical shores. The other most important coconut producing countries in the world are Ceylon, Malaya, Indonesia, Philippines and the South Sea Islands in the Pacific. On a small seale it is cultivated in East Africa, West Indies and Central America. In India it is mainly reported from Travancore, Cochin, Malabar, S. Kanara, East Godavari and Tanjore districts in Madras, Puri and Cuttack districts in Orissa, Ratanagiri and N. Kanara districts in Bombay and Mysore, Tumkur and Hassan districts in Mysore.

MEDICINAL USE : The root is diuretic, astringent and used in uterine diseases. Coconut water and milk are cooling, useful is thirst, fever and urinary disorders. The flowers are astringent. Fruit is sweet, diuretic and aphrodis, oil is used in local application in alopecia, and in loss of hair after fevers and debilitaling diseases.

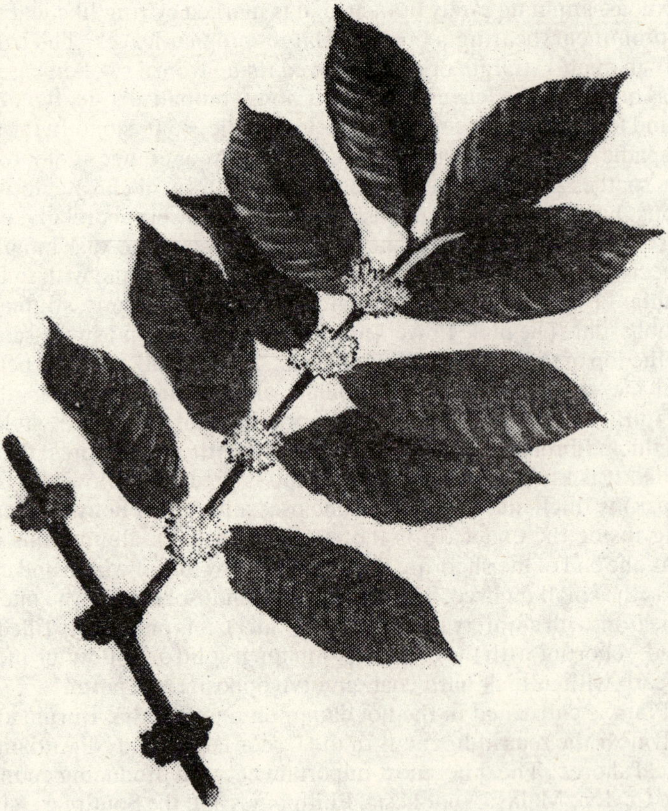

RUBIACEAE

COFFEA ARABICA LINN

HINDI- COFFEE., **BENG.-** KAFI., **ENG.-** ARABIAN COFFEE

Arabica type constitutes 80 per cent of the total production of coffee. Brazil (South America) itself produces 80 per cent coffee of the total world production. It is the only polyploid (tetraploid 4x=44) species. An evergreen shrub or small tree attaining a height of 15-30 ft. under cultural conditions in India it is kept pruned down to a height of 4-5 ft. It has a main stem or trunk with lateral branches which grow in pairs opposite to each other or in whorls around the stem. The branchlets are compressed. The leaves are also opposite, thin coriaceous and bright green in colour; opposite rarely in three, stipules (broad). Flowers are :- In a fasciele or eyme or solitary white or yellow scented; bracteoles often connate. The flowers are boarned by a single plant 2 or 3 times in a year. Calyx-tube short; limb short, often glandular, persistent. Corolla-tube short or long, lobes 4-7, spreading, twisted in bud. Anthers 4-7 sessile on the corolla-tube or throat, narrow, often recurved and twisted or any 2-celled; style filiform, smooth, branches linear or subulate, ovules 1, peltately attached to the Septum in each cell. Fruit:-are small, fleshy drupes, bright green when young changing to yellow and later to scarlet red with ripening. Drupe :- With 2 plano-convex or ventrally concave corxiceous or Cartilaginous pyrenes. The fleshy mueilaginous pulp of the drupe encloses two oval greenish grey seeds or beans, each covered by a thin membrane, the silver skin, and both are enclosed in a common husk-like membrane or parchment. The number of seeds is normally two but may sometimes be one or three when only one develops, the seed is called peabeny. Seeds plano-convex, concave or grooved ventrally, albumen horny, embryo short towards the base of the seed, curved, cotylodens thin cordate, radicle inferior.

Species about 20, in the tropics of the old World. C. ARABICA is considered to be a native of Abyssinia and was introduced into India through Arabians. At present it is cultivated in South India, Java, West Indies, East Africa, Brazil and other South American States and accounts for nearly 90% of the Worlds supply of Coffee.

The most popular varieties of C. ARABICA are C. CHICKS; C. COORGS; C. KENTS; C. MARAGOGIPE, C. BOURBON, C. AMARILLO (goldendrop), Blue-mountain. Besides these there are a no of hybrids.

MEDICINAL USE :- (1) The presence of a stimulative alkaloid in coffee makes it a much wanted beverage. It relieves fatigue and stimulates the physical and mental activities. There is no bad after-effect, such as is found with many other stimulants.

(2) It is of medicinal value. It is used for curing digestive disorders, blood pressure, etc.

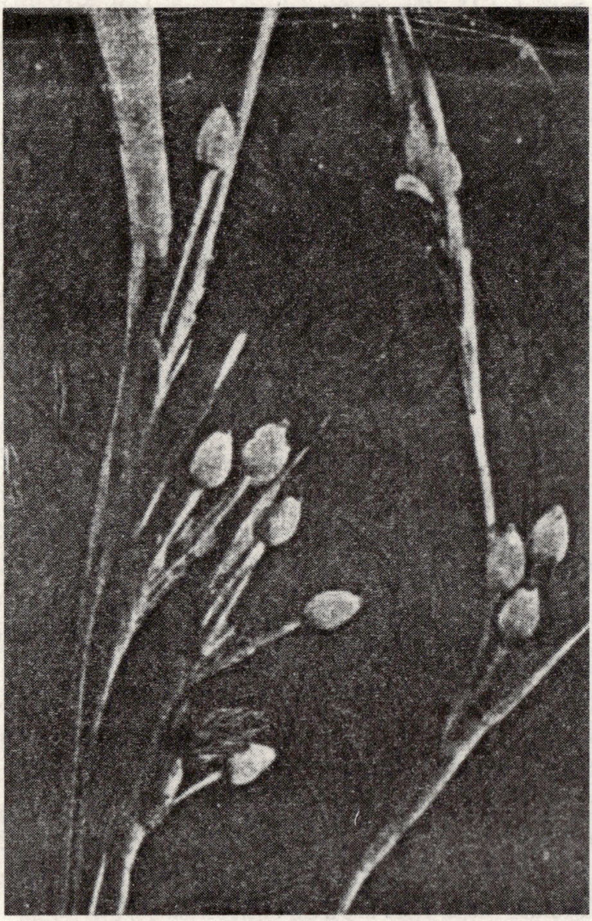

GRAMINEAE

COIX LACHRYMA LINN
SYN. C. LACHRYMA JOBI LINN.
SYN. C. ARUNDINACEA LAMK
C. AGRESTIS LOUR
LITHOGROSTIS LACRYMA-JOBI GAERTN.

SANS.- GAVEDHU, JARGADI., **HINDI**- GURLU, SANKRU., **BENG.**- GURGUR -BOM KASSATBIJA., **PUNJ.**- SANKIEE., **TAM.**- NETPAVALAM., **ENG.**- JOB'S TEARS., **KHASI HILLS**- SOHRIU., **MAR.**- RANMAKKAI.

A tall, erect annual grass, 3-6 ft. high with broad leaves. It is monoecious and bears large, shining, pear shaped fruits showing a fanciful resemblence to tears, and containing a whitish or light brownish grain similar to rice. Stem 3-5 ft.; stout, leafy, rooting at the lower nodes. Leaves : Are long and broad; 4-18 by 1-2 inch, wavy, base cordate; sheaths smooth; liqule very short, glabrous. Spikes numerous, axillary and terminal; Lower spikelets solitary. 2-3", subereet peduncled, male spikelcts 2-3 nate at each node of the rachis, one sessile and one or two pedicelled, lanceolate; glumes 4, I and II subequal, empty, rigid or herbaceous; I keeled along the inflexed margins, III & IV hyaline, paleate, triandrous or empty. Male spikelets 3 or 2 with an imperfect one, 1/3" long; gl. 1 narrowly winged. Female enclosed in and at length hardened polished nut like braet, through the apex of which the pedicelled male portion protrudes.

Female spikelets ovoid, acuminate; glumes 4, I chariaceous; II-IV successively thinner; IV paleate; staminodes minute, lodicules 0, ovary ovoid, styles 2; free slender. Fruit:-ovoid or spherical 1/4 -1/3 inch long, bluish gray. Grain:-orbicular, ventrally furrowed, enclosed in the hardened globose ovoid or cylindrical involucre.

It is found throughout the hotter and damper parts of India, wild or cultivated (not wild in Ceylon) Tropical Asia, cultivated in Africa and America.

MEDICINAL USE : The seeds are used as tonic and diuretic. Root is used in menstrual disorders. In Tongking grains are considered blood punifier and diuretic.

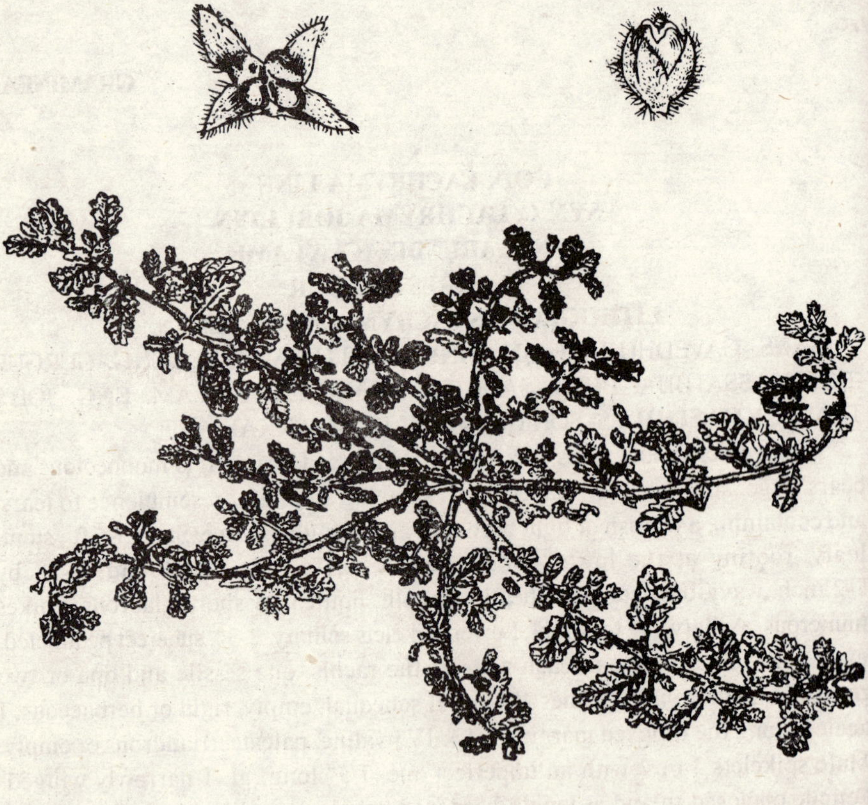

BORAGINACEAE

COLDENIA PROCUMBENS LINN

HINDI- TRIPANKHI & TRIPUNGKI., **BO.**- TRIPAKSHI., **SANS.**- TRIPAKSHEE., **TAM.**- SANPADI., **TEL.**- HAMSAPADU., **GUJ.**- BASARYIO, AKHRAD.

A procumbent, deep rooted, hairy herb with trailing stout stem lying flat on the ground. The leaves are 2.5 - 4 x 1.- 1.5 cm, crisped or thickly haired Obovate-oblong, coarsely serrate or subpinnatifid. Flowers white small, solitary and axillary. The fruit is drupe pyramidal subtended by Calyx, four lobed, separating into four, one seeded pyrenes. Flowers and fruits - May and June.

It is found common during summer months in abundance in the water dried areas which are moist where it spreads in abundance and alongwith other plants forming a sort of felt on the ground.

It is found throughout India in moist places and is considered a weed.

MEDICINAL USE : Fresh leaves, ground and applied to rheumatic swellings. Dried plants with equal part of fenugreek seeds is rubbed to a fine powder and applied warm for causing suppuration of boils.

Dried plant powder mixed with trigonella powder in equal parts is used as a remedy for Baltoe (a wound caused by pulling the hair out).

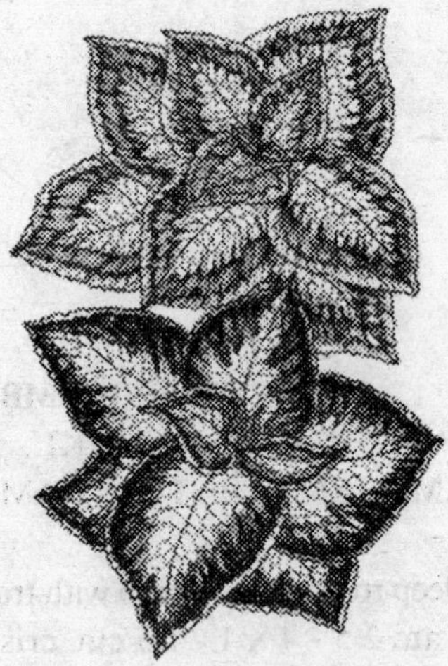

LABIATAE

COLEUS AMBOINICUS LOUR
(SYN. C. AROMATICUS BENTH)
(SYN. BORAGO OFFICINALIS LINN)

B- PATERCHUR., **BO. + H.-** PATHAR CHUR AMRODA., **S-** ?ASHANABHEDI., **TAM.-** KARPURAVALLI., **MARATHI-** PATERCHUR., **ENG.-** NDIAN BORAGE.

It is a glamrous hairy aeromatic herb or plant. The whole plant is considered ıs juicy. The leaves are aeromatic and pungent. The flowers are small and blue in :olour. The smell is due to an oil containing carvacrol.

It is cultivated in the gardens throughout India wild in Rajputana.

MEDICINAL USE : Leaves in urinary diseases, vaginal discharges juices of eaves- mixed with sugar acts as a powerful aromatic, carmin. given in collic and lyspep.

C. BLUMEI BENTH

(SYN. C. VERSCHAFFELTIC LEM) C. SCUTELLARIOIDES BLUMEI MIQ. It s popularly known as Flame nettle plant.

It is a perennial herb or undershrub. The leaves are multicolour and the flowers re dark blue or white. The foliage is often large coloured rose, pink, crimson and ronze. The busy plants of nettle like leaves are upto 45 cm (18 inch) tall. Flowers re in spikes.

It is cultivated in gardens.

MEDICINAL USE : Decoction of leaves given internally for dyspep. (Burkill, 635).

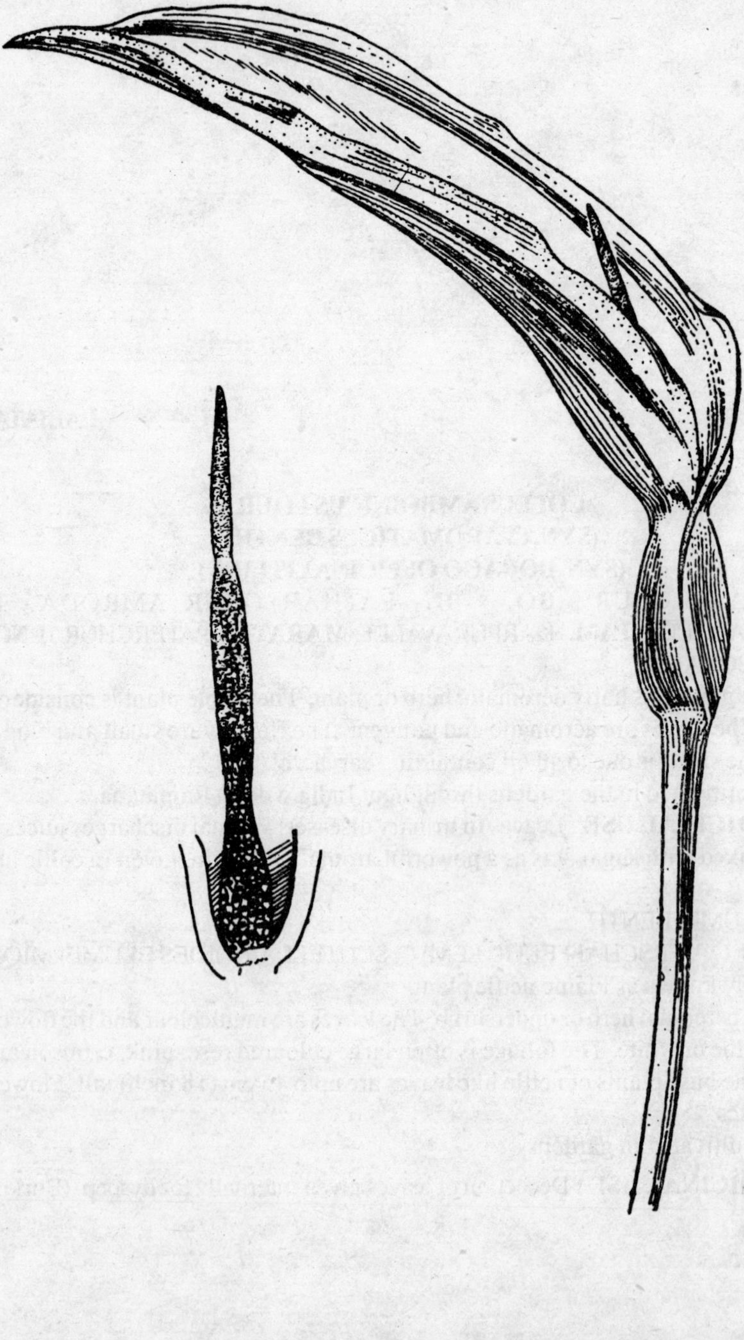

ARACEAE

COLOCASIA ESCULENTA (LINN) SCHOTT
(Syn. C. ANTIQUORUM (LINN) SCHOTT)
(SYN. ARUM/ESCULENTA L.)
Syn. C. ESCULENTA VAR. ANTIQUORUM HURB & REHD.

BENG.- KACHU., **SANS.**- KACHU., **HINDI.**- ARVI, KACHALU, GHUIYAN., **MAL.**- SHEMBU., **MAR.**- KACHMALU, ALU., **TAM.**- SHEPPAN-KIZANGU, SHAMAKKI-LANGU., **TEL.**- CHAMADUMPA, CHEMAGADDA., **BOMB.**- KACHUALU., **ARAB.**- QULQAS., **KAN.**- KACHCHI, SHAMAGADDE., **URIYA.**- SARU., **ENG.**- TARO, ARUM, TARO, DASHEEN., **LOCAL NAME**- ARVI, GHOYAN, KACHALU.

They are commonly and popularly called as aroids and Elephant's Ear. A perennial tuberous plant. The stem is modified into a large fleshy underground rhizome, root stock or a corm. It bears nodes, internodes, scaly leaves, axillary and terminal buds, The plant consists of a big tuberous rhizome or with a stout short caudex flowering and cafing together; leaves : Stoutly petioled, peltate ovate chordate; 6-16", dark green, dull sometimes clouded with black; petiole stout; 3-4 ft. green or voilet. Peduncles solitary or clustered and connate much shorter than the petioles. Spathe: 8-18 inch, caudate-acuminate, errect pale yellow, stoutly peduncled, tube thick acerescent, persistent, mouth constricted, limb erect, decidous. Spadix : Shorter than the spath stout or slender; male and female inflorecence with usually interposed flat neuters; appendage cylinderical subulate or 0; female inflorencence as long as that of the standnodes, male inflorencenae longer very common and variable. Roxburghl distinguishes 3 varieties, they are 1, a dark one from wet places in which the roots (base and stem 2) never swell, but send out many sukers and the leaves and petioles are more or less purple, it is much eaten; 2, one that grows under ground with dark purple or bluish coulds in the leaf; 3-one like the last but all green. Of nymphaeifolia which is described as having repand leaves. He says that the doubts if it is anything but a large aquatic state, abundant wild on boarders of lakes, with the subterraneous stem oten as long and thick as a man's arm, reddish petioles and leaves, narrower leaves and a short appendage; all parts are eaten. Ovaris and ovules as in REMCUSATIA, Berries obconic or oblong, Seeds oblong sulcate albumen copious; embryo axile.

The flowers of this plant are rare. They were observed only once in a Government Farm "Hatha" near Hindan River an Sept. 11, 1955.

The plant is considered to be a native of South Eastern Asia and Pacific Islands. Throughout the hotter parts of India (upto 7,600 ft. in the Himalaya) and Ceylon, in moist and dry places or cultivated-in all hot countries. Spier (1951) believes that the cultivated varieties originated in Assam or Upper Burma. Taro spread early in Japan, the West Asia and Northern Africa. In Africa it was common food in slave-trading time. Later they were carried to the New World along with the slaves. They are grown in almost all the warm tropical countries.

MEDICINAL USE : Juice of petioles is styptie, stimulant rubefacient whereas juice of corm is used in cases of alopecia and in Scorpian sting.

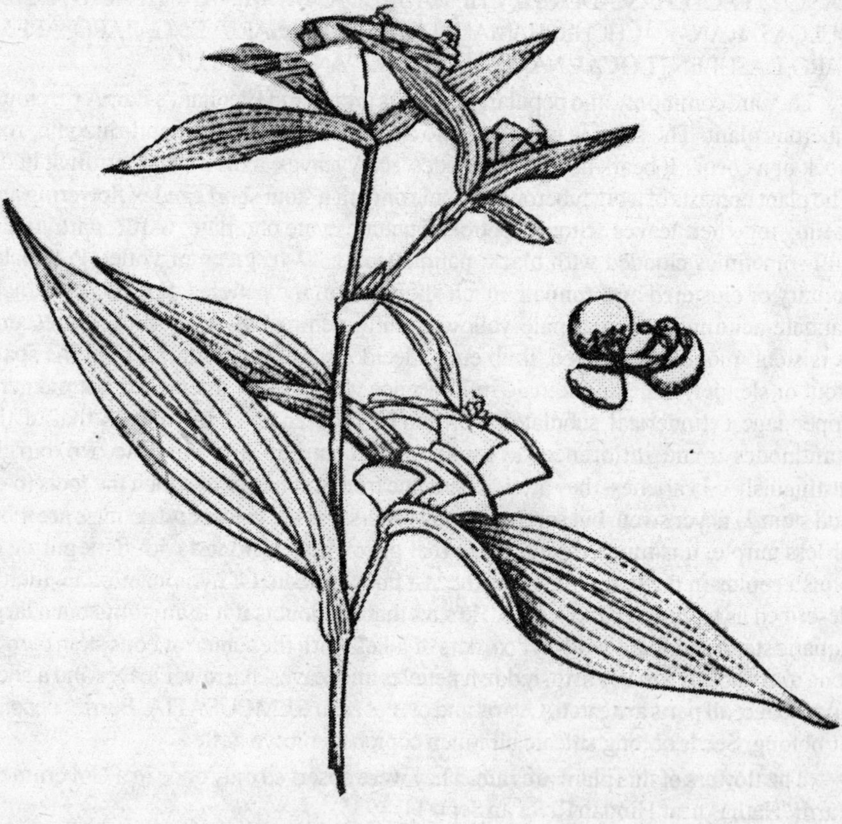

COMMELINACEAE

COMMELINA BENGHALENSIS LINN.

LOCAL NAME- KANTERI, KANVO, KANKAWWA, KANA., **HINDI**-KANCHARA, KANTERI., **SANS.**- KANCHATA., **BENG.**- KANCHARA., **TAM.**-KANAVAZHAI, KANANGAKARAI., **TELUGU**- VENNADEVIKURA.

*****

A branched, diffuse or straggling herb with dimorphic flowers, creeping and rooting below. The stems are fleshy with swollen nodes glabrous or pubescent. Leaves : 1-3 by 1/2-1- 1/2 sessile or petiolate. Alternate, entire basal sheaths encircling the stem; ovate to oblong, broader, obtuse, rounded, cuneate or Cordate at the base. Flowers in usually 2-fid cymes, emerging one at a time from a terminal complicate or funnel shaped or cucullate spathe. Aerial spathes 1-3 in the axils obeonic, funnel shaped or turbinate. Upper branch of cyme 2-3fid flowers of upper branch being cyme small, decidous; of lower fertile; fruiting pedicel and capsule retracted within the spathe. Flowers blue; sepals 3 membranous green, 2 inner often connate at the base. Petals larger, one larger and often clawed. Aerial flowers sky blue to bluish-violet. Stamens 3 perfect, and 2-3 imperfect; anthers oblong and one usually largest. Ovary 3-rarely 2-celled, 2-celled 2 cells, 1-2 ovuled, third cell if present. 1-ovuled or empty. Capsule membranous, shining, dorsal value striolate. However, P. Maheswari reports that capsule is 5-seeded and seeds are wrinkled and pitted. According to Benthem and Hooker seeds are ellipsoid or angled, retriculate pitted or rugose. 1/4-1/2" long & broad pubescent or hirsute. Underground flowers bisexual, usually solitary in a pear-shaped-spathe. The fruiting and flowering season is from June to November, every year.

Found throughtout India; ascending to 6,000 ft. in the Himalaya-top. Asia and Africa. locally in rainy season it is found abundantly on the ridge as well as in the fields, gardens and waste places, on moist, shady situations.

MEDICINAL USE : The plant is found bitter, emollient demulcent, referigerating; laxative, beneficial in leprosy (J. Bombay nat. Hust. Soc; 1937, 362).

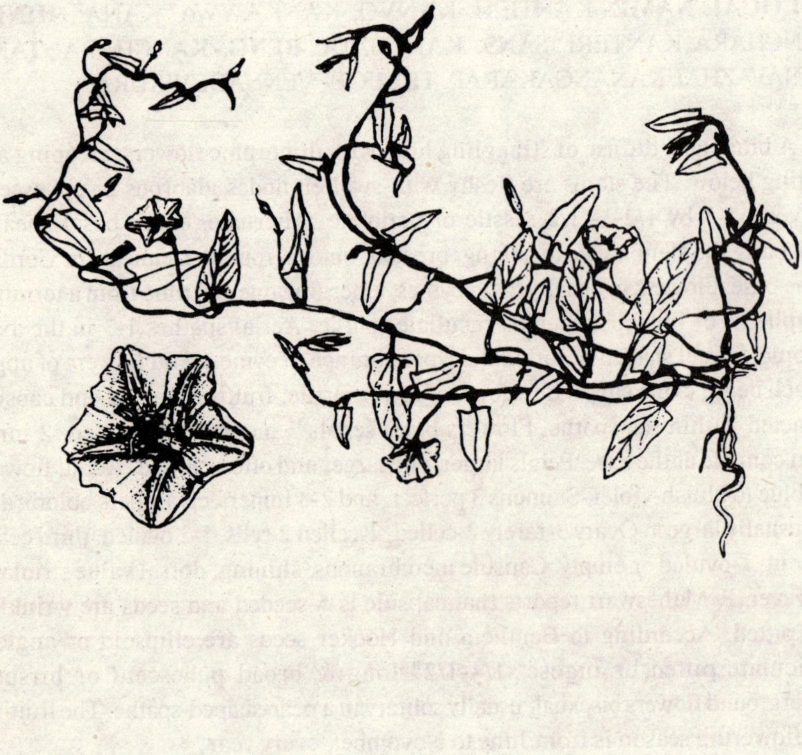

CONVOLVULACEAE

CONVOLVULUS ARVENSIS LINN.

PUNJAB-PORORANG, DODAK., **HINDI**-HIRANPADI., **BOMB.**-HIRANPAG., **BENG.**- GONDAL., **SANS.**-BHADRABALA., **P.**-HIRANPADDI., **LOCAL NAME**-HIRANKDHURI.

It is a trailing or twining, glabrous herb Spreading on the ground. Leaves ovate or oblong-lanceolate; base auriculate to hastate. Flowers pink or white, solitary, axillary, widely funnel- shaped, on long peduncles, capsules globose glabrous. Flowers and fruits July-October.

It is a common weed, cultivated all over India, ascending to 10,000 ft. in the Himalayas. Abundant in plains of Northern India and Bihar.

MEDICINAL USE: The juice of the plant caused a persistant fall in blood pressure of mammals. In larger doses it produced transient inhibiting effect in both force and rate of contraction of heart. Clinical studies reveal that with the decoction of the drug a gradual fall in blood pressure alongwith relief in symptoms was observed (Chaturvedi et al, 1966). Mudgel et al. 1972). states that maximum activity lies in leaves and flowers as compared to the roots and stem.

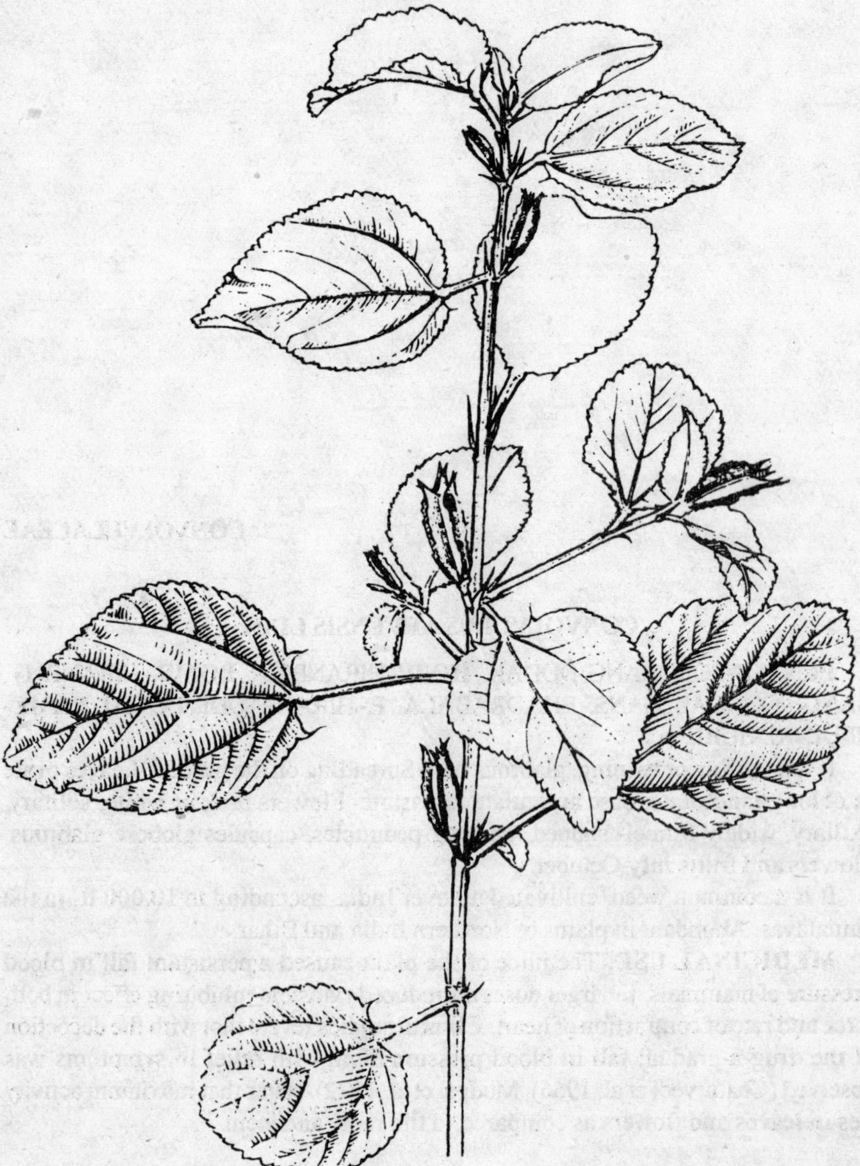

TILIACEAE

CORCHORUS ACUTANGULUS LAM.
(SYN. C. AESTUANS LINN)

B-TITAPAT., **LOCAL NAME**: CHONET.

An ascending, sub erect or erect, having annual leaves suborbicular to ovate-oblong, hairy. Flowers yellow peduncles 2 to 3 flowered, capsule 6 angled, 3 winged, short, stout, flowers and fruits-August-October.

Common in fellow and cultivated fields. Also found on the ridge, in waste localities along the hedges of gardens. It is found throughout the hotter parts of India.

MEDICINAL USE: Stomachic, in pneumonia.

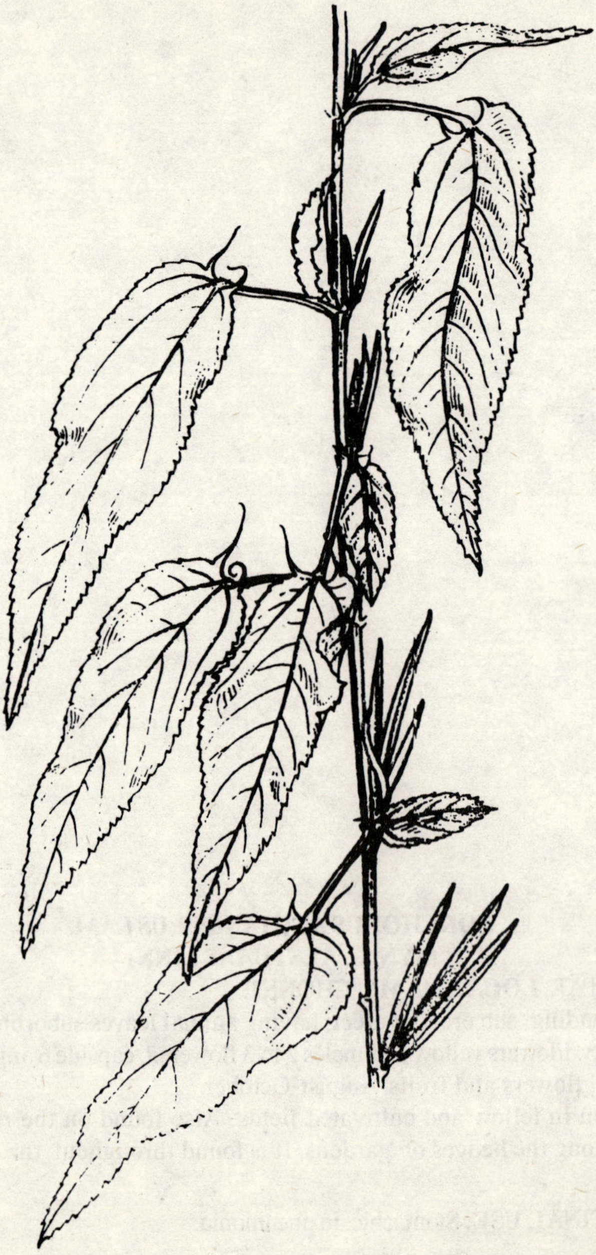

TILIACEAE

CORCHORUS TRILOCULARIS LINN

MARATHI- KODUCHHUNCH., **BO.**- KADUCHHUNEHLI., **GUJARATI**- KADVICHHUNCHHDI., **HINDI**- KADU KASTA., **S.**- DIRGHACHANCHU., **LOCAL NAME**- KOWWA- TORAI, KAG ROTI.

A diffuse undershrub, branching from near the ground, pilose. Leaves oblong, elliptie- oblong or ovate oblong, Shining with or without basal lobes. Flowers yellow. Capsules 3-6.5 x 03-0.4 cm, straight or curved, 3 to 4 angled, scabrous, beak short; flowers and fruits- August- October.

Common during the rainy season, usually found in moist, shady places, and as a weed infields. It is also reported from Bihar, Deccan and Carnatie of Madras and Bombay States, Khandesh, Gujarat, Cutch, sind and Baluchistan.

MEDICINAL USE- Seeds in fever and obstruction of the abdominal visera. Musilage-demulc. (Chopra et. al. 1956) and Nadkarni, 1954).

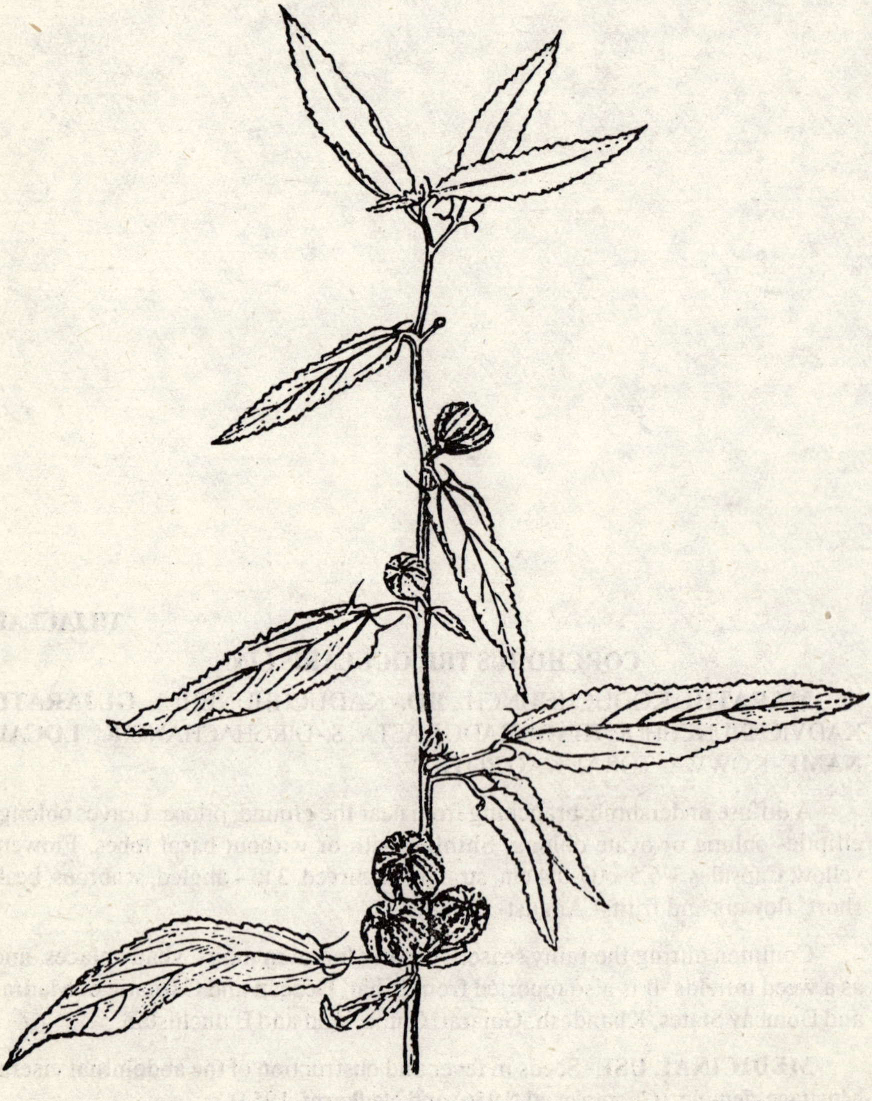

TILIACEAE

CORCHORUS CAPSULARIS LINN

ASSAM- TITAMARA., **S.-** KALASAKA., **BENG.-** NARCHA, TITAPAPP., **LOCAL NAME-** KHARENTI., **ENG.-** JUTE., **GUJ.-** CHUNCHDO., **HINDI-** PAT SINGHIN., **MARATHI-** KURRU CHANTZ., **TAM.-** PIRATTAIKEERAI., **TEL.-** PARINTA.

An erect or sub erect, glabrous annual. Leaves ovate lanceolate. The two lowest serratures produced into awns. Flowers yellow. Capsules globose-depressed, ridged and muricated. Flowers and fruits- September- October.

Found along fields hedges and along canal banks. It is found throughout the hotter parts of India. Cultivated in most tropical countries.

MEDICINAL USE : Infusion of leaves demule, stomach,lax, carmine, stim; to increase appetite, bitter tonic, in dysentry fever, dyspep. liver disorders.

Decoct. of root and unripe fruit in diarr.

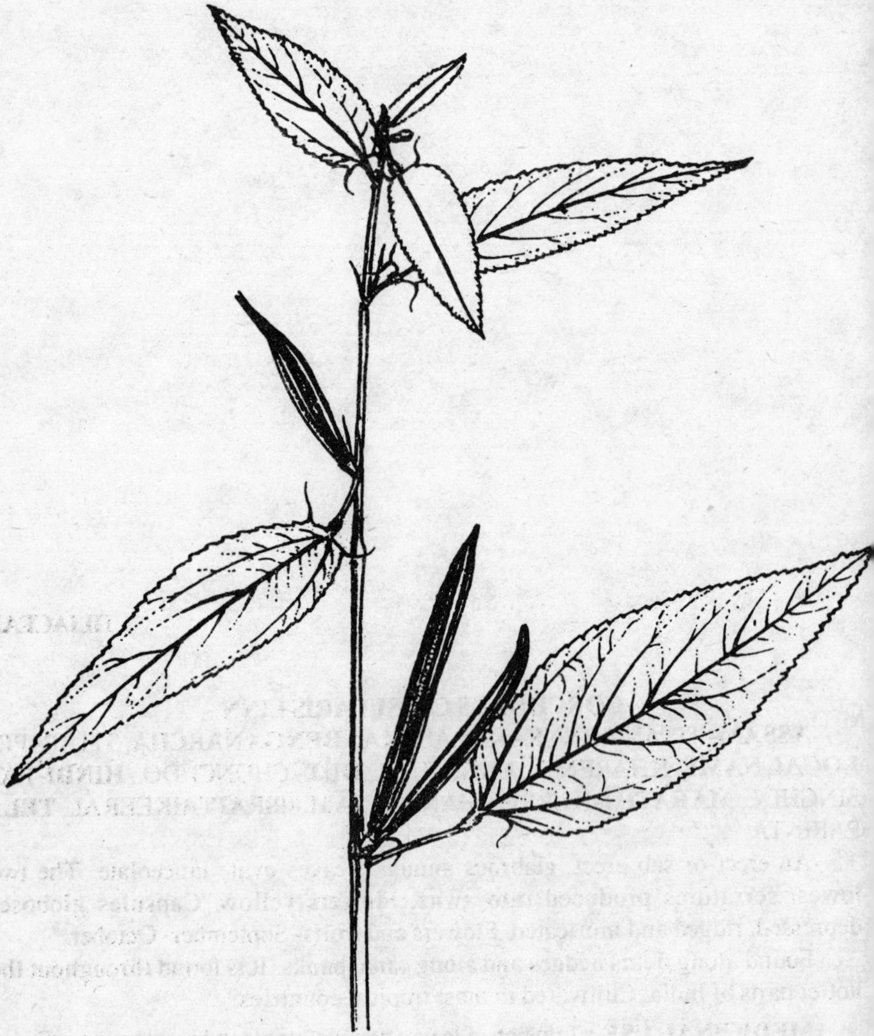

TILIACEAE

CORCHORUS OLITORIUS LINN

HINDI- KOSHTA., **BOM.-** TANKLA., **BENG.-** LALITAPAT, NALITAPAT MITHAPAT., **TAM.-** PERATTI., **TEL.-** PONINTAKURA., **MARATHI-** TANKLA.

An erect Shrubby plant. Stems very fibrous, Leaves upto 15 x 7cm, the basal two serratures produced into filiform appendages, Peduncles 1-3 flowered, flowers yellow capsule 10 ribbed, glabrous, beek long. Flowers and fruits September-October.

Found in moist, shady places in fellow and cultivated fields. Wild in many parts of India but not in Bengal. It is the predominant species grown in the districts of Hooghly, 24 parganas and Nadia in West bengal.

MEDICINAL USE : Leaves demulc, tonic, diur, useful in chronic cystitis, gonorr. and dysuria.

Infusion of leaves- tonic febge. Seeds purgative, fruits rich in Vita. C. (Philipp, J. Sei, 1934, 379).

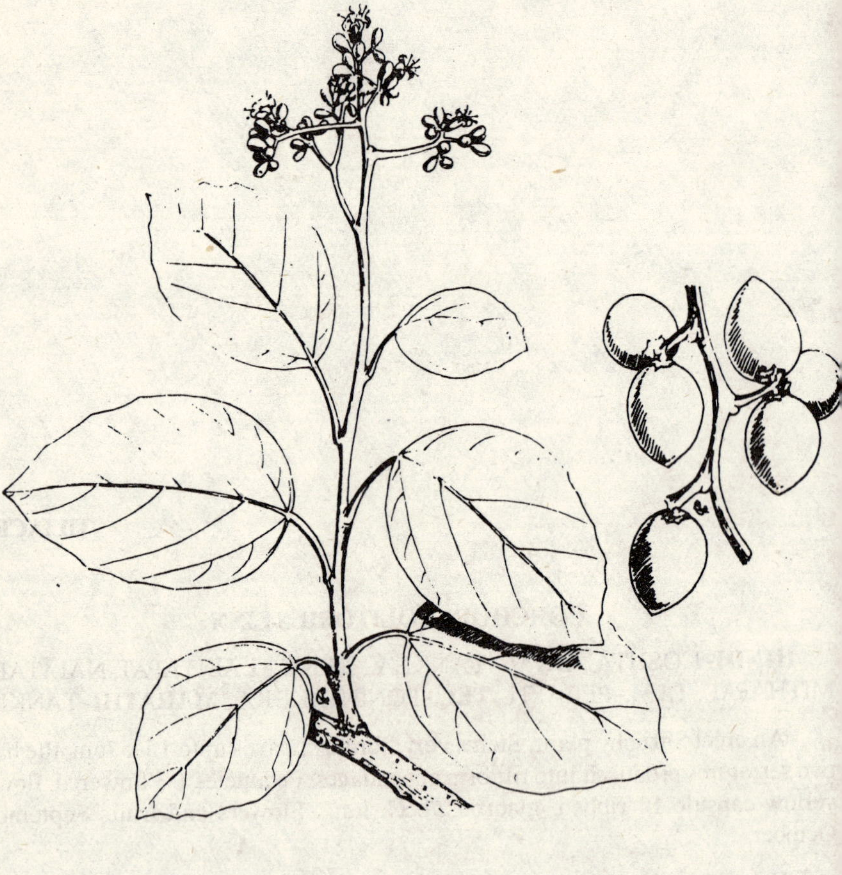

BORAGINACEAE

CORDIA DICHOTAMA FORST. F
(SYN. C. MYXA ROXB. NON LINN)
C.OBLIQUA WILLD

BENG.- BUHUL., **HINDI**- LASORA, CHOTA LASORA CHOKARGOND, B-BUHUL, BOHODARI., **MARATHI & BOM.**- GONDAN., **TAM.**- NARUVILI., **TEL.**- CHINNA NAKKARU., **LOCAL NAME**- LASOORA, LIASAURA., **ENG.**- SEBESTEN, CLAMMY CHERRY, INDIAN CHERRY.

It is a small or medium sized, deciduous tree. Trunk usually crooked. Bark grey, brown or shining whitish. Leaves alternate broad ovate, elliptic to suborbicular with basal nerves, 8-15 x 6-10 cm leathery. Flowers white, in lax terminal and axillary cymes, calyx accresent, Style terminal, fourfiet. Fruit-a drupe ovoid, cream coloured, apiculate flowers-Jan. April, Fruits May to July.

Found wild on the ridge and in waste places around villages Also planted in gardens and shrubberies for its fruit. It is common throughout India wild and often planted.

MEDICINAL USE : Fruit astringent, anthelar, diur. demulch, expect, used in inffections of urinary passages, diseseases of lungs and spleen.

Juice of bark- in gripes.

Decot. of bark- used in dyspep and fevers. Kernels- remedy in ringworm. Leaves application to ulcers and in headache.

Plant in snake- bite (Chopra et al. 1956). Bark contains 20% tanin (Indian for leaft. No. 72, 1944, 8).

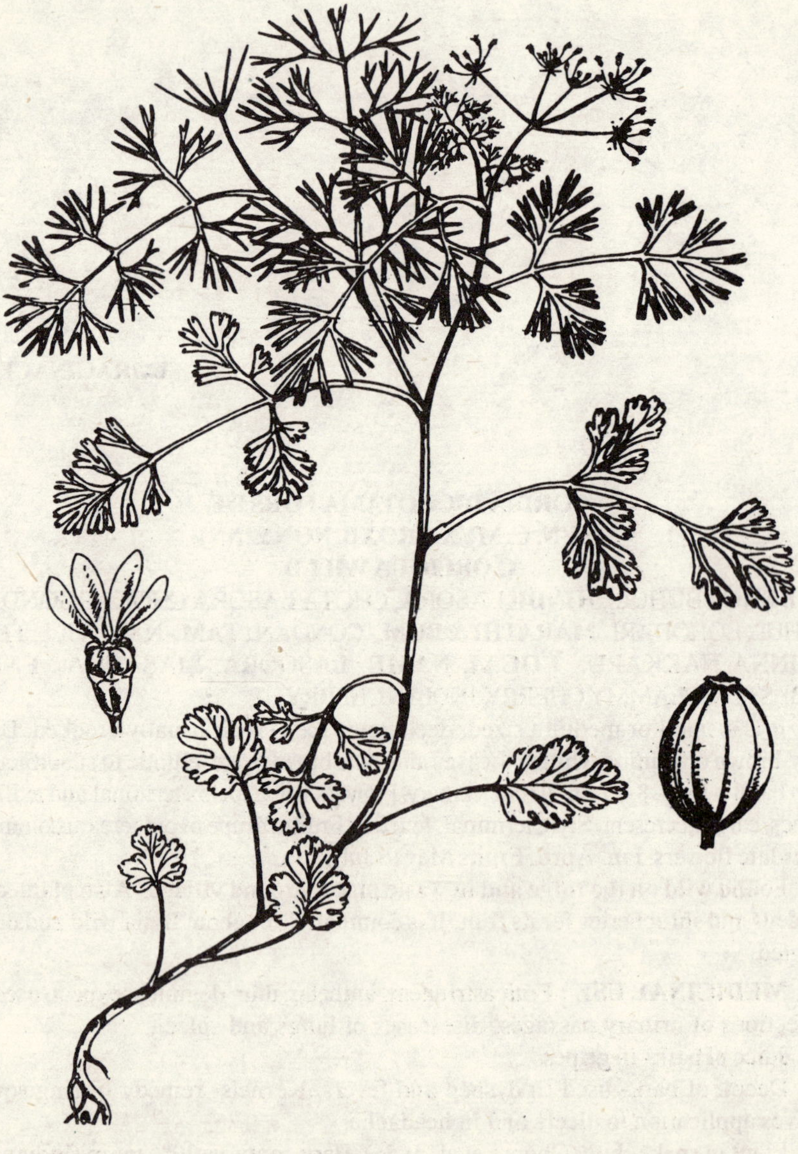

UMBELLIFERAE

CORIANDRUM SATIVUM LINN

It is popularly known as Coriander. Being strongly smelling Aromatic Herb.

SANS.- DHANYA, KUSTUMBURI, DHANYAKA., **HINDI-** DHANIA, DHANYA., **BENG.**-DHANE., **GUJ.**-KONPHIR., **MAR.**-DHANNA, KOTHIMBER., **TEL.**- DHANIYALU., **TAM.**- KOTHAMALLI., **KAN.**- KOTHAMBRI., **MAL.**- KOTHUMPALARI., **ENG.**- CORIANDER., **LOCAL NAME-** DHANIA.

An annual aromatic herb; branched; glaberous; 1-3 ft. high. Leaves : decompound; ultimate segments of the lower leaves ovate or lanceolate of the upper linear. The lower leaves are broad with crenately lobed margins, while the upper ones are narrow, finely cut with linear lobes. Flowers purplish or white, in compound umbels; rays few; outer ones zygomorphic; bracts 0, or small linear; bracteoles few, filiform; Calyx teeth small, acute, often unequal. Petals-obovate, emarginate, white or purplish, of the outer flowers unequal, often radiant carpels slightly concave on the inner face, commissure distinctly 2-vittate; carpophore 2-partite. Fruit : subglobose; ridges not prominent, dorsal primary and adjacent secondary strongest lateral primary and secondary obscure; vittae obscure, solitary, under the secondary ridges. Flowering and fruiting season in Delhi is December to April.

It is found all over throughout India. Cultivated. It is widely cultivated. Grown in the hills up to 3,000 m. as a herb; that exported from Lahul is especially highly regarded. (0. Polunin; Adam Stainton, 1984). It is considered as a native to the Mediterranean region and is now culivated chiefly in M.P., Maharashtra, Rajasthan, Andhra Pradesh, Tamil Nadu, Karnataka and Bihar.

MEDICINAL USE : Fruits are used as stimulant, carminative, stomachic, diuretic, antibilious, retrigerant, aphrodisia and heart tonic. The stem, leaves and fruits have a pleasant aromatic odour. The seeds are chewed to conceal the odour of other medicines and to correct the griping qualities of rhubarb and Senna (U.S.D., 329). The seeds also help in lessening the intoxicating effects of Spirituous liquors. The aromatic odour is due to the oil present in the seeds. The water extract of seeds mixed with crystalised sugar is taken to reduce irritation & burning in urinary tract.

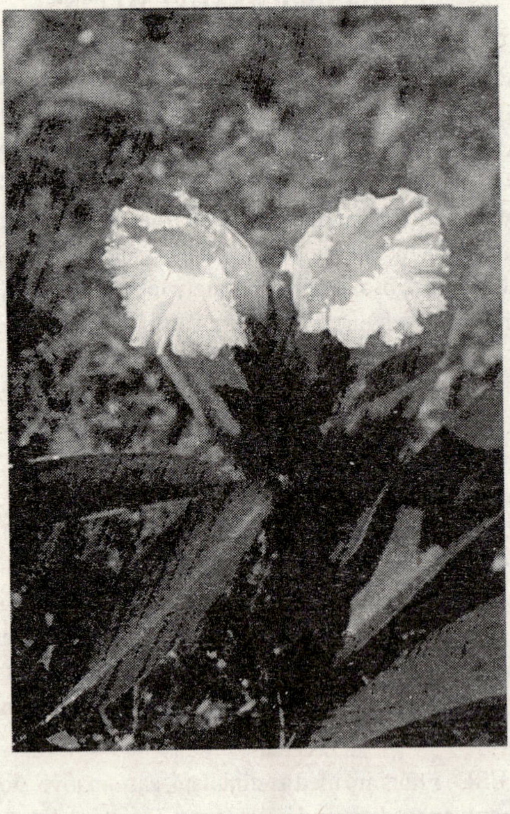

ZINGIBERACEAE

COSTUS SPECIOSUS (KOWN EX. RETZ.) SM.

BENG.- KEN., **HINDI**- KEN, KEMUKA., **BO.**- KEMUKA, KOSHTAM., **H & B.**- KEU., **SANS.**- KUSHTHA., **MAL.**- CHAMAK KOVA., **TAM.**- KURAVAM, KOTTAM., **TEL.**- KASHNAEERAMU., **KAN.**- CHANGAL KOSHTA & PUSHKANGMODA., **MAR.**- PENVA.

It is an aromatic herbaceous plant with fleshy braned underground rhizome and with axial stems. Flowers white, funnel shaped, with contrasting large bright red bracts, numerous in very dense cylindrical spike 5-10cm. long, borne on a stout red leafy stem 1-2 m. Flowers C-4 cm bracts ovate 1.5 - 4 cm. long calyx with 3 oral lobes, corolla tube shorter than calyx with unequal petals 2.5 - 4 cm. lip white with an orange red center, rounded 5-8 cm. forming a funnel with margins incurved and meeting. leaves, oblong acute, sheathing at base, 15-30 cm. capsules red, crowned with persistent calyx.

It is found more or less throughout India upto an altitude of 4000 ft. Particularly common in Bengal Assam, North Bengal, Khasi, Jaintia Hills and Konkan. Often cultivated as an ornamental plant. It is also reported from Uttar Pradesh to Sikkim, India, Burma to 1500 mtr. Forests and shrubberies.

MEDICINAL USE :- Root - bitter, astrin, pung, depurative stim, tonic, anthelm, used in snake bite.

Root rich in starch (Burkill I, 671). Tuberous roots are considered as raw material for commercial production of diosgenin, precursar of steroids including sex harmones and oral contraceptives.

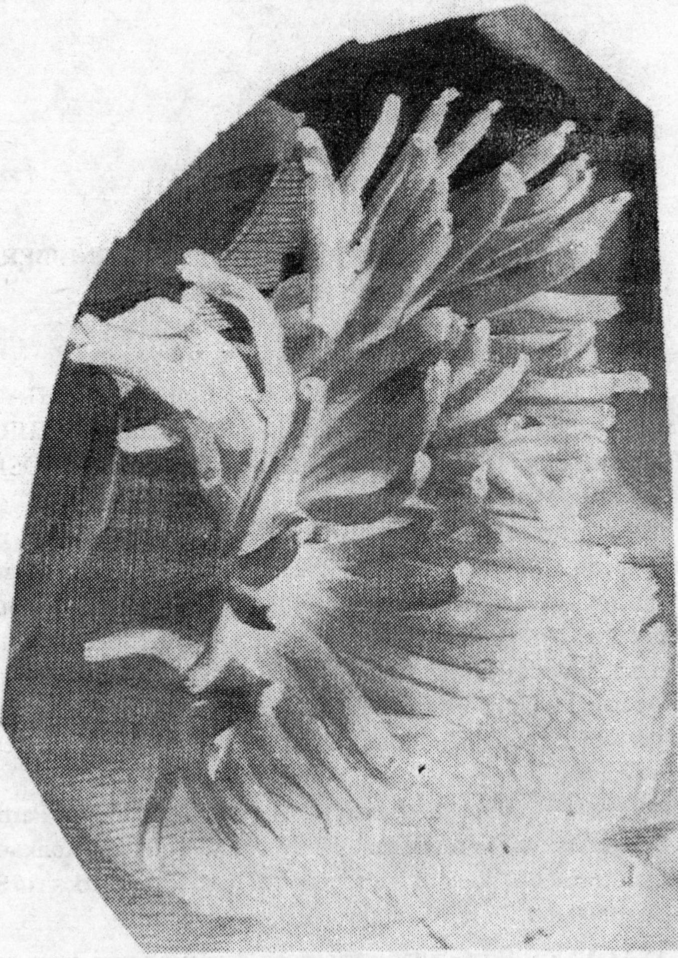

LECYTHIDACEAE

COUROUPITA GUIANENSIS (AUBL) ANJAL

ENG.- CANNON BALL TREE.

It is popularly known as cannon ball tree. It is distributed in South America, West Indies and frequently found in Botanical gardens in India.

MEDICINAL USE : Bark and leaves are mainly used in medicine. Leaves are used in skin diseases.

Note:- No report available on other aspects.

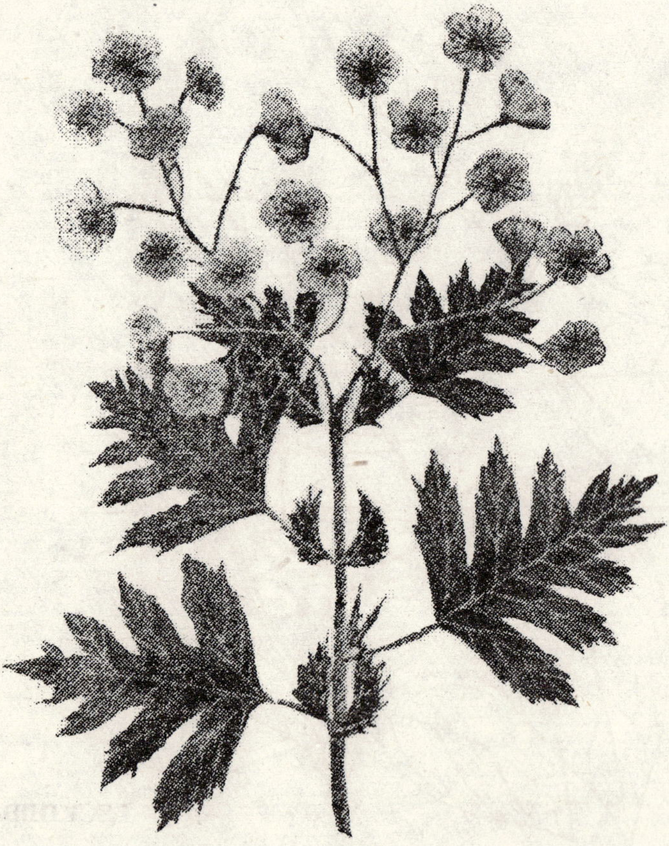

ROSACEAE

CRATAEGUS OXYCANTHA LINN

ENG.- HAWTHORN., **P.**- BAN - SANGLI, RING-RIGNO, FINDU K., **BAN.**- SANJALI.

It is a thorny large shrub or a small deciduous tree. It grows approximately as tall as 8 m. with greyish branches, deeply and sharply lobed leaves, and laxflat - topped clusters of white flowers. Flowers 1 to 1,5 cm. across, long stalked; Calyx cooly - haired below. Leaves deeply cut to two-thirds their width into nearly parallel sided lobes with coarse acute teeth; blade broadly ovate or rhombic in outline 3-5 cm, leaf stalk nearly as long. Fruit red, globular and flashy with 1-5 nuts.

It is reported from North -Western temperate Himalayas from Indus to Ravi, 6000 - 9000 ft.

MEDICINAL USE : Liquid extract of fruits - cardiac tonic, remedy for organic and functional heart diseases such as dyspnoea, hypertrophy, valvular insufficiency and heart oppression.

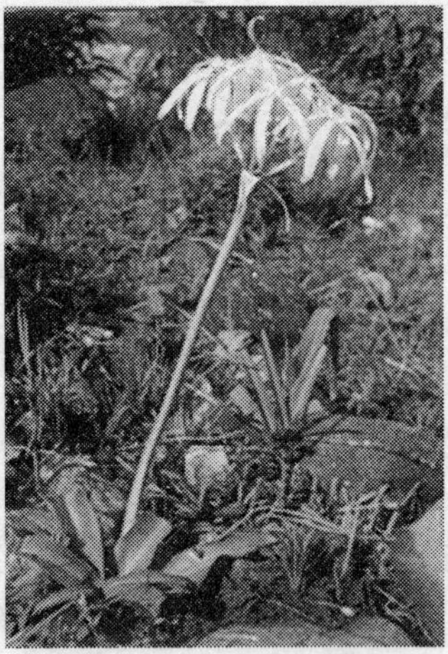

AMARYLLIDACEAE

CRINUM ASIATICUM LINN
(SYN. C. DEFIXUM, C. LATIFOLIUM LINN, C. BRAETEATIUM WILLD) C. TOXICARIUM ROXB. AMARYLLIS ZEYLANICUM LINN)

HINDI- PINDAR, CHINDAR, SUKHDARSHAN., **B.**- BERAKANUR, NAGDAUN., **S.**- NAGADAMANI, VISHAMANDELA., **BO.**- NAGDOWN., **TAM.**- VISHAMUNGIL., **TEL.**- VISHAMUNGALI & KESARICHETTU., **M.**- VISHAUANGIL., **LOCAL NAME**- SUKHDARSHAN., **BENGALI**- SUKHDARSHAN., **ENG.**- POISON- BULL., **KAN.**- VISHAMOONGULI., **KON.**- KIRTMARI., **MARATHI**- GADANI- KANDA.

A large bullbous leafy herb or undershrub. The leaves are large linear entire and deciduous. Flowers are large white funnel- shaped, borne in an umbel which is surrounded in bud by a papery spathe. Petals linear- lanceolate 6 fused into a corolla tube at the base. Filaments free. Anthers linear fruit subglobose, flowers October-December.

It is Commonly planted in hedges around gardens and near temples, etc. It is found wild or cultivated throughout tropical India.

MEDICINAL USE : Bulb is used as tonic and laxative in biliousness and other urinary troubles. Fresh root as emetic and diaphoretic, contains alks. Drug crinamine seeds are pergative. Leaves-expect. applied to skin diseases and to reduce inflamation.

Bulbs are also used for the treatment of burns, whitlow, carbuncle etc. The juice of the leaf is used in earache, bulbs when crushed and roasted are used as rubefacient and in rheumatism.

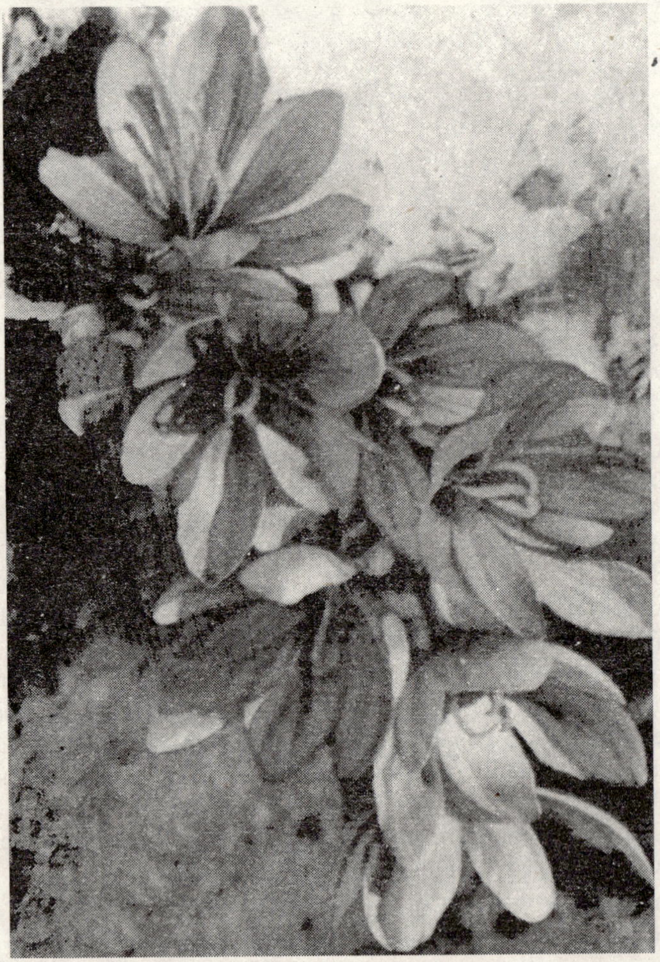

IRIDACEAE

CROCUS SATIVUS LINN
SAFFRON.

SANS.- KESHARA., **PERS.**- ZAAFARAN., **ARAB.**- JAFRANA, ZAAFARAN., **HINDI**- KESAR, ZAFRAN., **BENG.**- JAFRAN., **GUJ.**- KESHARI., **MAR.**- KESARA., **TEL.**-KUNKUMAPUVU., **KAN.**- KUNKUMA KESARI., **KASHMIR**- KONG., **TAM.**- KUNGUMAPU.

Root stock a sheathed corm; stem 0. Leaves radical, narrowly linear, channelled, margins recurved. Flowers solitary or fascicled, subsessile; basal spathes 1-3 or 0 hyaline, floral embracing the ovary and sometimes a narrow hyaline bract. Perlanth funnel shaped, tube very slender; limb subsequally 6-lobed in two series. Stamens on the throat of the perianth, filaments short, anthers longer, basifixed. Ovary 3 celled; style filiform, stigma slender subentire lobed or laciniate; tips stigmatic. Capsule oblong, membranous, loculicidal. Seeds subglobose. The flowers are deep blue voilet, funnel shaped, stalkless and flowering in autumn with the leaves. Styles range, stigmas brick red cultivated for its styles, which when dried form saffron, which is very highly prized.

Flower bloom in autumn and are considered as a native of S. Europe and W. Asia cultivated in the Kashmir Valley, especially in Panpur. 1300 cm. October. It is cultivated in Spain, France, Italy, Greece, Turkey, Persia, India and China. In India, it is also reported from Bhersar and Chaubattia in U.P. (Dic. of Eceo. pl. India, Umarao Singh et. al. 1983).

MEDICINAL USE : Dried stigmas and Tops of the styles-used in fevers, melancholia and enalrgement of liver, stim., stomach, in Catar affections, and in snake bite.

The plant contains many alkaloids of which crocin is the most important one, which is used medicinally.

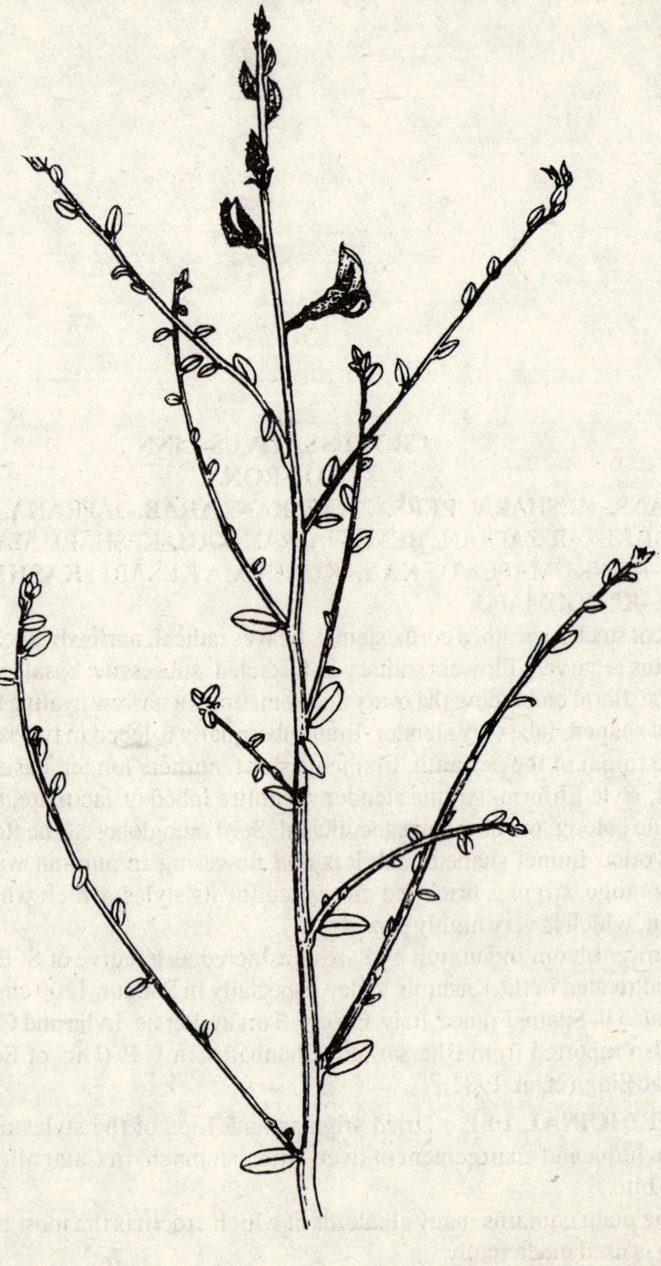

PAPILIONACEAE

CROTALARIA BURHIA BUCH-HEM

P- MEINI, SIS., **BO.-** SIS, SISSAI., **MARATHI-** GHAGARI., **LOCAL NAME-** JHAMO, KHIP, KAURIALA.

An erect or diffused, much branched xerophitic, undershrub. Leaves simple oblong or lanceolate. Flowers yellow with reddish veins. Pods oblong, villous. Flowers May- September.

Locally found in sandy and rocky areas near villages in the district. It is also reported from Sind, Baluchistan, Punjab, Upper Gangetic Plain, Rajputana, Cambay, Gujarat, ascending upto 4000 ft.

MEDICINAL USE : Leaves and branches- used as a cooling medicine.

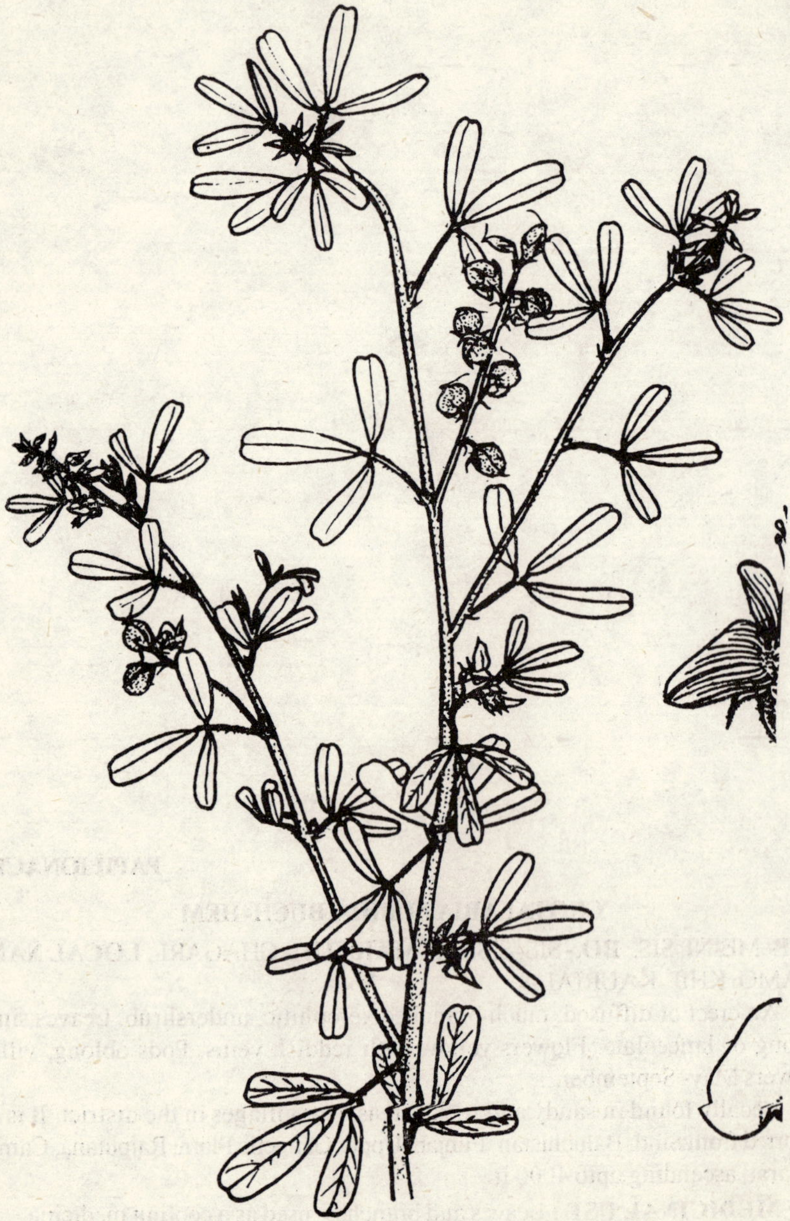

PAPILIONACEAE

CROTALARIA MEDICAGINEA LAMK

H & P - GULABI., **MARATHI**- JENJARU., **LOCAL NAME**- GULABI, JHOJHRU., **GUJ.**- RAMMETHY.

An erect, perennial herb or undershrub with several, ascending branches. Colour of roots like that of turmeric. Leaflets variable in shape. Flowers yellow, in many flowered erect often leaf opposed recemes. Pods obligquely subglobose, 5x5 mm 2 seeded, seeds polished. Flowers and fruits July- Nov.

Locally it is common in the fields of Jawar (Sorghum vulgare Pers). Gawar (Cyampsis tetra gonoloba Tauh. Sun hemp (Cotolaria juncea) and other crops; absent on ridge; occasionally found in lawns fellow fields; in waste places and alongroad sides.

It is found throughout India from the West Himalayas to Ceylon and Burma. Grows wild in South India.

MEDICINAL USE : Seeds contain fat, protein and carbohydrates used for medicine (Proc. Ind. Sci. Long, 1944; 126).

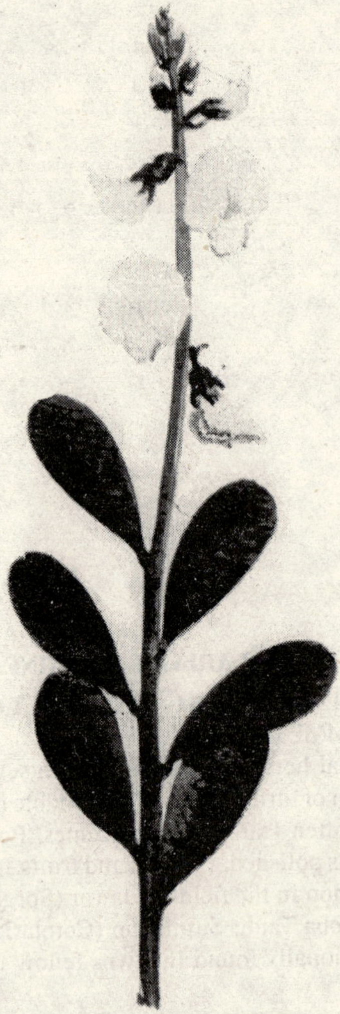

PAPILIONACEAE

CROTALARIA RETUSA LINN

BENGALLI- BIL- JHUNJHUN, **BO.-** GHAGRI., **HINDI-** GHUNG HUN IAN., **TAM. & TEL.-** POTTU- GALI GISTA., **MARATHI-** GHAGRI.

Grows in South India, in the tropical regions of India from Himalaya to Ceylon and also occasionally cultivated.

MEDICINAL USE: Used in Scabies and impetigo (Chopra et. al, 1956; Nadkarni, 1954).

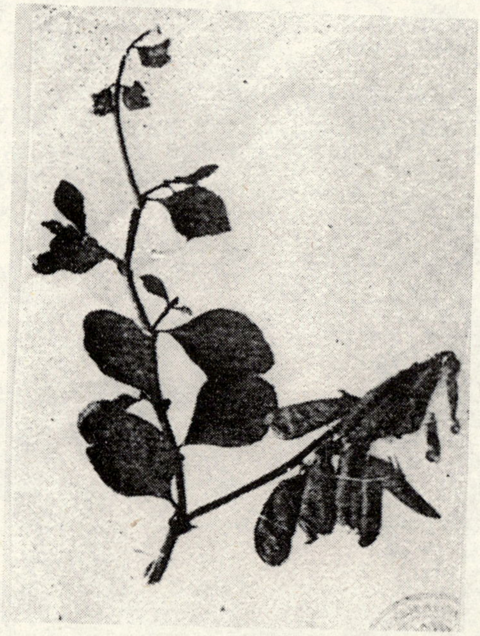

PAPILIONACEAE

CROTALARIA VENUCOSA LINN

S.- SHANAPUSHPI., **H.**- BANSHANA, JHUNJHUNIA., **BENGALI**- JHANI JHANA., **MARATHI & BO.**- TIRAT., **TEL.**- GHELEGHERINTA., **TAM.**- VILTAKILLU.

It is predominent in South India. Also it is found in the tropical region of India from Himalayas to Ceylon.

MEDICINAL USE : The juice of leaves used in scabies and impetog. Considered efficacious in diminishing salivation, when used internally as well as externally (Chopra et al. 1956 Nadkarni 1954).

The genus CROTOLARIA is of interest because of the presence of pyroolizidine alkaloids which are known to have anti tumour, hypotensive and mutagenic properties. They are quite toxic and affect the liver and hence are known as liver toxins.

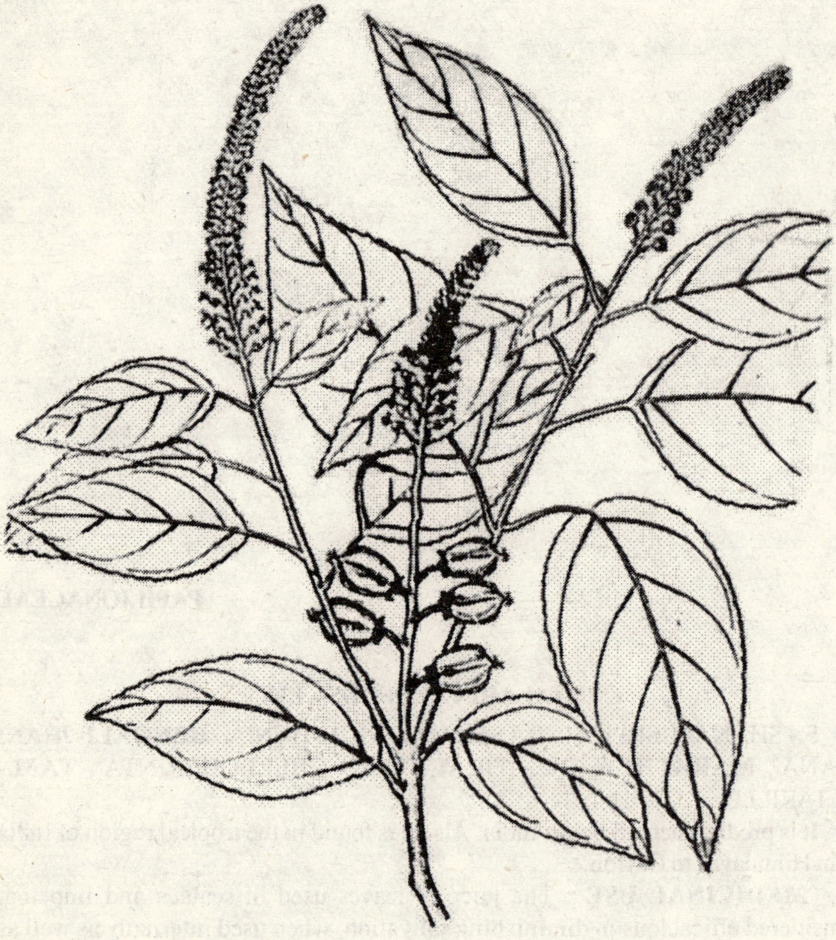

EUPHORBIACEAE

CROTON OBLONGIFOLIUS ROXB.
(SYN. C. ROXBURGHIL BAL. NOM. NOV.)

B.- BOROGACHI., **HINDI**- CHUCKA., **BO.**- GANASUR., **S.**- BHUTAN KUSA., **TAM.**- MILGUNARI, RAILPOONDU., **TEL.**- BHUTAN KUSAMU., **KON.**- GHANSURANG., **MAL.**- KOTE PUTOL., **MIR.**- GHANSURANG., **HINDI**- CHUKA.

It is a even, diffuse branched annual-30-90 cm. high Stems bear multi-armed trichomes, becoming sympodial. Leaves are crowded at the top of branches simple, ovate, lanceolate and (two) 2 glandular at the base. Inflorescence terminal, erect and andiogynous spike; male flowers are pale white and above female ones. Female flowers possess two extra floral glands at the base of the pedicels. Stamens vary from 12-16, capsules three angled hairy stellate and roundish. Seeds spongy oblong shiny with a white spot. Fruits are from June to September.

Found in Bengal, Bihar, SouthIndia, Deccan, Burma and ceylon.

MEDICINAL USE : Bark and root are alterative and cholagogue Seeds are purgative (Nadkarni1954).

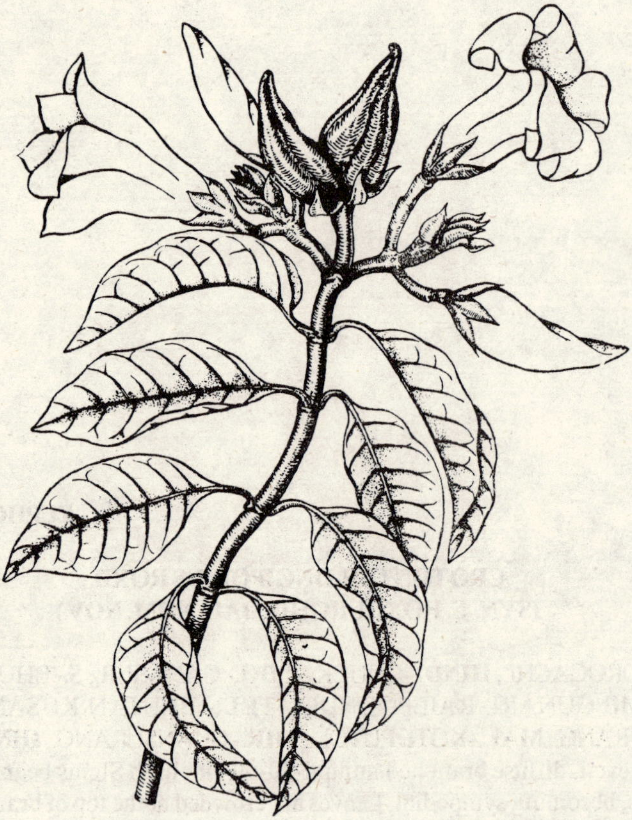

ASCLEPIADACEAE

CRYPTOSTEGIA GRANDIFLORA (ROXB) R. BR.

BO.- VILAYTI- VAKHANELI., **TAMIL**- PALA., **MAL.**- PALA., **MARATHI**- VILAYATI- VAKHANDI., **LOCAL NAME**- RUBBER KI BEL AAKSAN., **CHALUK-CHARI.**

It is a large straggling or climbing shrub. Leaves elliptic or oblong, glossy. Flowers large, pale purple or rosy, filaments free, pollinia grannular Follicles woody 2 winged. Flowers June to September.

Locally naturalized on the ridge, growing as liana or the branches twining among themselves. Initially it received attention as a source of vegetable rubber. Attempts were made to produce rubber from It. Hence its local name.

Largely cultivated in garden throughout in India. Though it has become naturalized in Bombay and Madras States and certain places in the Punjab, Uttar Pradesh, Delhi, etc.

MEDICINAL USE : Leaves are toxic, Plant contain rubber. An aqueous extract of the leaves was found to have hypoglycaemic activity in both normal and alloxan dibetic rabbits (Bapat et al. 1970).

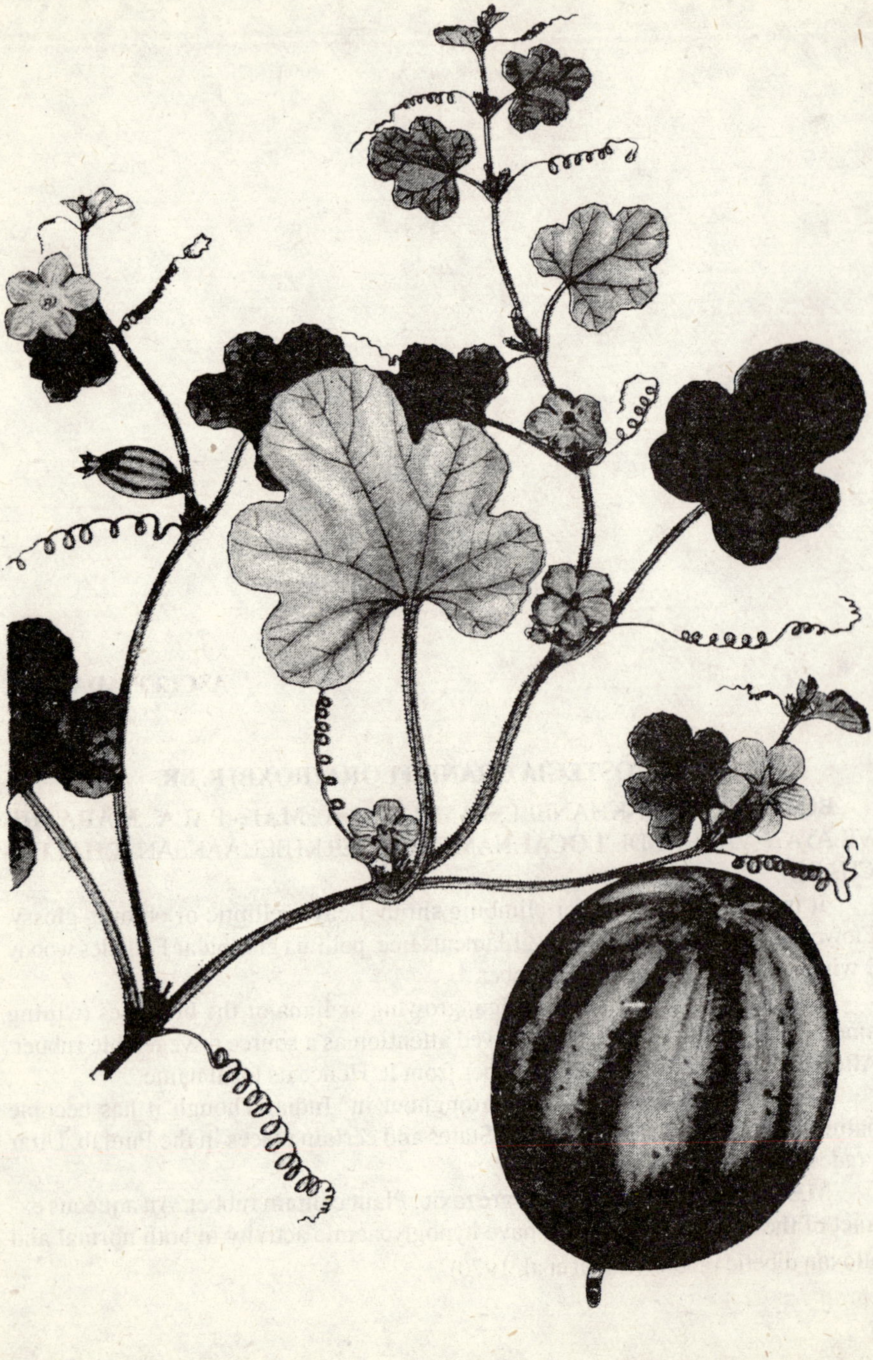

CUCURBITACEAE

CUCUMIS MELO LINN

ENG.- MUSK-MELON., **ASSAMESE**- CHIRAL., **BENG.**- KHARMUJ., **ORIYA**- KHARABHAJA, KASTURBA TARABHAJA., **TELUGU**- KARBUJA DOSA., **TAMIL**- MALAMPAZHAM, KA KKIRA KAI., **MALAYALAM**- THAI KUMBALOM., **KANNADA**- KAKKARIKA., **MARATHI**- KHARBUZ., **GUJARATI**- SAKKARTETI., **HINDI**- KHARBOOJA., **PUNJABI**- KHERBOJA.

It is a creeping hispid annual. Leaves scabrous-flowers yellow in facicles. Fruits variable in shape, spherical, ovoid, elongate or contorted; flowers and fruits are available from June to September.

Melon is a native of North West India. The primary centre of origin seems to be the region between. Iran and North West India. And from there it seems to have spread to China, Japan, Iran, Turkey and Asia. In India it is mainly in Uttar Pradesh and Punjab and in general all over India.

MEDICINAL VALUE : The fruit is highly relished and is used as a dessert fruit and also eaten alone. Musk melon is a good source of vitamins A, B and C. It has a cooling effect and is very wholesome and health giving. It also prevents constipation, seeds cooling nutritious diuretic. Pulp of fruit is diuretic useful in chronic exzema.

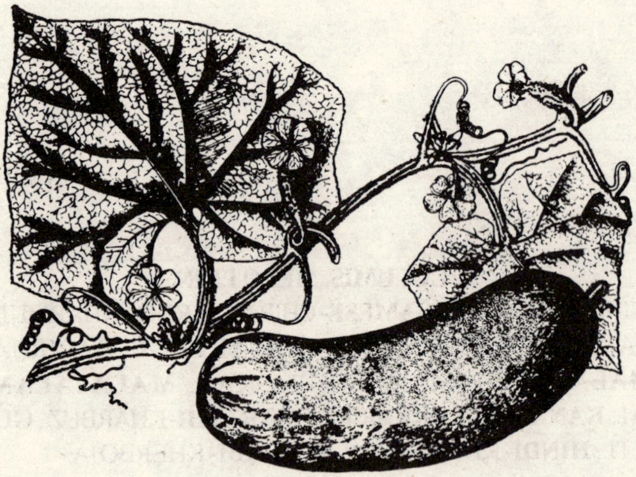

CUCURBITACEAE

CUCUMIS SATIVA LINN

ENGLISH- CUCUMBER., **ASSAMESE-** THIU., **BENGALI-** SHASHA., **ORIYA-** KAKUDI., **TELEGU-** DASA KAYA., **TAMIL-** VELLARTIKAI., **MALAYALAM-** VELLARIKKA., **KANNADA-** SAVATHI KAYI., **MARATHI-** KAKDI., **MALAYALM-** VELLARIKKA., **GUJARATI-** KHIRA, KAKKADI, DOUBLE BEEJ, **HINDI & PUNJABI-** KHEERA.

It is scabrous creeping annual, leaves 3-5 lobed, chordate very rough flowers yellow; male ones in axillary clusters and female solitary of facicled; Fruits ovate or oblong (veryable in shape and sizes, seeds numerous white cultivated flowers and fruit May to September.

Cucumber is a native of India and from here it has spread to Asia. Africa and from thance to Europe. It is also cultivaterd in Europe. France and England. It is an important crop, especially in the hills and tracts of North India. The fruit is eaten raw with salt and pepper at the immature and mature stage.

MEDICINAL USE : The fruit has a cooling effect and prevents constipation. Fruit nutritous, demulchant, seeds cooling tonic, diuretic, fruits contains vitamis B & C, proteolytic enzymes, asceorbic acid oxidase, succinic and malic dehyrogenases.

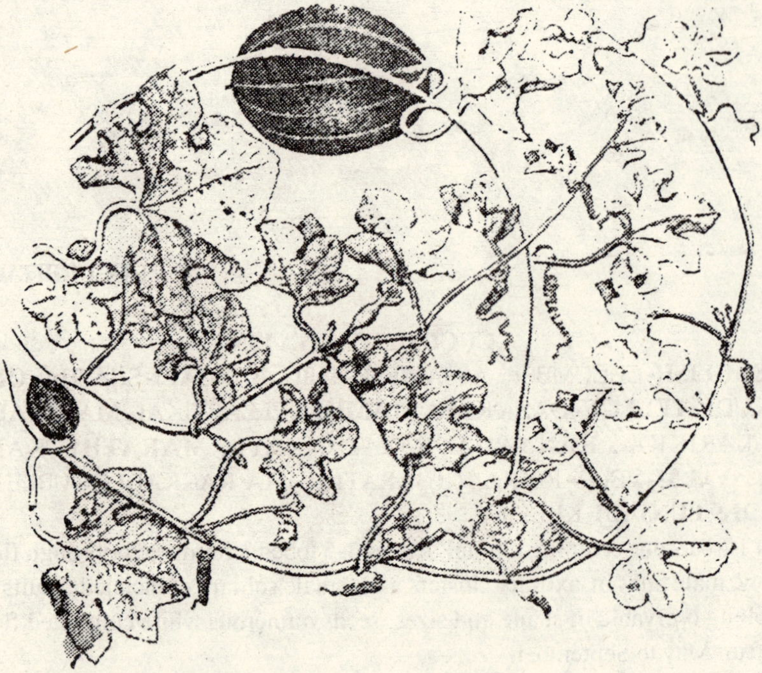

CUCURBITACEAE

CUCUMIS PROPHETARUM LINN
(Syn. VAR C.MIMORDICA DUTHIE + FULLER)

HINDI- KHARINDROYAN., **MAR.-** KANTEINDRYAN., **SANS.-** AINDRI., **GUJ.-** KANTALANINDRANAN., **LOCAL NAME-** PHUNT, KACHRA.

Climbing herbs, stem scabrous; tendrils short and simple. Leaves:- Petioled, palmately 3-7 lobed, or 5-angled or entire, dentate or serrate; 1-1½" reniform, subtriangular much lobed ½ - 1". Flowers:- Yellow monoecious, males clustered in the axils, females solitary, all shortly peduncled. Peduncle less than ½ inch stout. Male: Calyx tube top shaped or companulate lobes 5. Stamens 3; anthers free, one 1-celled, two 2-celled, cells conduplicate or much flexuouse, connective produced in a crest. Female: Calyx and corolla as in the male; ovary ovoid, style short, with three obtuse stigmas; ovules very many, horizontal placentas 3; fruit fleshy pale green, with paler vertical stripes and covered with short spines; indehiscent large or small, spherical or elongate, smooth or tuberculate. Seeds very many, oblong, compressed, mostly smooth.

There are 25 species of which half are African, a few in the tropical, regions of Asia, Australia and America and several widely cultivated are of doubtful origin.

MEDICINAL USE : The plant is emetic and purgative. A bitter resinous body, myriocupuri, which produces nausea and is slightly purgative, is present-in-the fruit pulp. It is highly toxic to animals whether given orally, subcutaneously or intravenously (Walt & Breyer, Brandwijk, 181, U.S.D., 1376).

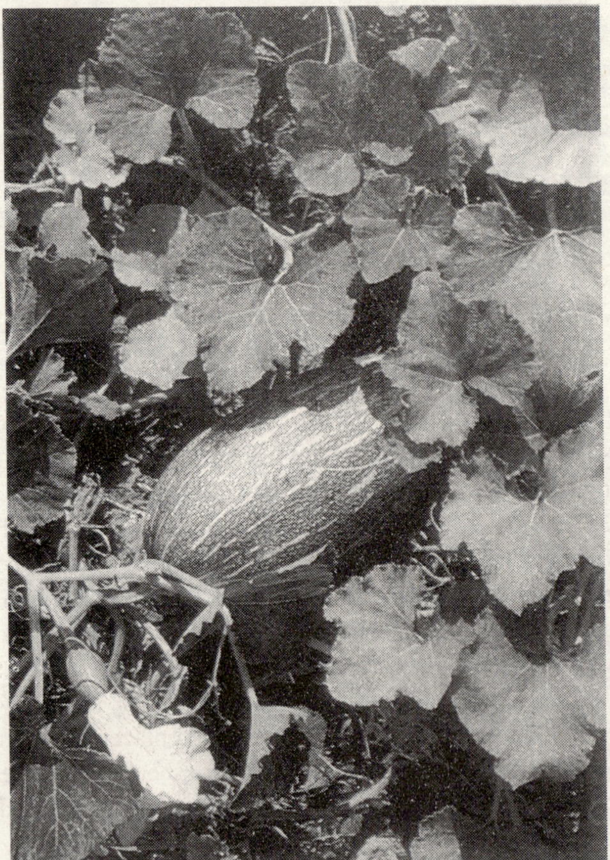

CUCURBITACEAE

CUCURBITA MAXIMA DUCH

ENG.- RED PUMPKIN., **ASSAMESE**- RUNGALAO., **BENG.**- MISTI KUMRA., **ORIYA**- BORTI KAKHARU., **TELGU**- TIYYA GUMMANADI., **TAMIL**- PARANGIKAI., **MALAYALAM**- VELLARI MATHAN., KAUNADAN-SEEGUMBALA., **MARATHI**- TAMDABHOPLA., **GUJARATI**- BHURA KOHALA, SAKAR KOHALA, SAKAR KOHALA., **PUNJABI**- WALATI HALWA KADU., **HINDI**- KADOO, SISTAPHAL.

It is an annual, soft and round leaves reniform; serrate not lobed or chordate with every deep SYNS; occasionally with white bloches fruit variable dull or brightly coloured. Seeds plumb, smooth not seperating easily and cleanly from the pulp.

Its varieties are known as 'Mammoth', 'Hubbard', delicious, and butter cup.

Originally it is recorded from PENI. but now it is cultivated all over India and practically it is utilised by every Indian tribe.

MEDICINAL USE : Seeds anthelmetic used as taenicide, diuretic and tonic; oil verve tonic. Fruit pulp is used as poultice, applied to burns, inflammations and boils.

Seed oil mixed with kahu oil and coconut oil in equal ratio when applied to scalp stops hair falling.

The seeds are cooling and in summer forms one of the important ingredient of the popular drink Tandai. Another variety C. PEPO L. has similar properties.

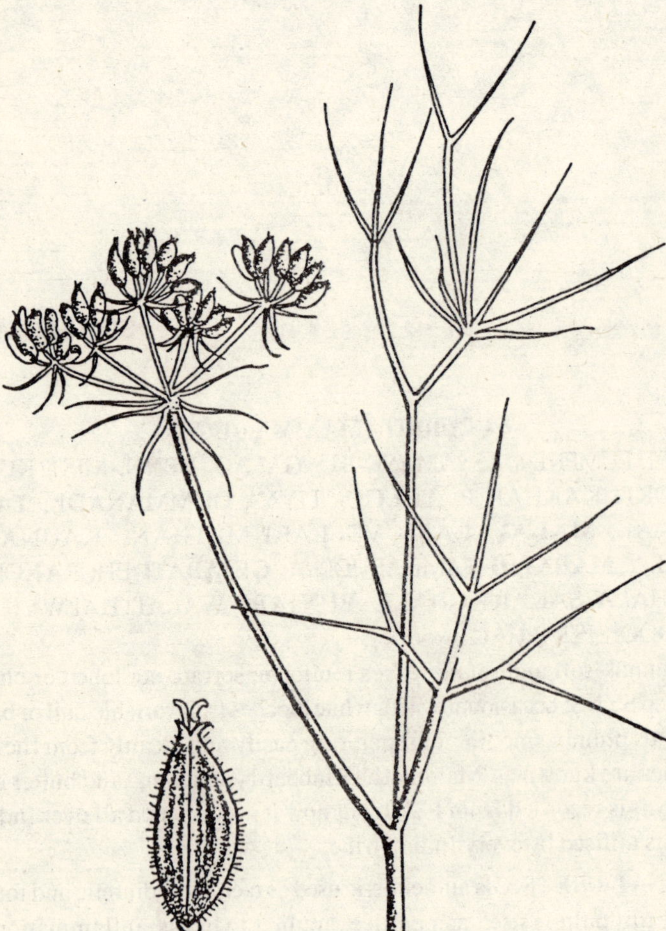

UMBELLIFERAE

CUMINUM CYMINUM LINN.

S.- JIRAKA, JIRA., **ARAB.**- KAMUNA., **PERS.**- ZIRA., **HINDI**- JIRA, ZEERA, ZIRA., **BENG.**- JIRA., **MAR.**- JIREGIRE., **TAM.**- SIRAGAM., **TEL.**- JILAKARA, JIRAKKA., **KAN.**- JEERIGE., **MAL.**- JOREKAM., **PUNJ.**- ZIRA-SUFED., **SIND.**- ZERO., **ENG.**- CUNIN CUMIN., **LOCAL NAME**- ZIRA.

A small slender annual herb about 1 ft. high, with a much branched angular or stiated stem. The leaves are bluish green in colour having sheathing bases. They are linear, twice or thrice, 3-partite, ultimate segments filiform. The flowers are white or rose coloured borne in compound umbels. Umbels:-rays few, bracts and bracteoles several, linear rigid. Calyx-teeth small, subulate, unequal five toothed petals oblong or obovate, emarginate, white, often unequal. 5, epigynous. Stamens five, epigynous; ovary inferior, 2-celled, disc 2-lobed; styles 2, stigmas capitellate ovules 1 in each cell pendulous. Fruit:-cylindrical, tip narrowed, primary ridges filiform, distinct; secondary usually hispidulous; vittae large solitary under each secondary ridge; canpophere 2-partite or 2-fid.

It is grown extensively in South-eastern Europe, and North Africa bordering the Mediterranean sea, and in India and China. It is cultivated in almost all the states in India except Bengal and Assam. The chief areas are reported to be U.P. and Punjab. It is also reported from Jaipur, Khalsa territory, Bombay, Gujarat, Madras, Coimbatore, Cuddapah and Kurnool districts.

MEDICINAL USE : In indigenous medicine, cumin seeds have long been considered stimulant and carminative. They are stomachic, astringent and useful in diarrhoea and dyspepsia. They are now chiefly used in veterinary medicine.

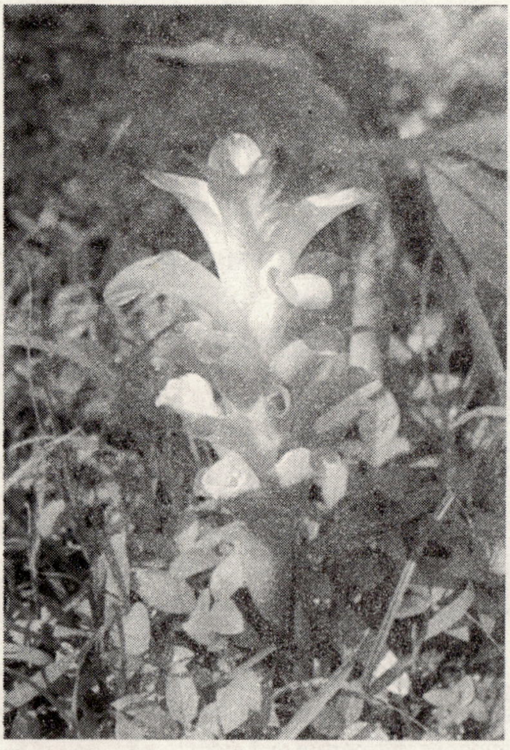

ZINGIBERACEAE

CURCUMA LONGA KOENIG NON.LINN
(Syn. C. DOMESTICA VAL.)

BENG.- HALUD., **ENG.**- TURMERIC., **GUJ.**- HALDDER., **HINDI & PUNJ.**- HALDI., **KAN.**- ARISINA., **KASH.**- LIDAR., **MAL.- & KON.**- HALAD., **TAM.**- MANJAL., **TELEGU**- PASUPU.

It is a perennial, 2-3 ft. high with a short stem and tufted leaves; the rhizomes which are short and thick, constitute the turmeric of commerce.

Root stock is large, tuberous, bearing sessile and long stipitate tubers; being bright yellow from inside. Stem none or neglegible. Leaves in a tuft 4-5 ft. high; leaves larger oblong narrowed to the base, petiole as long as plain green blade, which is 1-1½ ft. by 4-8" broad. Peduncle ½ ft. or more, hidden by the sheathing petiole flowers in dense compound spikes crowned by a coma of coloured enlarged bracts; lower bracts ovate, memberanous, enclosing several bracteolate fugitive flowers which open in succession. Flower bracts pale g reen, those of the coma tinged with pink, flowers pale yellow. Flower bracts pale green, ovate 1-1½"; those of the coma Pale pink. Flowers as long as the bracts. Spikes autumnal 4-6" by 2" in diameters. Calyx short cylindrical, minutely toothed. Corolla-tube funnel-shaped segments usually ovate or oblong, upper,longer and more concave. Lateral stamindoes oblong, petaloid, connate with the short filament; another not crested, cells contiguous, spurred at the base, lip orbicular, tip deflexed. Ovary 3-celled, many ovuled; style filiform; stigma 2-lipped; lips cilliate. Capsule globose, membrannous, finally 3-valued. Seeds ovoid or oblong, usually anillate.

It is widely cultivated in Bengal and other parts of India. Clarke considerd it to be indigenous on Parasnath, in Bihar, altitude 4-5000ft, distributed and cultivated through the tropics (Benthem and Hooker). It is grown on a large scale in India, China and East Indies. It is cultivated in almost all the states in India, particularly in Madras, Bengal and Bombay.

MEDICINAL USE : It is used as a stomach, tonic and blood purifier, as an antiperiodic alterative; with warm milk it is said to be beneficial in common cold. The juice of fresh rhizome is used as an antiparasitic for many skin affections. Externally, it is applied to indolent ulcers and a paste of rhizome with lime forms a remedy for inflamed joints. Decoction of rhizome relieves the pain of purulent opthamia. In large doses it acts as anti-spasmodic inhibiting excessive peristalic movements of the intestines.

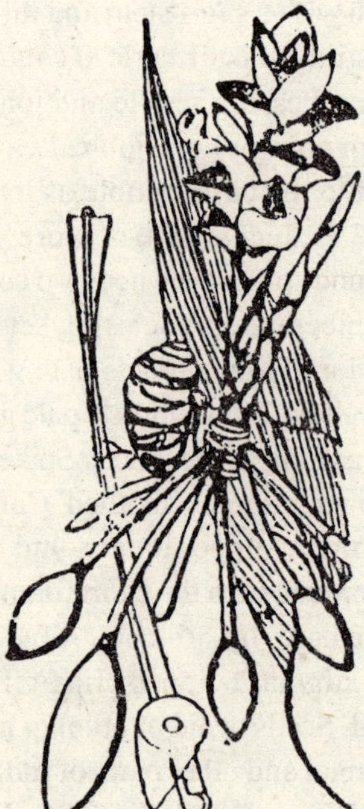

ZINGIBERACEAE

CURCUMA ZEDOARIA ROSE

SANS.- SATI., **TAM.**- KICHILI KIZHANGHU., **TELGU**- SHETTY, KACHORAN., **SANS.**- KARCHOOR., **HINDI-** KACHOOR., **MAL.**- PULA, KIZHANNAI., **BENG.**- KACHOOR., **BOM.**- KACHURA., **MAR.**- KACHORA., **GUJ.**- SHUT KACHOOR., **FA.**- JUNGKHAD., **ENG.**- ZEDORARY., **LATIN**- CURCUMA ZEDOALTIC.

This plant resembles Haldi or Ginger plants. The leaves are long from 1 ft to 2 ft. The leaves are of green colour but bearing red colour spots. The seeds are thin and long.

It is said to be wild in the eastern Himalayans and in the moist deciduous forests of the costal tracts of kanara, cultivated more or less throughout India.

MEDICINAL USES : Stomach, cooling diurnal, aromatic stimulant carminative, applied to bruises and pains, decoct. alongwith pepper and cinnamon and honey beneficial for cold and cough.

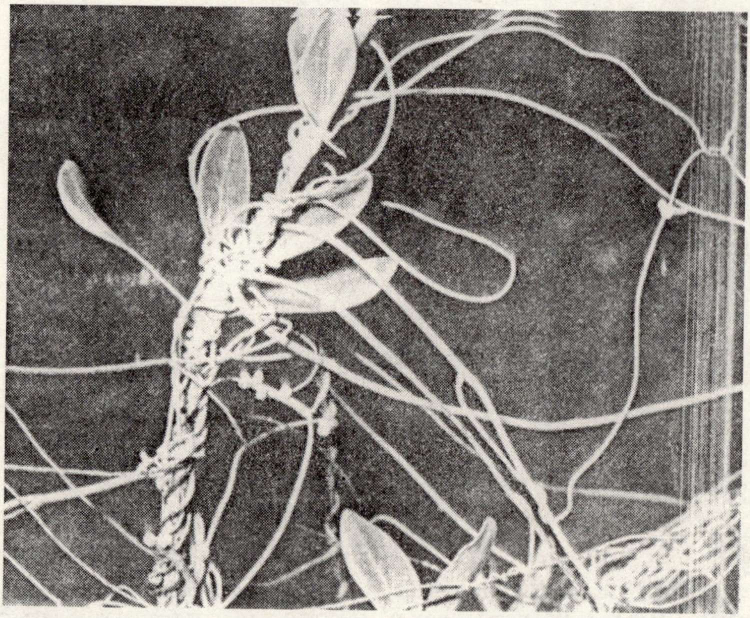

CONVOLVULACEAE

CUSCUTA REFLEXA ROXB

BENG.- ALGUSI., **MAR.-** NIRMULI., **ENG.-** DODDER., **PUNJB.-** NILATHARI+AMIL., **GUJ.-** AKASBEL., **TAM.-** AKASHAAVALLI., **HINDI-** AKASBEL., **TEL.-** SITOMA PARGONALU+SITAMIMA POGUNALU S-AMARAVELA.

It is a herbaceous parasitic climbing plant with leaves reduced to scales. It has no underground root but only grows as a parasitic twiner on other plants. It grows during rainy season and every year the growth is fresh on the same plant.

It is mainly a climber on shrubs and multiply in late monsoon. It forms dense interlacing masses of stout yellow to purplish stems with small fleshy bracts andwith lax clusters of very fragrant white to pink flowers, clusters 2.5- 10 cm long; flowers bell shaped, 6-8 mm long, with short tirangular reflexed lobes, calyx-lobes surrounded, pale green; stamens yellow; fruit fleshy 4-seeded.

It is commonly found through the plains of India, ascending the hills upto 8000 ft. It is also reported from Afghanistan to S.W. China, S.E. Asia 600-3300 m. It is aboundant in Bengal.

MEDICINAL USE : The plant is alterative, purgative and anthelmintic, seeds are carminative and anodyne. Stem is purgative (Nandkarni, 1954).

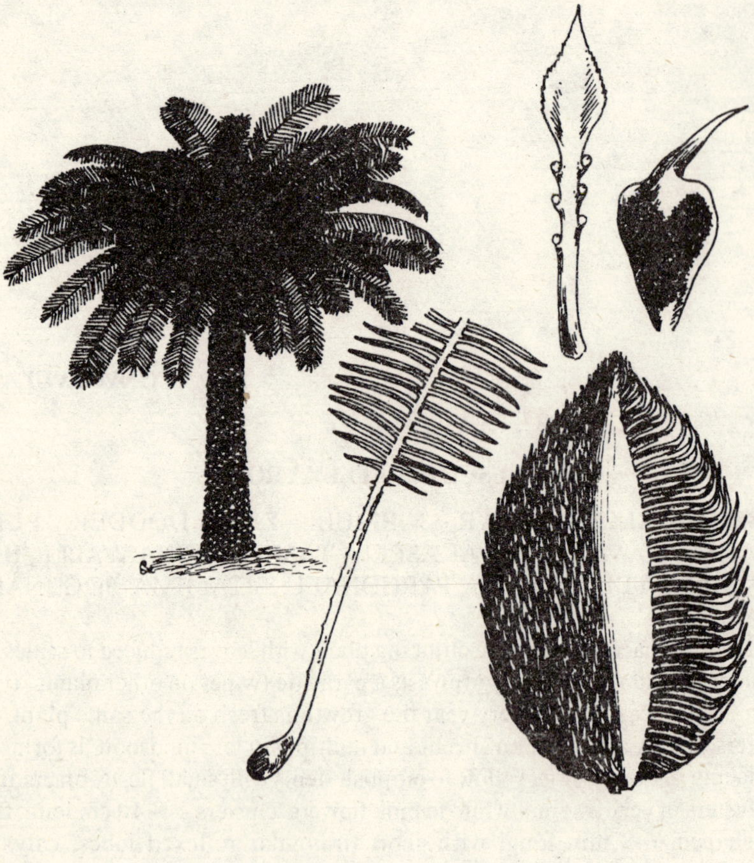

CYCADACEAE

CYCAS CIRCINALIS LINN
SYN. C. THOUARSII R. BR.

SANS.-VARAGUNA., **HINDI**- JANGLI-MADAN-MAST-KA-PHUL., **TAM.**-CANNINGAY, MADANGAMA., **TEL.**-KAMKSHI., **MAL.**-INTALAPPANA., **ENG.**-FERN PALM., **KAN.**- MUNDIKALU., **MAL.**- INTALAPPANA.

An evergreen dioecious palm-like tree, 15 ft. and up wards, rarely forked when old, glabrous throughout. Trunk cylindrical clothed with the woody bases of the petioles. Leaves : In terminal crowns, linear oblong, pinnate; leaflets linear, nerved, quite entire, involute in venation, lower often reduced to spines, 5-9 ft. long, petiole 18" to 2 ft., with short distant slightly deflexed spines near the base; leaflets 10-12 in long, about 1/2 inch wide, elongate-linear-lanecolate, subfalcate, acuminate. Male cones-apparently terminal peduncled, scales cuneate, closely imbricate, apex often long accuminate, anthers ellipsoid, in groups of 3-5, shortly peduncled, often 1-1/2 ft. long, cylindrical ovoid; antheriferous scales 1-1/2-2" long, 1/2-3/4" wide, obovate-deltoid, prolonged into an upward curved subulate acumen about 1" long, clothed with a brown tomentum externally, glabrous above, Carpophylls numrous, crowded round the apex of the stem, densely woolly, appressed into an apparently terminal cone, then spreading, elongate, flattened, dilated above into an entire crenate or pectinate blade. The blade of carpophyll ovate or lanceolate tapering into a long acumen or crenate or more or less. Spinous toothed throught, about 1 ft. long, long stalked, with 3-5 pairs of ovules above the middle ferruginous-tomentose blade 3-4" long, 1- 1-1/2 inch wide. Ovules :- 1-5 ft. in notches on either side of the stalk of the carpophyll, distant, alternate or opposite, nearly erect; seeds ellipsoid or globose; about the size of a pigeon's egg.

Reported from : Malabar Coast Orissa, Rheedle, Buchanan. Dry hills in West Madras to 3,500 ft. Beddome, Ceylon to 1,500 ft. Thwaites. Distribution to East tropical Africa, Comoro Islands, Madagascar, Sumatra, Java, Occassionally groom in Indian Gardens.

MEDICINAL USE : The bark and seeds ground to a paste with coconut oil, are used as polutice for sores and swellings. The juice of the tender leaves is said to be useful for flatulence and vomiting. The pollen is narcotic (Bierkill, I, 721). The stem yields a gum (Gamble 721).

The seeds contain a toxic glucoside, Pakoeins phytosterin and a reducing sugar. The continuous use of Cycas starch is said to cause intestinal troubles. (Burkill, I, 720, Wehner, I, 1).

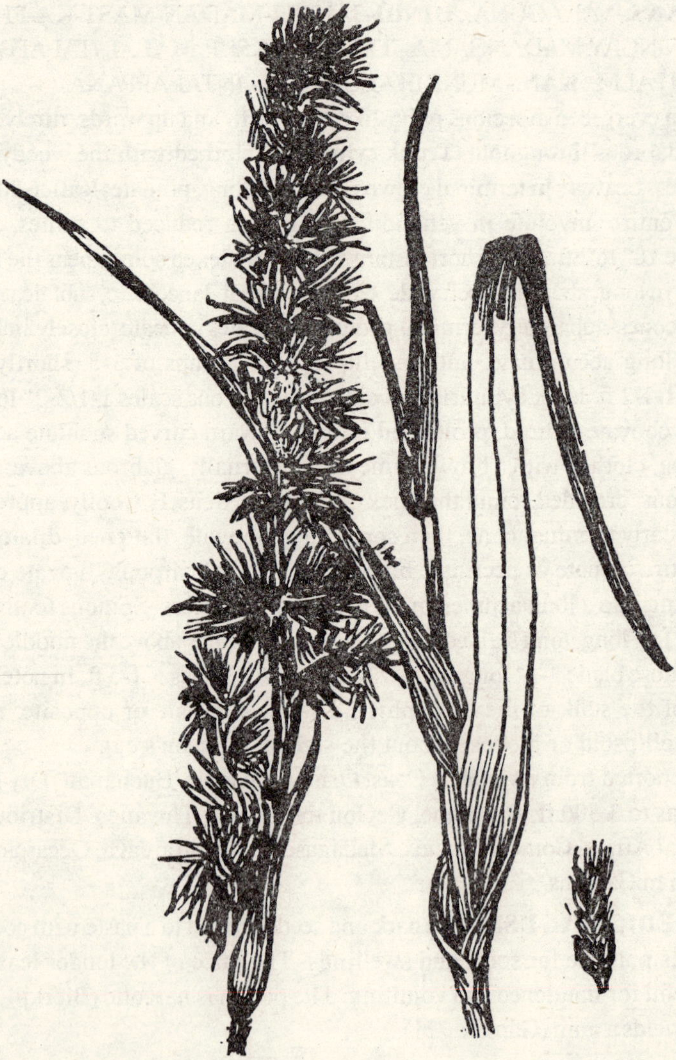

GRAMINEAE

CYMBOPOGON CITRATUS STAPT
SYN. ANDROPOGON CITRATUS DC.
WEST INDIAN LEMONGRASS.

SANS.- BHUSTRINA., **HINDI**- GANDHATRINA, AGINGHAS., **BENG.**- GANDHABENA., **MAR.**- HIRVACHA, OLECHA, VASANAPILLU., **GUJ.**- LILICHA., **TEL.**- NIMMAGADDI., **TAM.**- VASANAPPILLU., **KAN.**- MAJJIGE - HULLU., **MAL.**- VASANAPPULLA., **PUNJABI**- KHAWL., **PERS.**- CHAE KASHMIRI., **GUJ.**- GANDHA - BELA.

It is a tufted perennial grass with numerous stiff stems arising from short rhizomatous root stocks. It seldom flowers in cultivation. The plant tillers strongly, making large tussocks, leaf blade narrow, linear, glaucous, drooping, 50-100 x 0.5-1.5 cm, with scabrid margins, bigule truneate, 0.2-0.8 cm. long. Inflorescence rarely produced, a large loose panicle; spathe bracts long and narrow; sessile spikelets auwnless, linear - laneeolate, concave on lower part of the back.

It is propagated by root division when 4-8 months old, is subsequently harvested every 3-4 months and continues for about four years.

It is probably a native of Mfalosia or Ceylon and is not known in a wild state. It is now widely distributed throughout the tropies and is grown for oil extraction in the West Indies, Gratemley Brazil, the largo, Tanzania, the Malagasy Republic and Indochina. It cannot be produced systamatically grown in gardens in the punjab, Bombey and Baroda. Reported to grow wild in Mysore. It is abundant in Rajasthan & Kathiawad.

MEDICINAL USE : Infusion of leaves is sudorific and stimulant. Oil is carmiative and also given in Cholera. Lemon grass oil is one of the most important essential oils being widely used for the isolation of citral, which is used for the production of B. lonone; which is an intermediate in the commercial synthesis of vitamin A.

It is also used in fever, wormiform, asthma, intestinal disorders, constipation & heart troubles.

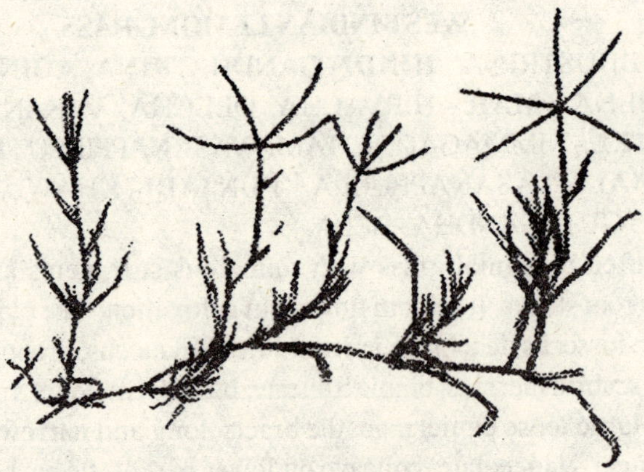

GRAMINEAE

CYNODON DACTYLON PERS

BENG-DUBH., **MAR**.-HARYALI., **TAM.**-ARUGAMPULLU., **HINDI**-DHUB., **TEL**.-HARVALI., **SANS.**-DOORVA., **KAN.**-GRIKE., **LOCAL NAME** : DOOB.

A perennial grass with an extremely creeping base. Culms slender, many noded, wiry, forming matted tufts. Leaves linear, accuminate; spikes 4-5, digitate, arcuate spreading, green or purplish, spiklets laterally compressed sessile, appressed, imbricate floral glumes boat shaped; fruits- throughout the year.

Common and abundant, forming a carpet in lawns extensively used as lawn grass. Grows throughout India upto 2600 m.

MEDICINAL USE : Decoction of root is diuretic, used in dropsy and in secondary syphilis. Infusion of roots is given for bleeding piles. Crushed roots mixed with curd is used in chronic gleet: Juice ofthe plant is astringent, used as an application to fresh cuts and wounds, diuretic and also used in dropsy and anasarca, in hysteria epilepsy, insanity, chronic, Diarrhoea and dysentery. It is reported to be useful in catarrah and opthalmia.

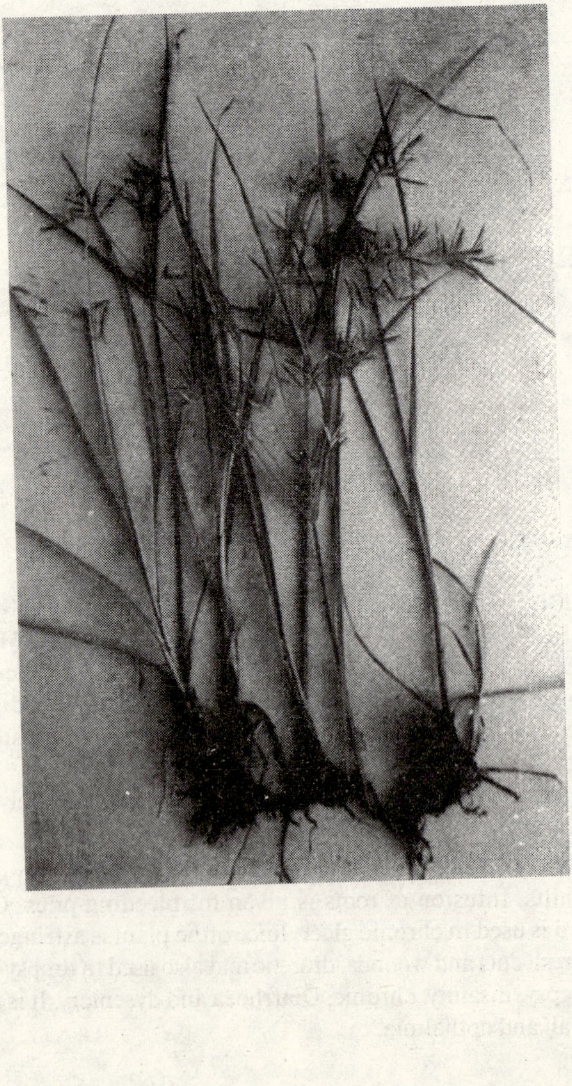

CYPERACEAE

CYPERUS CORYMBOSUS ROTTB (SYN. CYPERUS ROTUNDUS LINN)

S & B O-MUSTA., **B & H** - MOTHA, MUTHA, MOOTHOO., **TAM.**-KONAI., **LOCAL NAME**-MOTHA., **TEL.**-TUNGAMUSTI., **ENG.**-NUTGRASS., **GUJRAT**-BARIKMOTHA., **HINDI**- KORCHI-JHAR., **KON.**- BHADRAMUSTI., **MAL**-KARIMUTTAN., **KAN.**-TANGAHULLU, MUSTORA., **MAR.**-MASTA., **TAMIL**-KORAI.

It is an erect glabrous herb upto 50-60 cm high leaves linear usually shorter than the stem. Inflorescence an umble of more or less condensed spikes, bracts, foliar, generally three, exceeding the umbel. Spikelets pale yellow or brown, often with a reddish finge, Glumes decurrent below as hyaline wings, nuts obvoid-ellipsoid.

A common and variable weed during the rainy season in lawns unused ground and fields, growing in different types of habitats, often becoming abundant and dominating the vegetation. Flowers and fruits July-October. It is found throughout India. Common in waste grounds, gardens and roadsides in open spots and upto and elevation of 6000 ft. It is abundant in South India.

MEDICINAL USE : It is a stimulant, tonic, demulcent, diuretic anthelmintic, stomachie, carminative, diphoretic, astringent emmenagogue and vermifuge (Nadkarni, 1954). It is also found useful in disorders of stomach and irritation of the bowels.

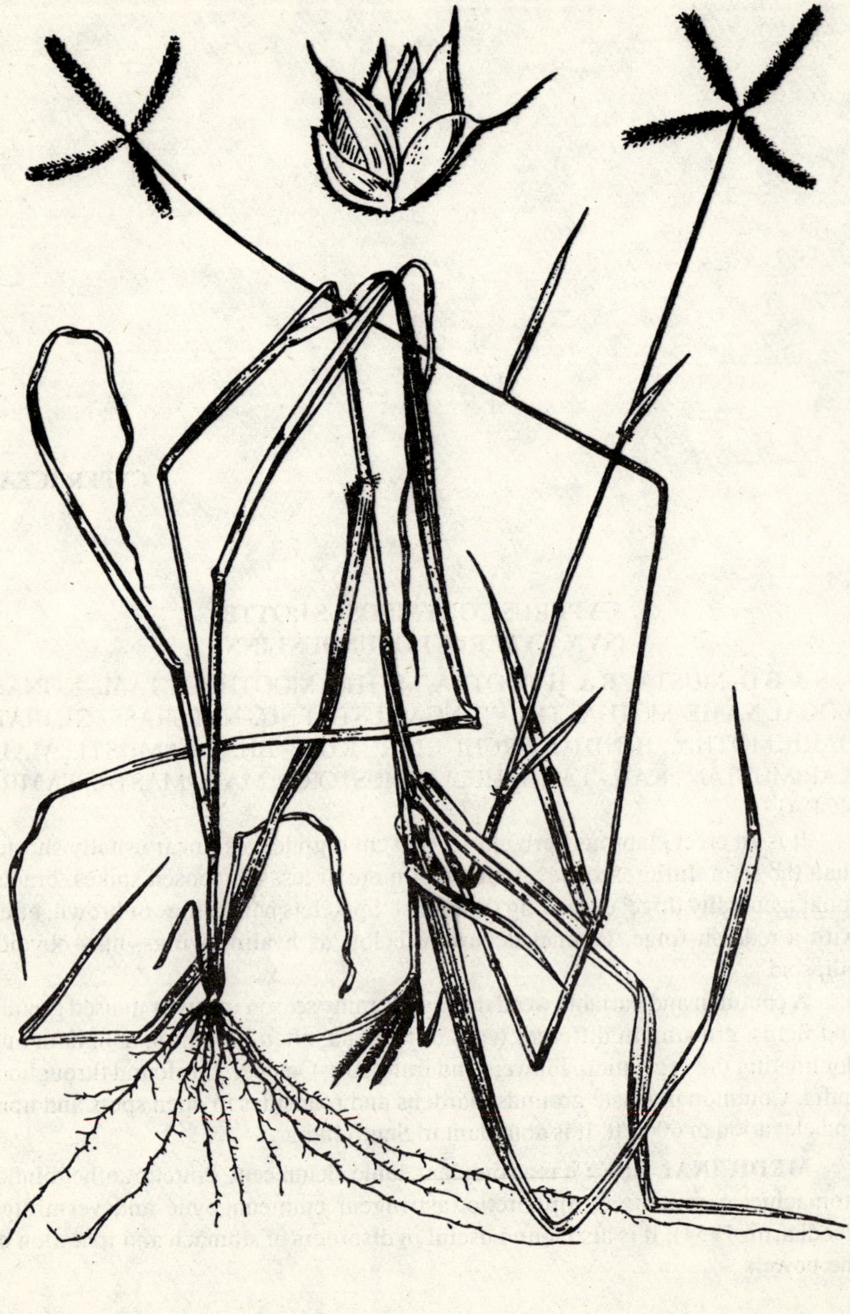

GRAMINAE

DACTYLOCTENIUM AEGYPTIUM (L.) P. BEAUV (SYN. CYNOSURUS AEGYPTIUS LINN. ELEUSINE AEGYPTIUS DESF.

BO.- MAHR., **H.** - MAKRA., **P.**- MADANA., **TAM.**- TAMIDA., **LOCAL NAME :** MAKRA.

An erect or decumbent annual, variable in habit. Culms rooting at the base and from the brand nodes. Leaves distichous, narrowly linear, flat. Spikes 2-6, digitately radiating, rachis, keeled, spikelets densely crowded, spreading at right angles to the rachis, -3 - 5x3mm Lower involucral glume cuspidate, upper awned, Floral glumes mucronate or awned. Grains obovoid - globose, rugose. Flowers and fruits - May to October.

Common during the monsoon period on the ridge in depressions and amongst bushes and shrubs and as a weed in cultivated fields and open places, often becoming abudant. Erect prostrate and decumbent types are known from the area. Srpead throughout tropical and subtropical regions of India.

MEDICINAL USE : Grains - perched and eaten by women who suffer from bellyache after child birth. Decot. of seeds renowned in Africa as an alleviator of pain in kindely region.

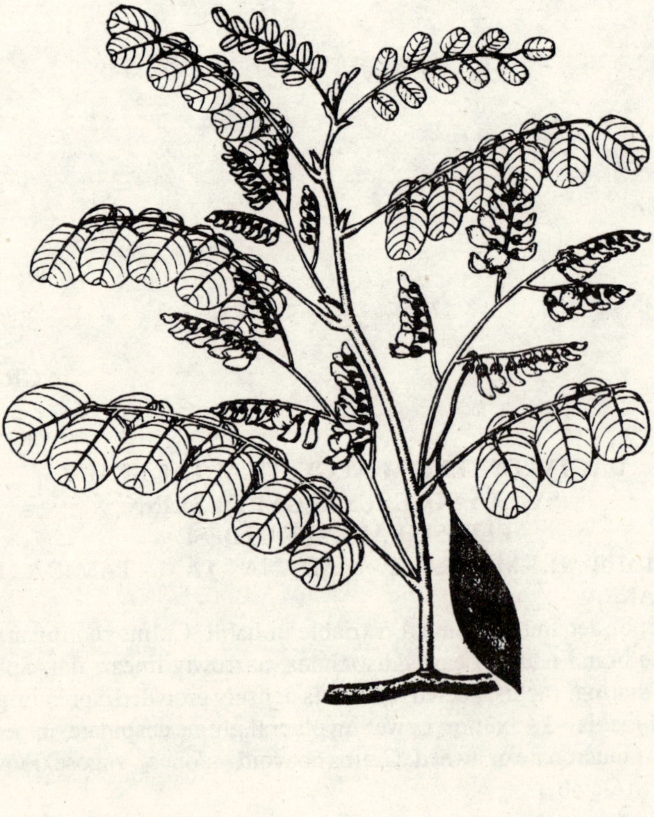

FABACEAE

DALBERGIA LANCEOLARIA LINN F.
(SYN. D. FRONDOSA ROXB.

HINDI- BITHUA, TAKOLI., **BOMBAY**- CHAKEMEDIA., **BO.**- TAKOLI., **TELGU**-ETHURPACEARI, PEDDASOPRA., **TAMIL**-NALVEL LANGUS EREGAE., **M.**- DANDUS, KORCHI., **KAN.**- BELAGA, KANAGA, HASURUGGANI., **MAL.**- MUNVITTI, PULARI., **SRI LNAKA**- BETURUBAI.

It is a tall leafy tree with a straight stem occupying an area of 2.1 m. The wood is yellowish white and granular. The leaflets are from 5-12 cm orbicular in shape showing a sort of depression at the top of mid rib. The flowers are axillary in position and arranged alternately. They are found in branched clusters and on maturing become yellowish in colour. The pods strap shaped and one seeded. It is also supposed to be an ornamental plant found in plains from western Himalayas down to Ceylon.

MEDICINAL USE : Bark alongwith FLACOURTIA RAMONKI is used as an external application during intermittent fever. It's infusion is given internally in dyspepsia. Seed oil is used in rheumatic infections.

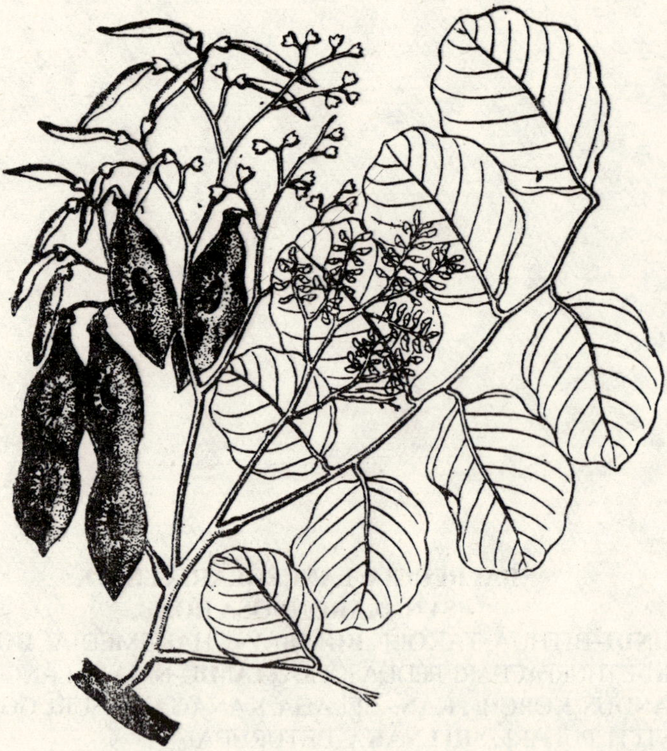

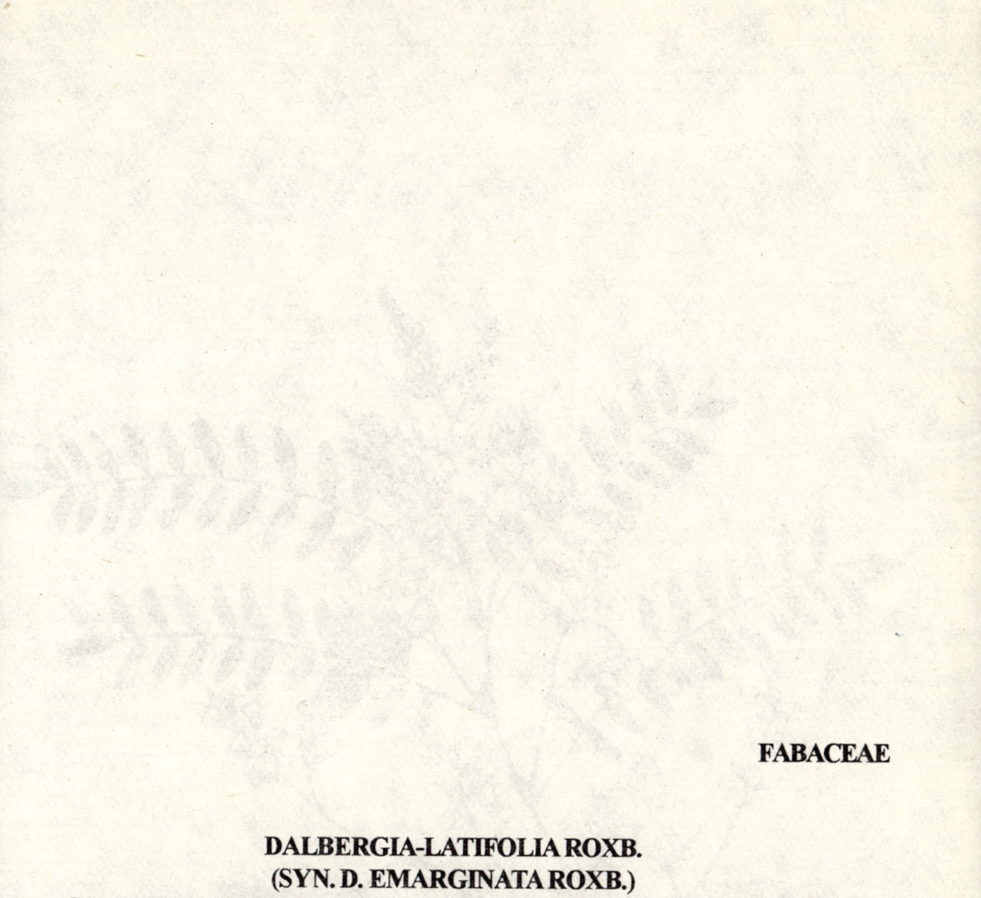

FABACEAE

DALBERGIA-LATIFOLIA ROXB.
(SYN. D. EMARGINATA ROXB.)

SANSKRIT- SHISHAPA., **BENGALI**- SITSAL., **TEL.**- CITTEGI, YERUGUDU JITIGE, JITANGI., **TAMIL**- ITI, TODAGATRI., **MARATHI**- SISHAM, SIU & KALORUKH., **ORIYA**- SISSNA., **KANNADA**- BITI, THODAGATTI., **HINDI**- KALA., **SHISHAM & ENGLISH**- INDIAN ROSE WOOD., **BOMBAY**- SITSAL, SAFED SAL., M.P SISWA, SISSOO, BOTHULA., **GUJARATI**- SHISHAM, KALAROOK, **MAL.** - ITTI, KOLEVITI, CAR, CTTI.

It is a large deciduous tree attaining a height of 24 mtr. with a girth of 30 - 37-5. metre. The tree is leafy and straight the top is spherical in shape. Leaflets 3-7cm broadly elliptic, orbicular, obtuse sometimes emarginate upto 7.5 cm long; Flowers are whitish; pods oblong lanceolate 1-4 seeded.

It is found in Maharashtra, Bengal Bihar, Sikkim, Madhya Pradesh and Western Peninsula.

MEDICINAL USE : It is a bitter tonic, stimulant, appetiser and stomachie. It is also used in dyspepsia, diarrohoea, leprosy, obesity, worms. etc.

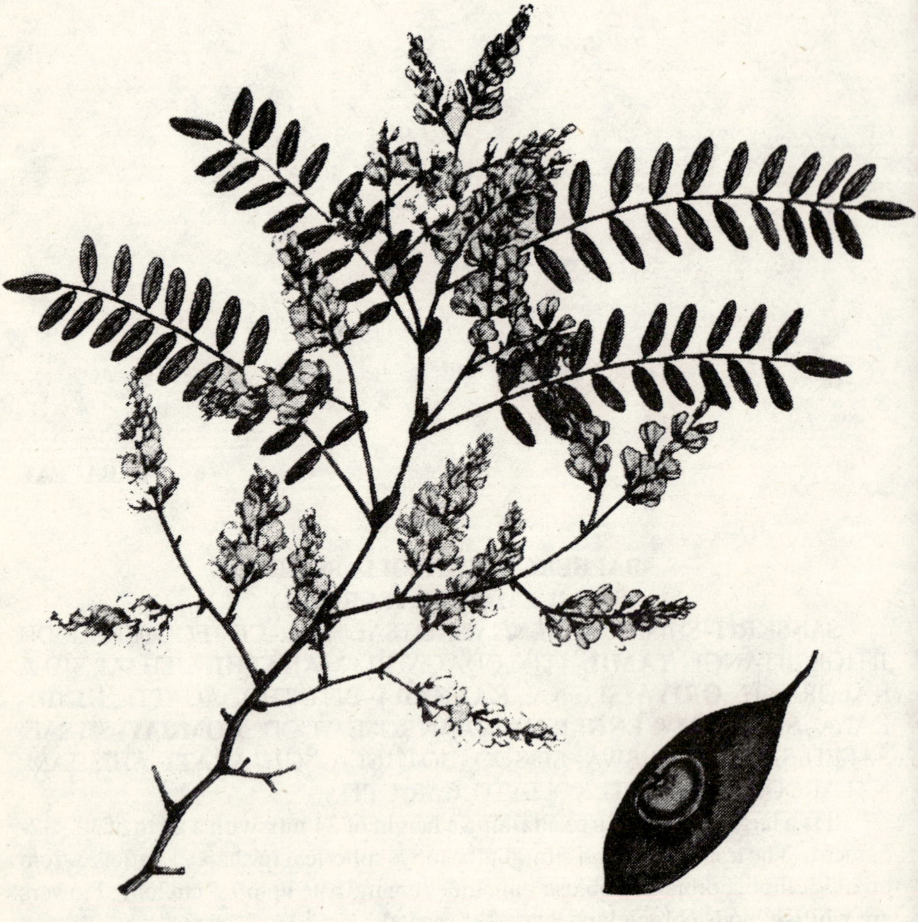

FABACEAE

DALBERGIA PINNATA (LOUR) PRAIN
(SYN. DELBERGIA TAMARINDIFOLIA ROXB)

ASSAM : KETI., **NEP**.- DAMAR.

D. PINNATA is a woody plant. The leaves of this plant are used as foder.

It is reported from Eastern Himalayas, Assam and Western Peninsula.

MEDICINAL USE : The root used in Indo-china as masticatary, anthelmic and responsible for killing worms. In Assam the bark of the plant is eaten with betal.

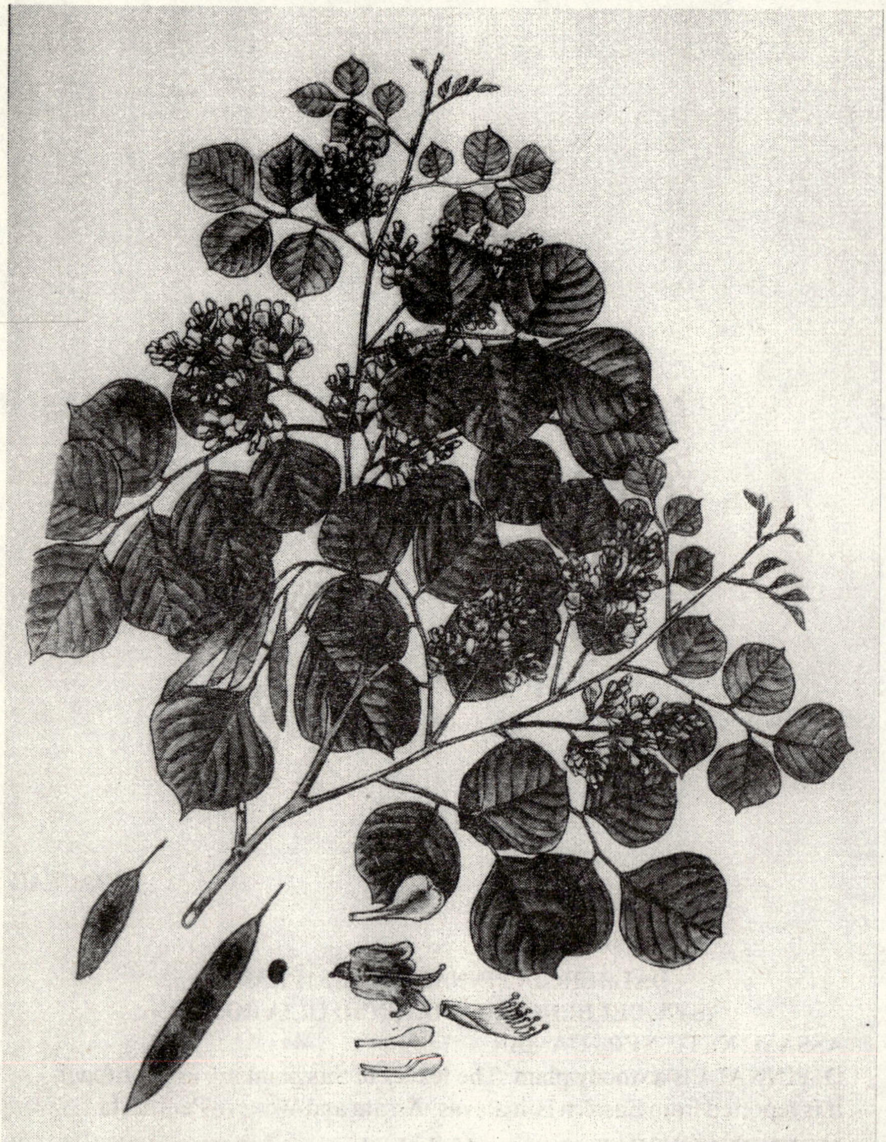

FABACEAE

DALBERGIA SISSOO ROXB

BENGALI- SISHU, SHISU., **ENGLISH** - BLACK WOOD., **HINDI-** SISAM, SHISHAM, SISSU, SISSAI., **MAR.-** TALI., **PUNJAB-** TALISAFEDAR, TALI, SHISHAM, SHISHAI., **TAM.-** NUKU KETTAI, SISU, ITTI, GETTE., **TEL.-** SISSUKARRHA, ERRASISSU, SINSUPA., **SANS.-** SHINSHAPA, AGURU, SHINGAHUDA., **GUJ.** - SISAM, TANACH., **MAL.-** IRUVIL., **KAN.-** AGARU, BIRIDI., **ORRIYA-** SISSU, SIMSAPA., **BOMBAY-** SISSU., **TRADE-** SISSOO, SHISHAM.

An erect deciduous tree, with finely grey - downy, branches bark is grey under favourable conditions, it attains a height of about 100 ft. a girth upto 8 ft. and a clear bole upto 35 ft. Leaves alternate subcoriaceous leaflets, leaf - rachis zigzag leaflets 3-5 roundish with a very distinct cusp, leaf - lets firm glabruscent, 1-3 inch long. Flowers in short axillary panicles with racemose - corymbose branches, pedicles short. Panicles much shorter than the leaves. The erect patent branches densely are pubscent. Calyx - companulate, teeth five, distinct 1/6 inch deep, downy, teeth very short, the lowest rather the longest. Lanceolate Corolla - exerted standard broad. Keel obtsue, with its petals only joined at the tip, yellowish, twice the length of the calyx, standard with a long claw and round limb. Stamens 9 (nine) monodelphous or the sheath slit down the keel, anthers minute basifixed with the cells back to back and the slit mostly short and apical Ovary stalked few ovuled, style short incurved glabrous, stigma capitate pod thin, strap shaped, pale brown. Glabrous 1.1/ - 4 by 4 by 1/4 - 1/2 obtuse wih a stalk twice as long as the calyx. Flowering period is March - June fruiting period is July to August.

It is found in the plains of India ascending to 5000 ft. in central Himalayas. It is also reported from Afghanistan Baluchistan, Sub Himalayans Track from Ravi to Assam, ascending upto 5000 ft. It is gregariously growing in elluvial forests and extensively cultivated in Punjab, U.P. Bengal and Assam.

Locally it is planted along roadsides in village and also introduced on the ridge.

MEDICINAL USE : Bark or raspings of the wood are alterative while the roots are astringent and leaves bitter and stimulant. A decoction of leaves is found useful in gonorrhoea. The wood has been found useful in leprosy, boils, eruptions and to allay vomitting.

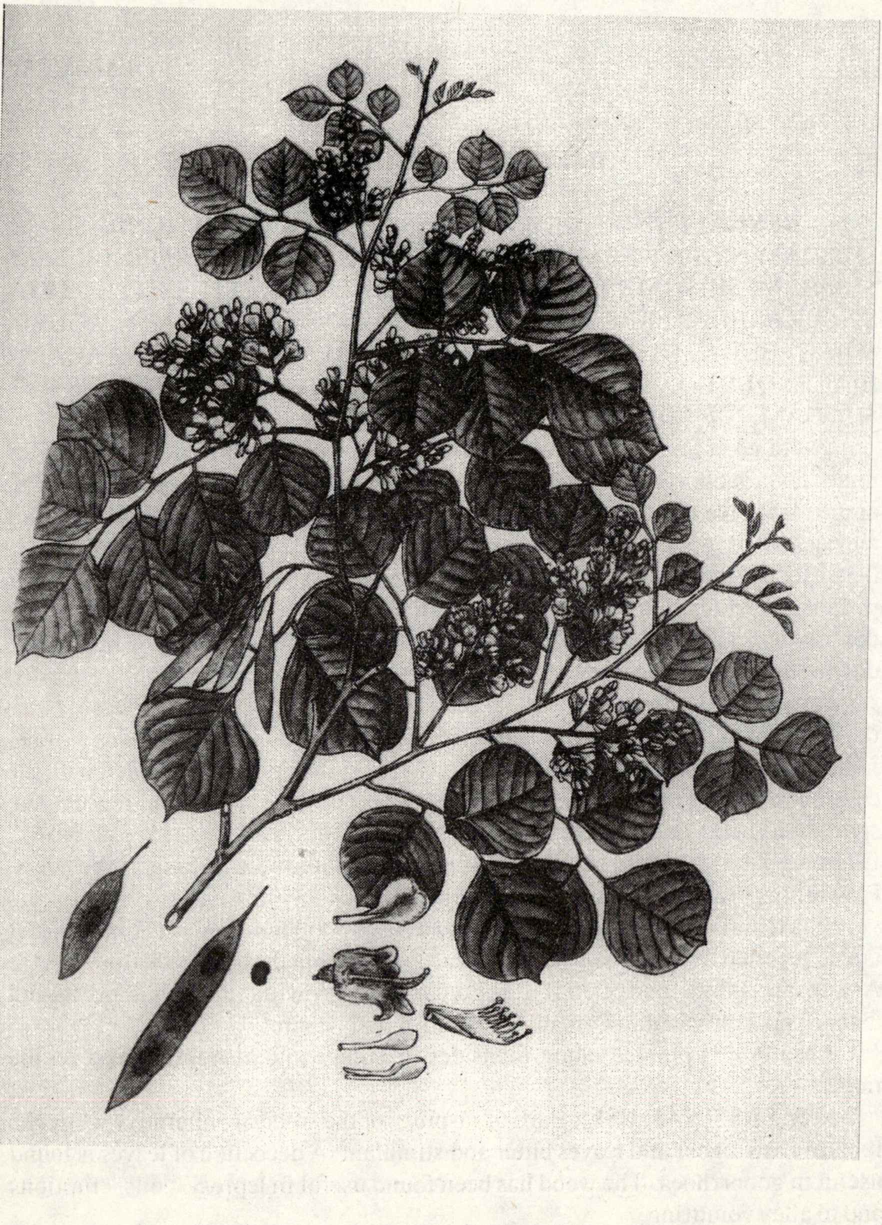

FABACEAE

DALBERGIA SCANDENS ROXB.
(SYN. DERRIS SCANDENS (ROXB.) BENTHS.

B.- NOALATA., **H.**- GANJ., **P.**- GUNJ., **T.**- TAKIL., **TEL.**- NALLA TIGE.

A large woody climber. Young parts rusty pubesent. Branches pendulous. Leaflets 9 - 13 flowers white, in long axillary racames. Pods thin, flat, indehiscent. Flowers - May - September. Fruits October - December.

It is reprted from N. Oadh, konkan,kanara,Madras,state from northern Circars southwards.and Bengal especially near Chittagong,Orrisa, somtimes, cultivated in gardens. grows wild in south india.

MEDICINAL USE : Bark is a cholagogae and used as a fish poison.it is also used in snake bite. Roots contain scanenin,nallanine and chandanin. (proce.indian acad.Sci.Vol.24a,1946,305,chem.Abstr.1944,81: Curr.Sci.1947,346)

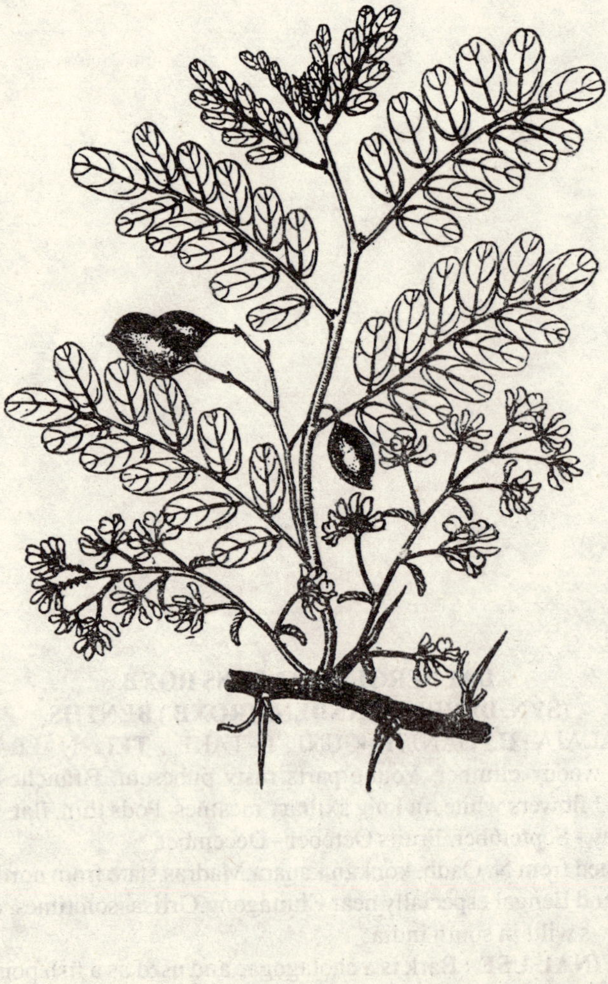

FABACEAE

DALBERGIA MELANOXYLON GUILL AND PERR.

ENGLISH- AFRICAN BLACKWOOD., **SUDAN-** EBONY DAXIY SENEGAL, SOODAIN, ABNOOSE, CHINI BLACK DARU.

It is a small tree. The main stem is having very prominent sharp thick and straight spines arranged alternately. The leaflets are ovate - orbicular showing a depression at the top of the mid rib. The leaf let branches are arranged alternatly. The flowers are in clusters and found in long stalks in axillary position on either side of a branch. The clusters are again in their turn borne on small stalks. Stipules are present. The pods are very small and single seeded.

It is distributed in Tamil Nadu. Karnataka, Maharastra and Bengal.

MEDICINAL USE : The leaves are used in curing pimples and mouth rash.

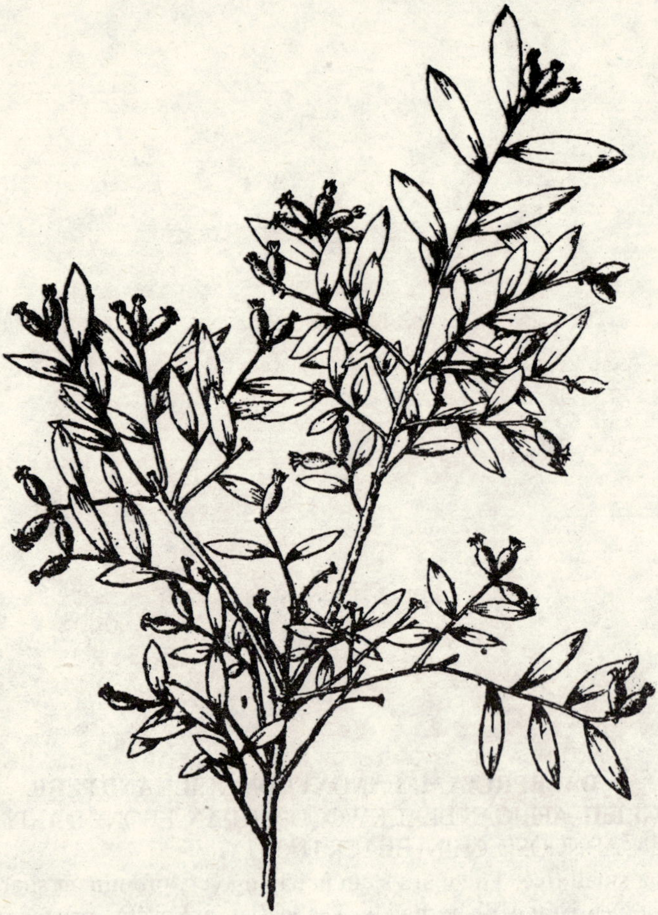

THYMELACACEAE

DAPHNE OLEOIDES SCHREB

MAR.- PECH., **PUNJ.**- MASHUR.

Habitat; Grows in western Himalayas at 1000-3000m Kanawar, Chamba, Bakichistan and Waziristan.

MEDICINAL USE : Root is purgative. Bark and leaves are used in cutaneous infections. Leaves or their infusion is given in gonorrhoea and applied to abscesses.

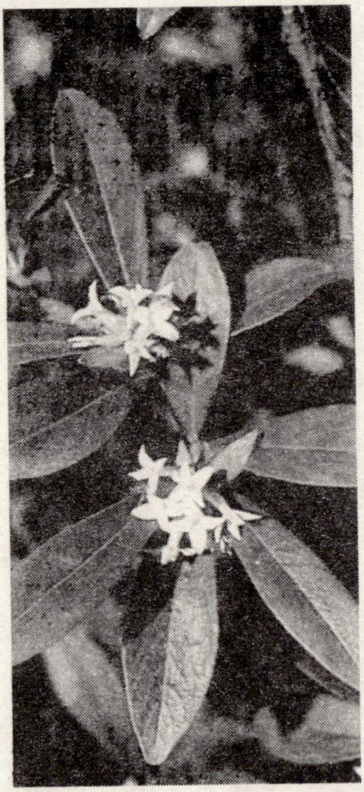

THYMELACACEAE

DAPHNE PAPYRACEA WALLICH EX. STEUD (SYN. D. CANNABINA LOUR EX WALLICH)

H.- SATPURA, SETBURBKU, SETBURUSA., **NEP.**- BHULLU, DANKOTAHA GAINDA, KHKEAGUTI., **P.**- JEKU, BHUTANS - DASHING., **PUNJAB:** NIGGI, JAYKU.

A much branched erect evergreen shrub with smooth grey bark, with dull green narrow lanceolate to oblanceolate leathery leaves and with scented white or greenish white flowers borne in terminal clusters with persistent hairy bracts. Flowers with tube 10-13 mm long, very downy outside and 4 acute spreading lobes c-8mm long, leaves 5-12 cm hairless, with veins inpressed above, stalk short and grooved , stems 1.25mm long. Fruit c 1.cmm fleshy at first orange than deep red when fully ripe.

It is reported from Temperate Himalayas; from Chamba to Bhutan 5,000 - 7-000 ft. in the West and also from pakistan to C. Nepal Forests 1500 - 2100m

MEDICINAL USE : The plant is bitter, purgative and feberifuge.

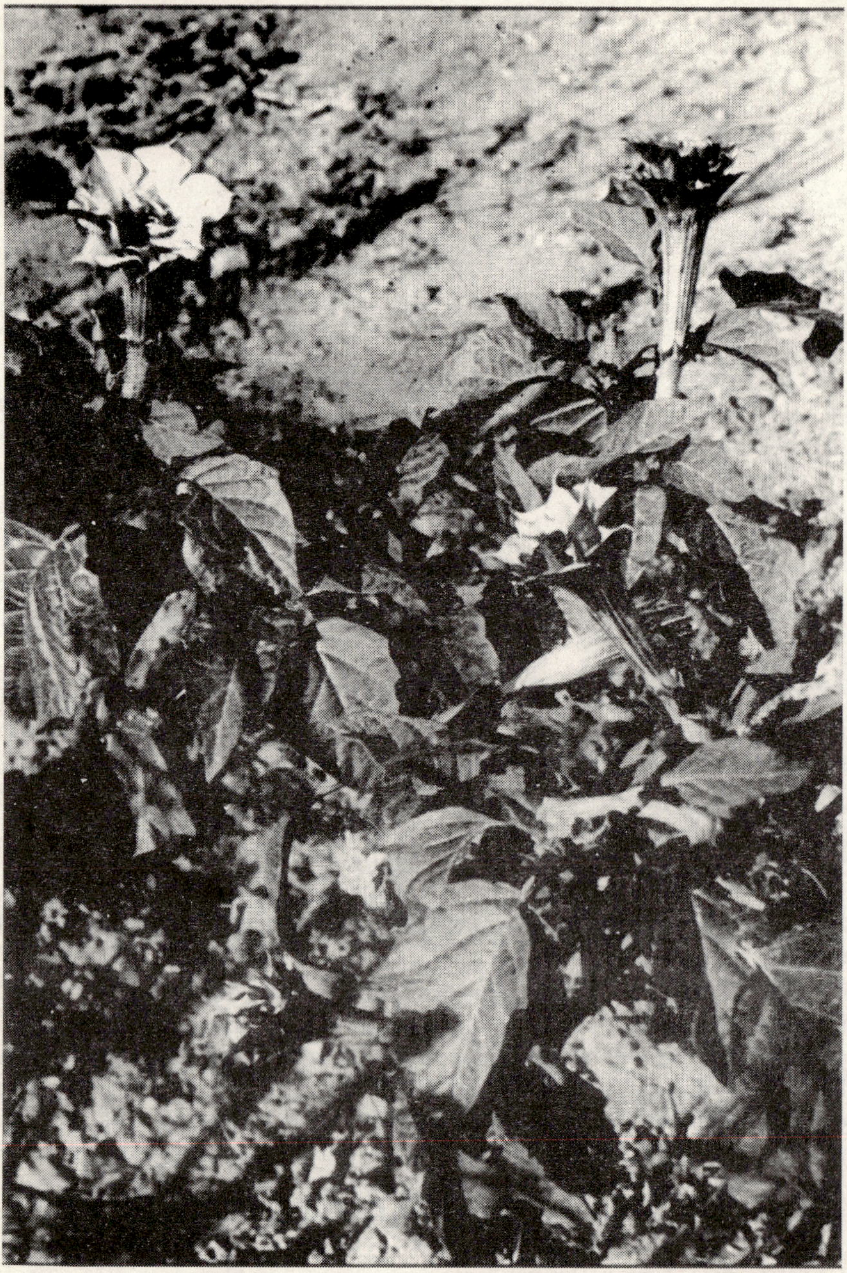

S0LANACEAE

DATURA INNOXIA MILL
(SYN. DATURA METEL LINN SIMS)

A short stout shrub with grey tomentum. Leaves ovate lanceolate to broad ovate, unequal at the base. Calyx reflexd in fruit, corolla white. Capsules globose, clothed with sharp spines. Flowers and fruits - November - January.

Common near graveyards and open waste places. A native of Mexico introduced into India and now found growing in Western Himalayas, the hilly regions of western parts of Deccan Pennisula and a few other places in India. In appearance the plant resambles D. METEL closely.

MEDICINAL USE : Similar to D. METEL.

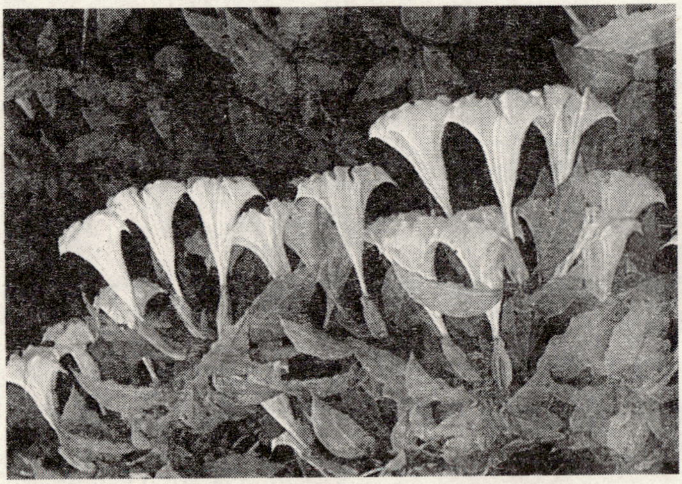

SOLANACEAE

DATURA METEL LINN
(SYN. D. ALBA NEES
(SYN D. FASTUOSA VAR. ALBA CL.
(SYN. D. ALBA RUMPH.

BENG.- DHATURA., **ENG.** - THORNE APPLE., **GUJARATI**- DHATOIRA., **HINDI**- SADHA DHATURA, SAFED DHATURA, KALA DHATURA., **KAN.**- UMARATTY., **KASHMIRI**- DATHII., **KAN.**- DUTRO., **MAL.**- UMMATUM., **MARATHI**- DHOTARI., **PUNJABI**- TATTUR, DATURA., **TAMIL**- UMMATAI., **TELEGU**- UMMATHA., **LOCAL NAME**- DHATURA.

A shrub like herb glabrous or subglabrous with dichotamous branches, 0.6 - 1.2 mm high older branches marked with scars of fallen leaves. Leaves ovate, sinuate, unequal sided at the base. Flowers large, funnel-shaped, white, dirty whitish, violaceous, reddish - purple or purple on the outside and white within. Calyx base persistent, reflected corolla 5 toothed, capsules, globose or tuberculate prickled, or armed with short spines on a short curved stalk becoming inclined or nodding, opening irregularly. Seeds light brown. Flowers and fruits - January - April.

It is found throughout India occasionally grown in garden. They also grow commonly in waste places throughout India from Kashmir to Malabar.

MEDICINAL USE : The plant has narocotic anodyne and antispasmodic properties, analogous to those of belladonna. It causes dilation of the pupil when locally applied as aqueous. solution. Dried seeds are thought to be more powerful for sudorific than the leaves. Uaidyas regard the drug as intoxicant, emetic, digestive, antispasmodic demulcent and anodyne and healing asthma & cough.

Properties and uses of this plant also resamble to D. INNOXIA MILL and are recognised in the N.P.E. under the name DATUPAE FOLIUM.

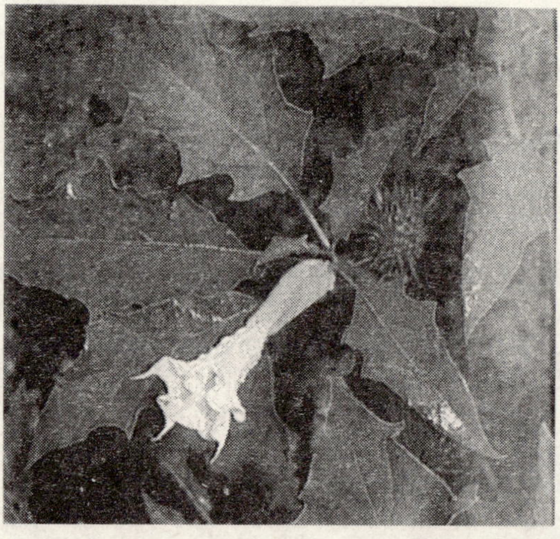

SOLANACEAE

DATURA STRAMONIUM LINN
(SYN. D. TATULA LINN)

BENGALI- SADA DHATURA., **SANSKRIT-** DHATURA., **PUNJABI-** TATTU DATURA., **MARATHI-** UMATA.

It is properly known as Thorne - Apple.

It is a strong smelling hairless annual, with a few large erect white or rarely voilet narrow funnel shaped flowers and with ovate, coarsely lobed or toothed leaves. Flowers 7.5 - 12 cm long by 2.5 - 7.5 cm across with 5 lobes and long pointed apices. calyx tubular, five ribbed and lobed, about 1/2 as long as corolla. Leaves C. 17 cm, stem 60 - 120 cm. Capsules ovoid, 4. valved, 3.5 to 7 cm. long. Covered with sharp slender spine, and with the enlarged base of the calyx below.

It is a native of tropical America. Naturalized in the Himalayas 200-2200 m cultivated areas, waste lands. March - April. Reported from Himalayas from Kashmir to Sikkim upto 9000 feet. Bulochistan hilly district of central and S. India.

MEDICINAL USE : Leaves and seeds antiseptic anodyne, narcotic fruits sedative and intoxicating. Juice of flowers for Earache. Juice of fruits is applied to scalp for curing dandruff and falling hair. This plant is also used in the making of atropine, hyoscine and hyoscymine. Drug consists of dried leves, flowering tops & seeds which are used in treatment of asthma. Kanaka Asava an Aryuvedic preparation contains STRAMONIUN as one of the main ingredient.

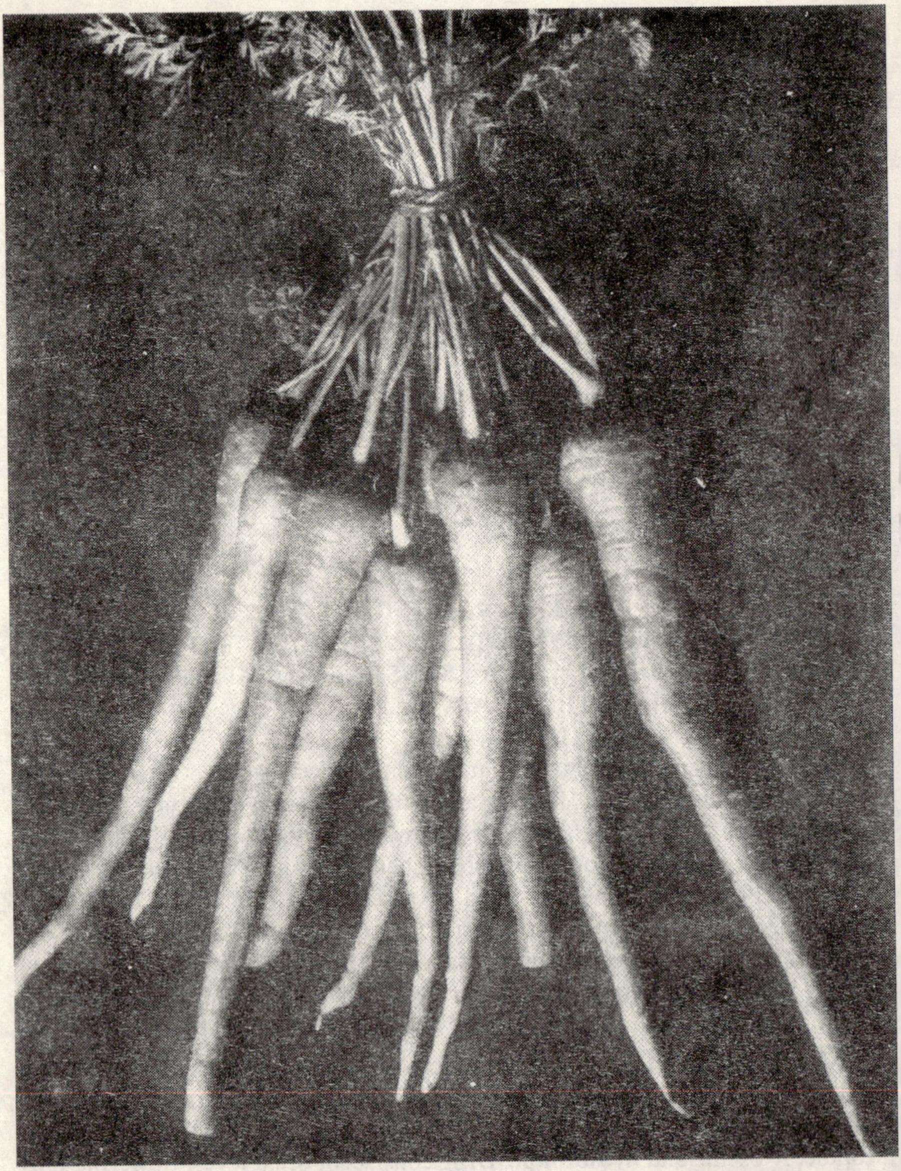

UMBELLIFERAE

DAUCUS CAROTA LINN
VAR. (D SATIVA D, C.)

S.- SHIKHAMOOL., **H. & B. & P.**- GAJAR., **M.**- GAJJARA & KELANGU., **ARBI.**- JAJAR, PITKAND., **FARSI**- JARDAK., **TEM.**- GAJJAR, GUDDA., **TEL.**- GAJAR KILLUNGU, KARATUKILLUNGU., **KAN.**- GAJERI., **LOCAL NAME**- GAJAR., **ENGLISH**- CARROT.

A hispid much branched herb. Leaves pinnetely decompound. Flowers white numerous in showy compound umbels. Outer flowers zygomophic. Frutis bristly along the secondary ridges, about 4x1 mm. It is extensively grown as a cold season crop for its fleshy, edible roots. Flowers and fruits - January - March.

It is probably originated in central Asia in the hills of the Punjab and Kashmir with a secondary centre of distribution in Asia, Europe and North Africa around the Mediterranean. It is cultivated through out India.

MEDICINAL USE : Seeds aromatic; stimulant, carminative useful in diseases of the kidney and in dropsy. nervine tonic. aphrodis, given in uterine pain.

Roots refrig. black carrots are used for making a beverage called kanji which is supposed to be a good appetizer. The orange coloured variety is rich in carotene, a precurser of Vit. A and contains apriciable quantities of thiamine and riboflavin Hence it is very good for eye diseases, hairs and skin, in general. Green carrot leaves are highly nutritive rich in protein, minerals and vitamins.

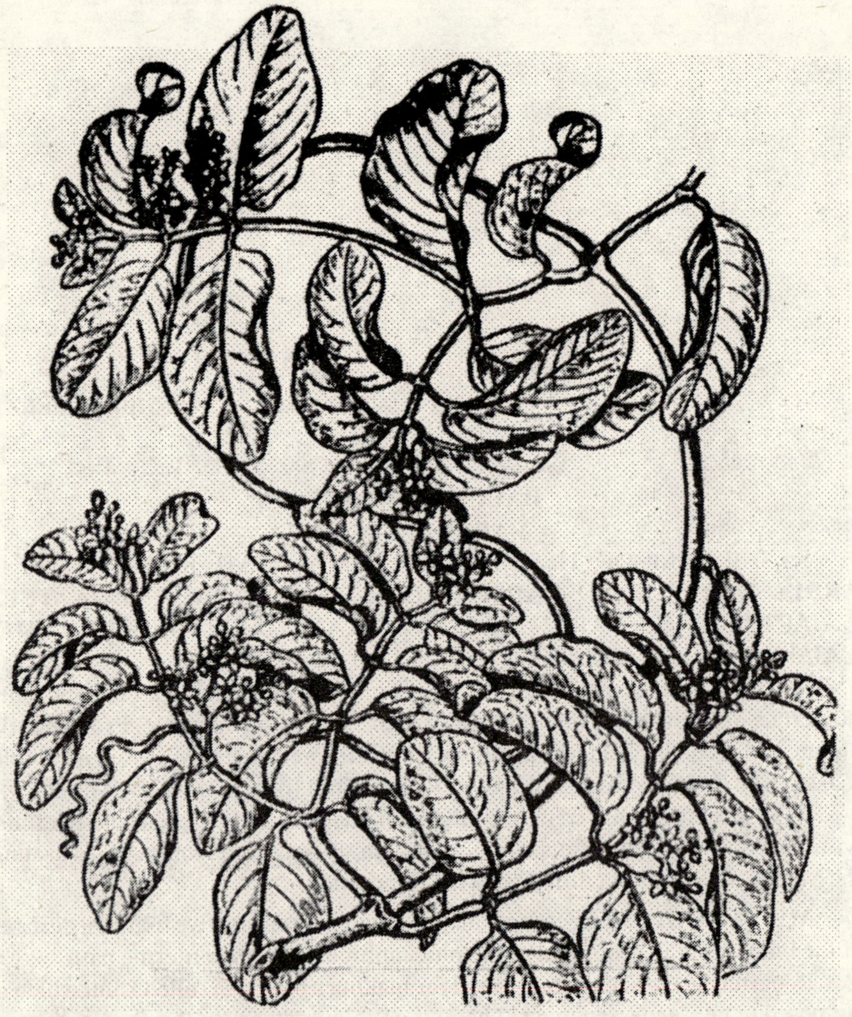

ASCLEPIDIACEAE

DECALEPIS HAMILTONII WIGHT AND ARN

TAMIL- MAHALI KIZHANGU., **KAN.-** MAKALI BERU.

It grows in the form of a hedge. The stem is jointed and knotty. The leaves are oval to accuminate, juicy and pulpy with 1-6 cm. radius. The roots emit a sharp pungent odour and are pungent in taste. It is considered as an agent in increasing the apetite and purifying the blood. It is reported from Deccan Peninsula and common in the forest areas of western ghats.

MEDICINAL USE : Roots are considered as an appetiser and blood purifier.

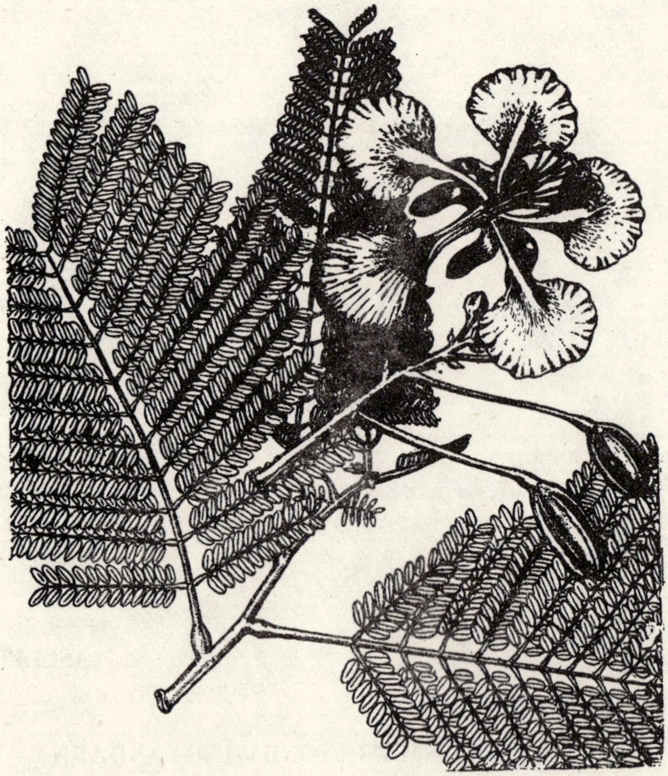

LEGUMINOSAE

DELONIX REGIA (BOJ) RAF
(SYN. POINCHIANA REGIA BOJ.EX. HOOK)

BO.- VAYNI., **TEL.**-VATANARAYANA., **TAM.**- VADANARAYANA., **LOCAL NAME :** GUL-MOHAR.

A magnificent tree with an umbrella shaped crown leaves bipinnate, feathery, 60cm long, leaflets about 1.2 x 0.5cm Flowers red or orgnage red.Pods 30x60x5 cm lated, seeds numrous, oblong. Flowers : April -September and fruit Nov-April. Commonly planted in gardens, squares and avenues for ornamental purposes and for the shade given by its dense foliage. The flowering period is irregular, almost throughout the year. The tree often produces vegetative buds after the 1st few showers. Very likely introduced in India. Reported to ocean in same parts of Kathiawar & South India and frequently planted as an avenue tree.

MEDICINAL USE : Leaves used for rheumatism and flatulense. Bark-In Indochina considered antiper; and febge.

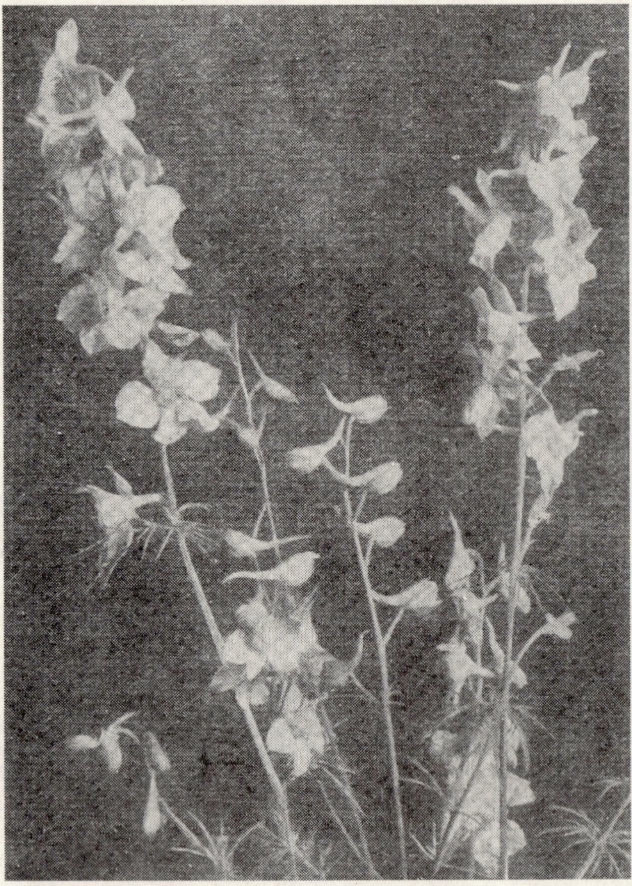

RANUNCULACEAE

DELPHINIUM AJACIS LINN

ENGLISH- LARKSPUR.

It is an annual or perenial winter plant visually it is a great pleasure giving plant. Many individual strains and mixtures are available. Colours include blue, purple, pink, white and red. Single or double flowers are produced on erect stems up to 30-120cms. (48 inch) tall. in long recemes. The plant spread to about 30 cms (12 inch) Delphinium is distinguised by its irregular flowers (symmetrical in one plain only) with 5 outer coloured petals, the upper most with a backward projecting spur, and 4 shorter inner petals, the upper two forming nector - secreting spur which are inserted in the outer spur. Leaves with rounded blade 5-15 cms. across hand shaped cut into 5-9 lobes with rounded blade. Stem leaves widely spaced up. stamens 8 follicles, usually 3. The seeds are squarish in shape, and are of buff or brown coloured.

It is commonly cultivated in gardens throughout india.

MEDICINAL USE : seeds insecticidal, in tincture form applied externally for the destruction of lice in hair. The seeds contain alkoloids and an oil. The insecticidal property is attributed by some of the oils and alkoloids.

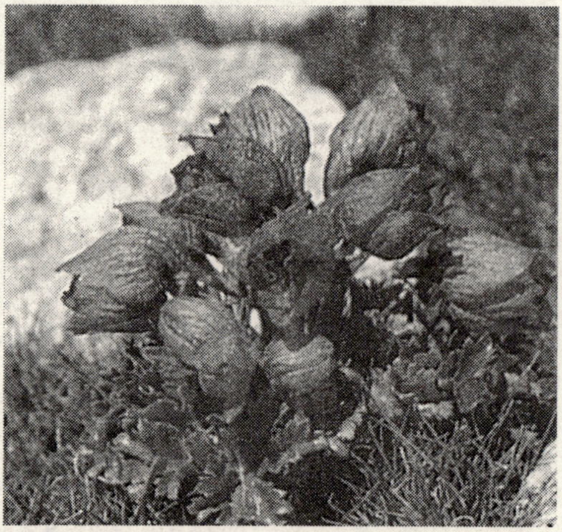

RANUNCULACEAE

DELPHINIUM BRUNONIANIUM ROYLE

PUNJABI- LASKAR., **ENG.-** MUSK LARKSPUR.

It is an annual herb ranging from 30 to 40 cm. distinguished by its large woolly- haired often conspicuously veined blue to purple flowers with broad blunt spurs, borne in small dense cluster on short stems to C.20 cm. Flowers 3-5 cm. including spur appearing inflated and rather papery. Inner petals blackish, leaf blade rounded in outline 3-8 cm. across lobed to 2/3 rds. The lobes toothed. Some plants with a strong musky odour, as also varying in degrees of hairiness. Follicles 4-5.

It is recorded from western Himalayas and Tibet, 13000 - 17000 ft, also from pakistan to east Nepal, S.E. Tibet 4300-5500 in stony slope, in drier areas July-Sept.

MEDICINAL USE : Juice of leaves used to destroy ticks in animals (J. Linn. Soc. Botny, 1881, 25).

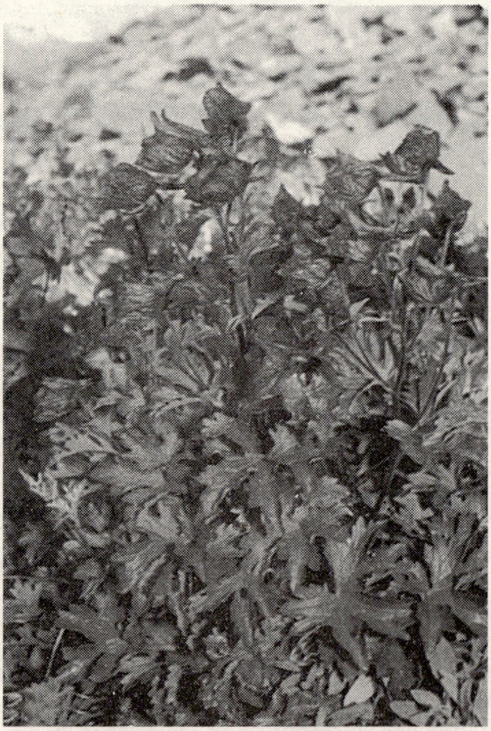

RANUNCULACEAE

DELPHINIUM CASHMERANUM ROYLE

It resembles D. BRUNONIANUM Royle but differs in not being glandular hairy in the upper parts and with smaller less inflated flowers mostly 2-3 cm, bluish - purple with a stout spine to 1.5 cm, hairy and veins. Flowers several long stalked, clusterd into a dense somewhat flat, topped head. Leaves deeply lobed, 3.5 across follicles 3-7.

It is recorded from West Himalayas, Kashmir and Tibet at 10,000 - 16,000 ft. also from Pakistan to Uttar Pradesh 27.00 - 4500 m. Alpine slopes, also in irrigated land in Ladakh August - September.

MEDICINAN USE : Roots used medicinally.

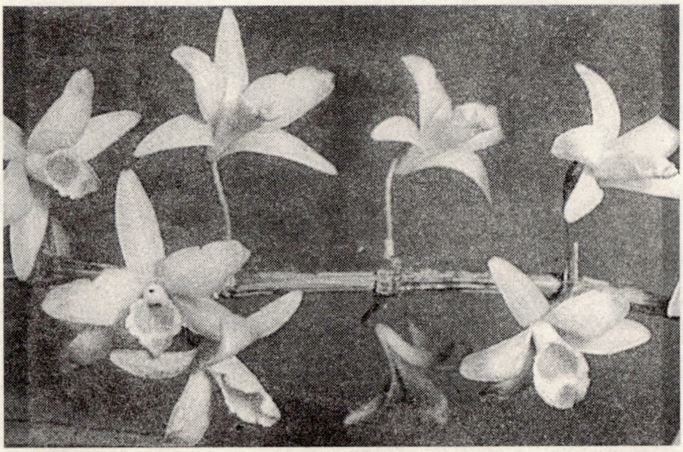

ORCHIDACEAE

DENDROBIUM MACRAEI LINDL. (SYN.DESMOTRICHUM FIMBRIATUM HOOK)

BENGALI- JABANTI., **MARATHI & SANK-** JIVANTI., **HINDI-** JAIVANTI., **BO.- H & S-** JIVANTI.

Flowers showy,brilliant yellow with a rounded wavy shortly fringed lip,sometimes with a large radish - brown central patch. Flowers 5-7.5 cm. across, in pendulous clusters of 7-12 borne towards the ends of the stemlike pseudo bulbs - flowering stem with sheathing bracts at base Leaves oblong - lanceolate long pointed, 9-15 cm. stem like pseudobulbs tapering upwards grooved, 60 - 150 cm.

It is also reported from C. Nepal to Bhutan. Burma 500.2400 m. Forest epiphyte April - May. A much branched plant often found in sikkim, khasia hills Konkan, Nilgiris and also common on hills of South India.

MEDICINAL USE : The whole plant is cooling, mucilaginous, light strengthening demulchant and tonic, given debility due to seminal discharges. The whole plant is used as decoction along with other drugs having similar properties. Used also in snake bite.

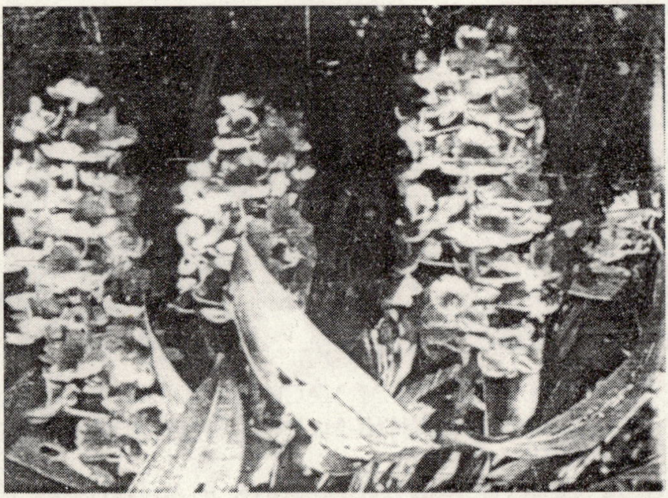

ORCHIDACEAE

DENDROBIUM CRUMENATUM SW.

It is reported from Andaman islands. Common Plant of the Malay Peninsula, found also in ceylon, Burma, Southern China, & East wards to Amboina & the Philippines.

MEDICINAL USE : Used by Malays for infections of the brain & nerves and a conserve of the flowers & leaves used for cholera & pounded leaves for poulticing boils and pimples.

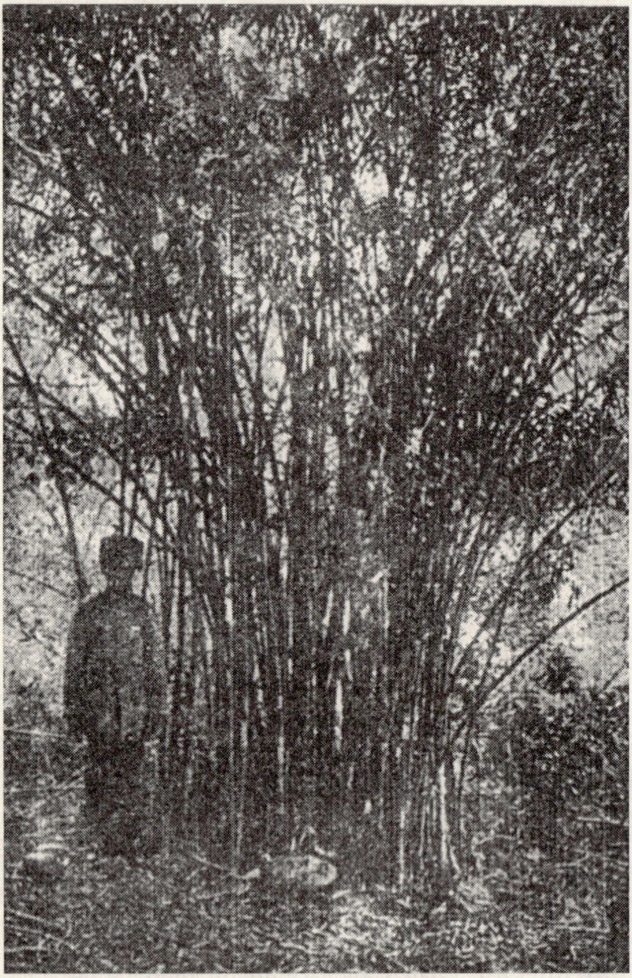

GRAMINEAE

DENDRO CALAMUS STRICTUS (ROXB.) NEES
(POUPULARLY KNOWN AS MALE BAM BOO-

S.-VANSHA., **TEL.**- SADANAPA BAS, S VEDMAU., **TAM.**- KALMUNGIL. **HINDI**- BANS- KABAN & B-KARAIL.

Forms densely packed clumps 7 - 15 mtr. high, of greyish green often blotched stems, with stiff spreading branches. Stem 5 - 8 cm. in diameter, internodes 10-25 cm. long, stem - sheaths hairless or with greyish - brown hairs, little shorter than the internodes. Leaves narrow lanceolate long. 10-25 cm. Final hairy on both sides, Flowers spiklets spiny tipped, in dense globular heads to 2.5 cm. borne along slender somewhat branched stems. braets hairy and with distinctive spiny tips, flowering sporadically.

It is reported from Pakistan to Burma. India to 1500 mtr. common around villages in Nepal. In deciduous forests and in dry or moderately dry regions practically all over India upto 3,500 ft.

MEDICINAL USE : Silicones better tonic, astrin leaves - Ecbolics to animals.

It secretes a substance known as Vansh lochan which is used for expelling stones from the body kidney and bladder making skin rich and healthy.

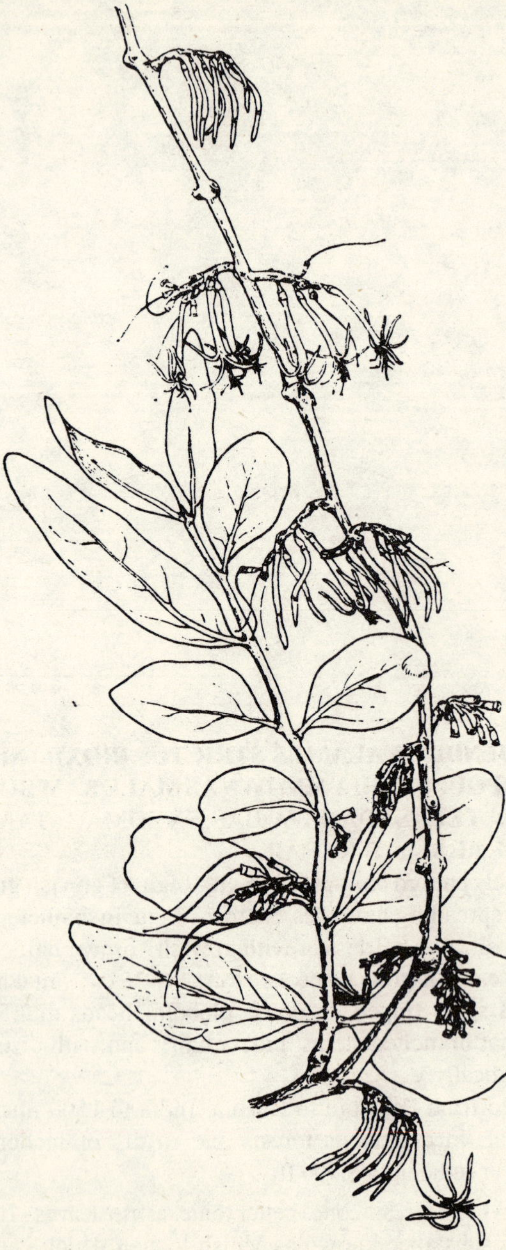

LORANTHACEAE

**DENDROPHTHOE FALCATA (LINN. F.) ETTINGSH.
(SYN. LORANTHUS FALCATUS LINN
L. LONGIFLORUS DESR.**

LOCAL NAME- BANDA, BARAMANDA., **H.**- BANDA., **GUJARAT**- VANDO., **P.**- BANDA., S.- VANDA., **TAM.**- PULLURI., **TEL.**- BADNIKA.

A much branched, stout leafy, partial parasite. Leaves opposite, 10-15 x 5.8 cms. Leathery, variable in shape 6-12 x 2.5 - 6 cm. brittle, dull coloured, midrib distinct in the lower part. Flowers vemllion or deep orange, 50 x 4 mm, crowded in short racemes on leafless nodes, bracteate, Stamens exserted stigmas knob shaped, Fruits ovoid oblong black when ripe. Flowers November - January and Fruits February - April met during cold season on the ridge and also in gardens, Decean pennisula.

MEDICINAL USE : Leaves used for checking abortion and for stones in the blader and kidney.

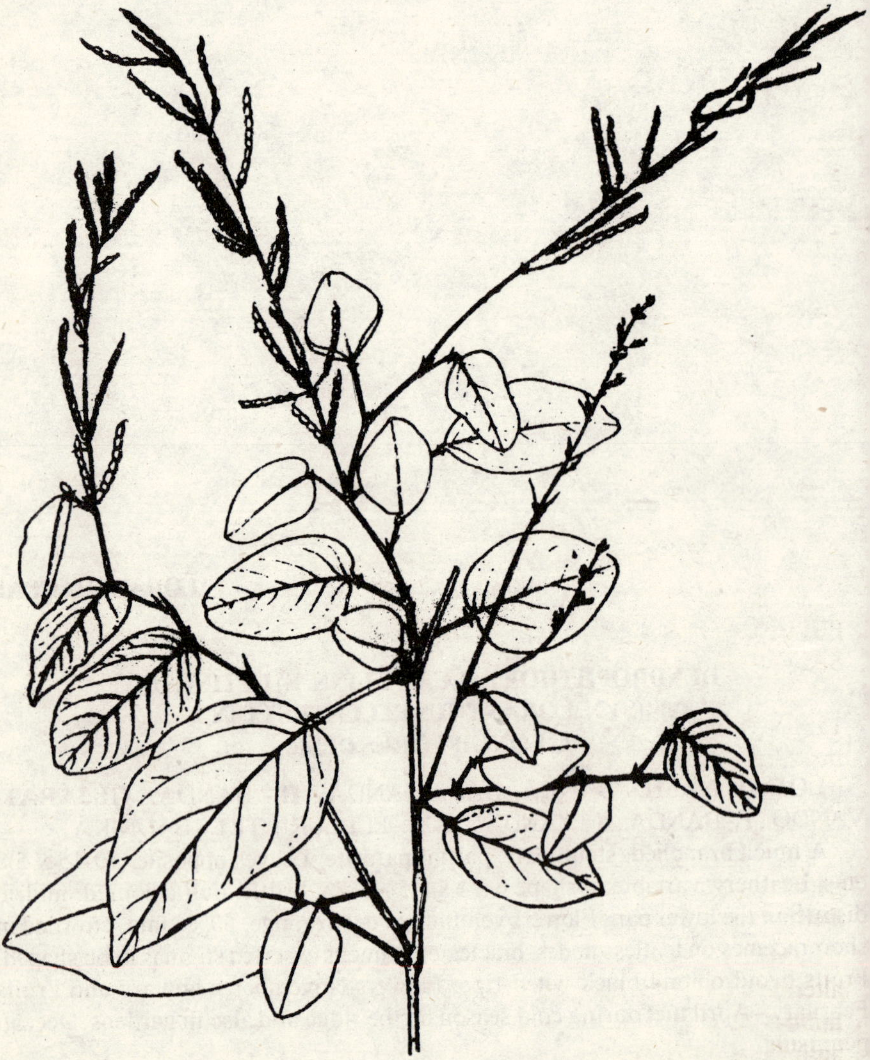

PAPILIONACEAE

DESMODIUM GANGETICUM DC.
(SYN. HEDYSARUM GANGETICUM LINN)

S. & BO.- SHALAPARNI., **HINDI**- SARIVAN., **BENGALI**- SALPANI., **TAMIL**- PULLADI., **TEL.**- GITANARAM., **KAN.**- SHALIPARNI., **MAR. KON & GUJ.**- SALVAN., **LOCAL NAME :** SALPALNI.

It is an erect or decumbent undershrub or shrub, 60-120 cm. tall. Leaves upto 15 x 8 cm, ovate - eliptic to ovate. Oblong, grey - puberulous beneath. Flowers lilac, in several fascicles arranged in racemes. Pods deeply indented on lower suture, indehiscent, hooked - hairy, 2.-2.5 x 0.3 cm. The flowers and fruits from August to November.

It is found common in the moonsoon and post monsoon period in open lands gardens and canal banks. Also found as an undergrowth in the fruits orchards of Delhi. Outer Himalayas, upto 5,000 feet and throughout the plains of India.

MEDICINAL USE : It is a bitter tonic, febrifuge, digestive anticatarrhal, alterative and tonic. The root of D. GANGETICUM is one of the ingredients of a famous Ayurvedic preparation Dasham cola kwaatha which is considered to be antipyretic, alterative and a bitter tonic. It is reported to be beneficial in the treatment of typhoid, billiousness and also as diuretic and aphrodisiac.

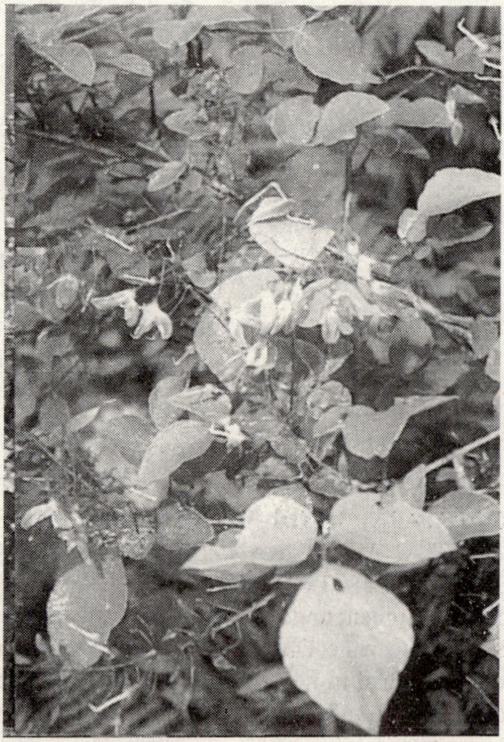

FABACEAE (PAPILIONACEAE)

DESMODIUM ELEGANS. D.C

It is a deciduous shrub with trifoliate leaves with broad leaflets, and with terminal spike - like clusters to 30 cm. long of pink to dark purple flowers. Flowers. 7 - 13 mm, borne on slender stalks. Standard, rounded; calyx 2-3 mm with blunt lobes, shaggy - haired. Leaflets rounded to mostly 2-4 cm paler and hairy beneath, the middle leaflet long - stalked; young leaves often densely silvery white haired. Stems 1.8 - 3mm, pod 3-6 cm long by 6mm broad, the lower margin conspicuously indented between the seeds, the upper nearly straight, hairless, or densely silvery - haired.

Mostly it is a subtropical plant reported from Afghanistan to South West China. 1200-1300 in Forests, shrubberies open slopes, common June - August.

MEDICINAL USE : Roots - carminative; tonic; diur. Leaves - galact. Decoct. of whole plant - given in stomach and abdominal complaints.

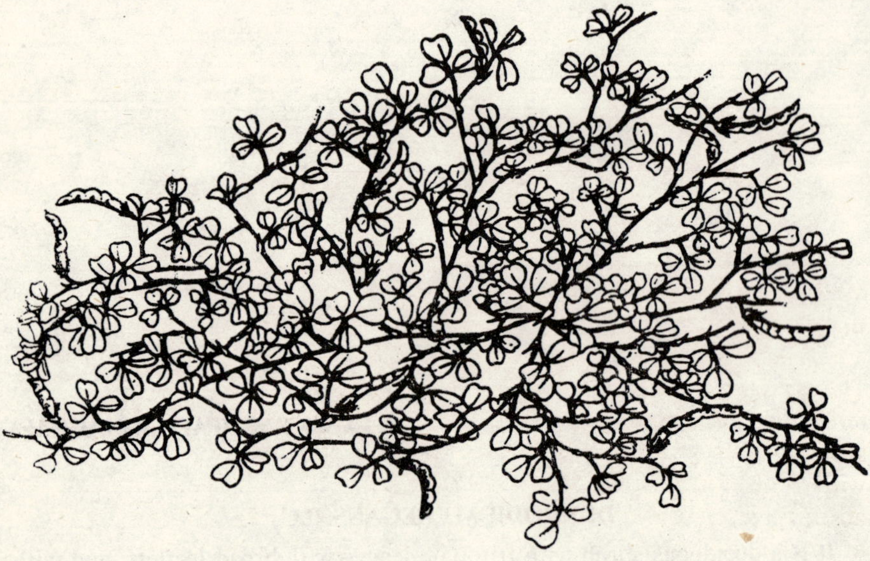

FABACEAE

DESMODIUM TRIFLORUM (L/D.C.)
(SYN HEDYSARUM TRIFLORUM L)

HINDI- KUDALIYA., **BENGALI-** KUDALIYA., **MARATHI-** JUNGALI-METHI & RAM METHI., **TEL.-** MUNTAMANDU., **TAMIL-** SIRUPULLADI., **BOMBAY-** JUNGLI METHI.

A much branched gregarious, wiry, trailing perenial herb rooting at the nodes. The plant roots and spread over the ground forms a close mat. Branches slender terete, finely downy. Leaves - compound, petiole 2-3 inch; leaflets thick, flexible, subcoriaceous, green, glabrescent above, more or less densely persistenly matted with whitish silky hairs beneath, ends are broad, obovate 12.4 with long entire or abscurely repand, base deltoid or rounded. Flowers are in racemes copious, lax, often a footlong axillary and terminal, the latter often copiously painted with lower branch again compound. Flowers pink or purplish 1-3 in the axils of leaves. Pedicls 1/4 - 3/8 moderately long braets, lanceolate, corolla large, joints many thinly clothed with adpressed silky hairs, ascending, finely downy, calyx 1/8, downy, teeth deltoid shorter than the tube. Corolla 3/8 - 1/2 pod 2-3 curved, flat indented on the lower edge 1/4 broad. joints 6-9 longer than broad, seeds brown. The flowering and fruiting season is during rains and early winter.

It is present all along the Himalayas from the upper Punjab to Tavoy, temperate, and tropical zones ascending to 4000 ft. Locally it is common in lawns and pasture fields.

MEDICINAL USE : The plant is utilized in indigenous medicine for a variety of purposes. Fresh leaves are applied to wounds and absecesses. They are also used internally as galaetogogue and for diarrohea.

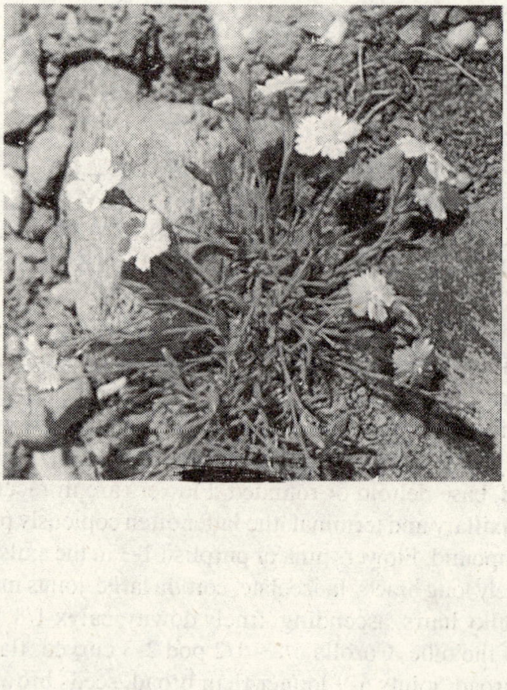

CARYOPHYLLACEAE

DIANTHUS ANATOLICUS BOISS
IND. BOISS - KANTURIYAN.

ENG.- SWEET WILLIAM., **IND. & BAZ.**- KANTUNIYAN.

It is a slender densely tufted perennial, with many ascending stems 15-25 cm. bearing one or more pink flowers C. 1 cm across. Petals with a broad toothed blade, without hairs on the upper surface calyx narrow cylinderical with 1-2 cm, bracts usually 6, broad and with a tooth like tip. Leaves linear, 1-2 cm, stiff with a thick midrib and margin.

It is distributed from West Himalayas to West Tibet and Kashmir. it is also reported from Pakistan to Kashmir. West Asia 1800-4500 on stony ground, common in Ladakh-July - August.

MEDICINAL USE : The plant is used as an antiperiodic in intermittant fevers.

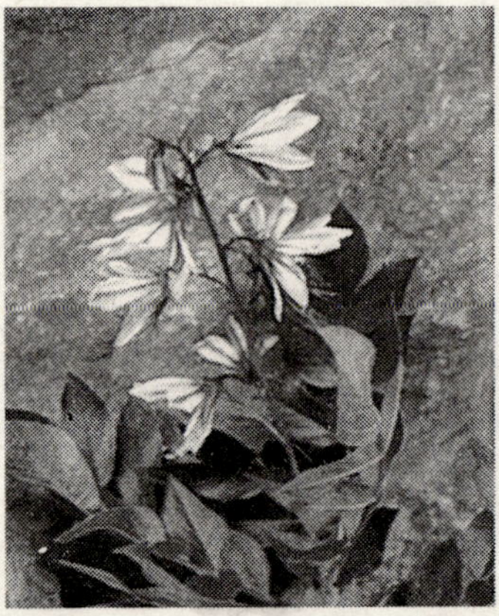

RUTACEAE

DICTAMNUS ALBUS LINN

It is popularly known as BURNING BUSH.

It is a strongly aromatic bushy perenial plant. Stems, bracts and sepals densely covered with conspicuous dark glands, which give a strong acid aroma when crushed. Leaves pinnate with 4-6 pairs of leathery, elliptic gland dotted finely toothed leaflets, stems robust, 30-60 cm. Inflorescence terminal, branched with a lax spike of large conspicuous pink or white flowers, Flowers irregular 2.54 cm, petels 4.5, lanceolate. Unequal to 2.5 cm. streaked and dotted with boilet, stamens 12-15, longer, with purple filament and green anthers. Fruit a capsale 1.5 cm, deeply divided into 5 segments which split at the apex, brightly glandular.

It is found in temperate West Himalayas, from Kashmir to Kunawar, 6,000 - 8000 ft. Common in Panaji.

MEDICINAL USE : Root bark aromatic, bitter, used in intermitent fever, nervous diseases and amenor; in Indo-China and Malaya a decoct. of the root given for scabies and other skin infections and hysteria.

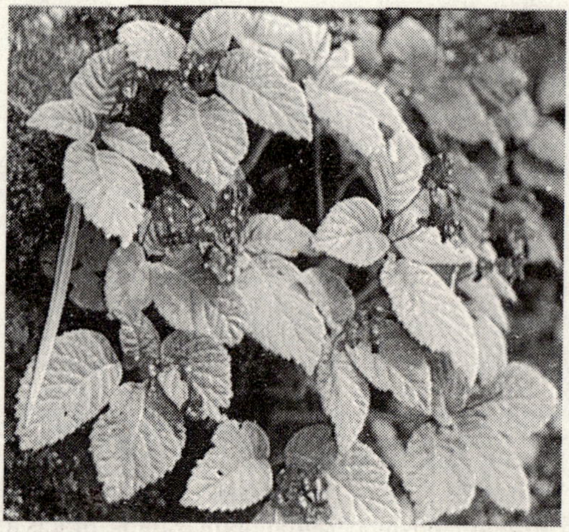

GESNERIACEAE

DIDYMOCARPUS AROMATICA WALL.
(SYN. D. PRIMULIFOLIUS D. DON)
(SYN. D. PEDICELLATA R.B.R.)

HINDI- PATHAR PHORIP, KUM KUMA.

Flowers, larger, dark purple C. 1. 6cm long and nearly hairless and pink. Calyx smaller, cup shaped C. 4mm, With shallow triangular blunt lobes, and glaudular hairy inflorecence, Several or many borne in a terminal branched cluster, corolla is cylindical tubular, tube one and twice as long as the red bell shaped, hairless calyx which has rounded lobes; bracts broadly elliptic fused below 4-6mm long. Leaves often in an apparent whorl of 4 borne at the top of the stem, or leaves opposite and arranged up stem, broadly elliptic to 10cms finely toothed; densely woolley haired above and often so beneath stem 4-30cm capsule are 2-4cm. Stigma oblong, notched; fertile stamens; stamens 2 and 2+3, rudimentary; It is found from utter pradesh to sikkim 2000-3000 in rocks in forests; sometimes epiphytic. June-July, It grows in sub-tropical western Himalayas from chamba to kumaon 100-200m.

MEDICINAL USE : leaves are used as a cure for stones in kidney and bladder.

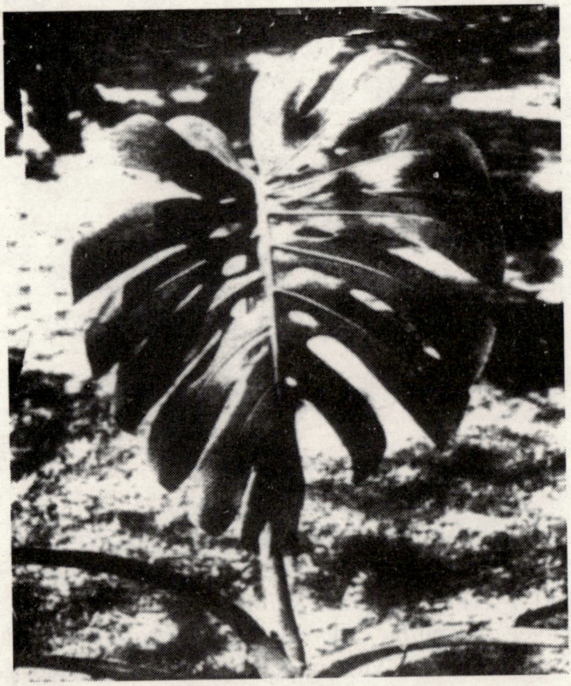

ARACEAE

DIEFENBACHIA SEGUINE (JACK)-SCHOTT

A genus of very wide variety of evergreen/climbers shade loving and fast growing which produce very decorative foliage and climb with the help of their aerial roots produced from the stems. It looks at its best if allowed to grow up at tree or trained on a log of wood covered with moss. The foliage is glossy and leathery of deep green colour, plain or variegated or mottled, with or without marked or shaded veins and with or without cut margins. There are species producing beautiful crimson coloured flowers.

It is reported from West Indies. Cultivated in India for ornamental purposes.

MEDICINAL USE : Juice of plant poisonous. Leaves used in Malaya for the treatment of rheumatism and swellings: they are either powdered and applied as poultice or boiled in oil and used as embrocation.

Rhizome contains calcium oxalate

(Burkill, I, 807, wehmer, I. 136)

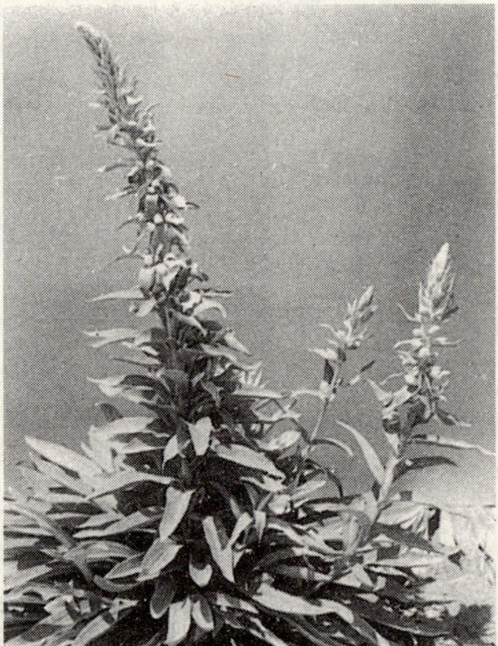

SCROPHULARIACEAE

DIGITALIS LANATA EHRH.

ENGLISH- GRECIAN FOXGLOVE, WOOLLY FOXGLOVE.

It's commercial name is Digitalis.

It is a perennial or biennial creeping herb, 2 - 3 ft. high, pubescent. The leaves are corwded in the lower portion of the stem which is about five feet in height. Leaves greyish green, somewhat hairy or glabrous, decurrent, sessile, oblong lanceolate often arranged in a rosette form at the base. Flowers are small and downy, creamy, yellow or purplish in colour and terminal in position. They are either axillary, solitary or fascicled, spikes, ebraceteolate. Calyx is companulate, 4-8 feet corolla. subrotate; lobes 4-8 spreading. subequal stamens as many as the corolla - lobes or one fewer; anthers sagitate, touching stigma capitate, Capsule membranous, compressed, loculicidal, valves septiferous, seeds few, plano - or coneavo - convex, regulose.

It is known as a native of Europe and Asia introduced into India and are cultivated for medicinal purposes. For medicinal purposes mainly in Kashmir, Utterpradesh, Ootacamund and some other mountaneous regions. the plant prefers altitude of 1500-2400 mtr. and a calcarious soil.

MEDICINAL USE : The therapeutic activity of dried leaf is due to cardiatonic glycoside digitoxin which strengthens weekened heart and allows it to function more effectively. It is also used in some ointments for application on burns and wounds. The leaves are dried and are the chief source of the drug digoxin, which is highly valued in medicine for its diuretic and cardiotonic effect.

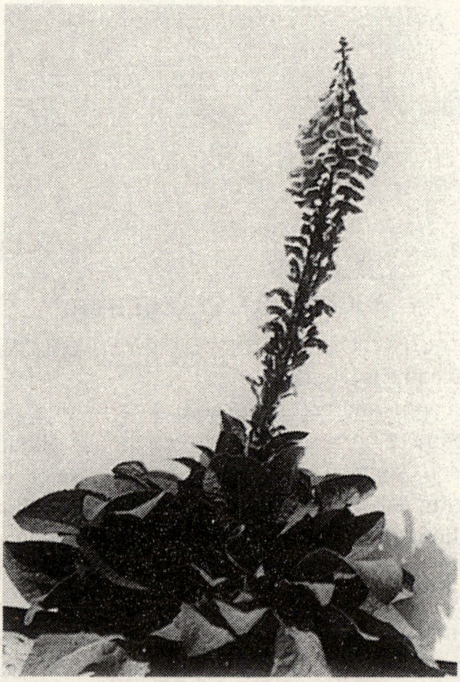

SCROPHULARIACEAE.

DIGITALIS PURPUREA LINN.
SYN. D. TOMENTOSA LINK AND HOFFMGG

ENGLISH- COMMON FOXGLOVE.

Grown as a biennial, they will thrive in a moist and shady place in the garden. It flowers in the year after sowing. Its excelsier hybrid strains - ornamental. It produces the familiar long spikes 1- 1.5 cm (3-5 feet) bearing tubular bell shaped flowers of marroon or purple blue, yellow and white only on one side and they are distinctly spotted in the throat of each bloom.

It is a biennial and sometimes perennial cultivated plant 60 - 180 cm. tall. In the 1st year Shrunken and soft hairy leaves arise in the form of rossets. Leaves are 15-30 cm long. oval to obovate linear. They contain long winged bracts. In the 2nd year one long straight flowering axis arise in which full and half leaves arise without bracts, only on one side.

Cultivated in Kashmir at Tangmarg and Kishtwary 6000-7000 ft. Darjeeling district and Nilgiris.

MEDICINAL USE : Leaves used for certain conditions of the heart mainly as a cardiac stimulant and tonic. D. PURPUREA LINN (Eng. Fox Glove)

Mainly cultivated in Jammu and Kashmir at 2000-3000 m. Darjeeling district and in the Nilgiris. In properties it is identicle to D. LANATA. It is one of the chief and renowned constituent in cardiac therapy.

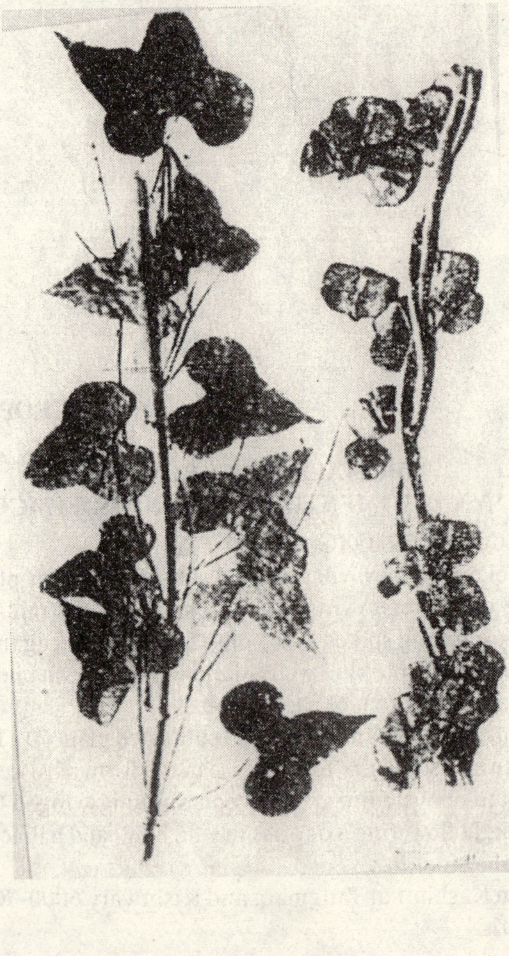

DIOSCOREACEAE

DIOSCOREA DELTOIDEA WALL EX KUNTH.

KASHMIR- KINS, KILOTI, **P.**-KNISS, KINTA.

It is distributed north-western Himalayas from kashmir to Punjab. East ward to Nepal and China at 3000 - 10000 feet.

MEDICINAL USE : Tubers yield cortisone, steroid harmone which is used in rheumatic diseases and opthalmic disorders. Also steroidal sapogenins are yielded which are considered as source material for manufacture of oral contraceptives.

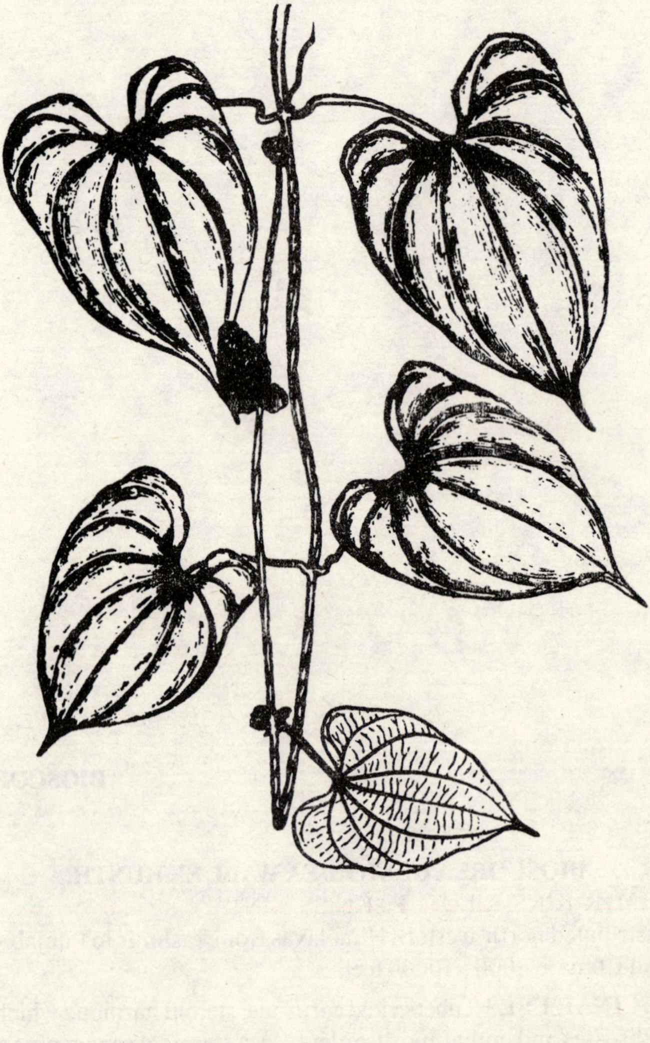

DIOSCOREACEAE

DIOSCOREA ACULEATA LINN

(SYN. D. ESCULENTA BARKITL., D. FASICULATA ROXB., D. SPINOSA ROXB., D. SATIVA L.

BENGALI- BHIRA SUTHNI, SUSNIALU., **BO.-** KANGAI., **TAMIL-** MUSILAM VALLI KILANGU, SIRUVALLI KILANGU., **TEL.-** SILAKADOMP TIPPATIGA, TIPP, TIGA., **K.-** MUDDUGAMOUS., **MAL.-** MULLOO, KILANGU, CHAROO., **MARATHI-** KANGAI., **ENG.-** LESSER YAM, KAREN POTATO., **HINDI-** SUSNIALU.

Found in Malabar. Coromondal coast in Dacan, Madhya Bharat, Uttar Pradesh, Bihar, Orrisa, West Bengal and Assam, ascending to 3000 feet in the eastern Himalayas. Also in Khasi, Nagahills, Garo Hills and Andaman Islands.

MEDICINAL USE : Grated tubers, used as application for swellings. Rhizomes contain sufficient quantities of diosgenin which may be exploited for manafaeture of precursors of steroid hormones.

DIOSCOREA BULBIFERA LINN

(SYN. D. CRISPATA ROXB.)

It is popularlay known as potato yam or Air Potato,

HINDI- RATALU, SUARALU, PITALU., **BENGALI-** BANALLU, KUKURALU GAICHA ALU., **MARATHI-** MANAKUND, KARUKARINDA, GATHALU., **TELGU-** CHEDUPADDY-DUMPA, MALAKAKA-YAPENDALAMU., **TAM.-** KODIKILANGU, PANNUKILANGU., **KAN.-** HEGGENASU., **MAL.-** KATTU-KACHIL., **LOCAL NAME-** RATALU.

A large unarmed climbing herbaceious perennial with long tuberous roots and claws with small globular tubers twining to the left. Tubers large, variable in form, stem slender green or purple, quite glabrous, stem terete bulbiferous. Leaves : Opposite and alternate, very variable in size attaining 14 inch in length and breadth, membranous dark green, usually very deeply ovate conate but sometimes with only a shallow broad sinus acuminate cuspidate or caudate 7-9 costate. Flowers small or minute, panicled racemose or spicate, always monosexual, male spikes slender panicled almost capillary 1-4 inches, flowers crowded or scatterd very variable in sizes, green or purplish, sepals 1-10-1/4 long fleshy, petals rather narrower, filaments much shorter than perianth anthers minute, didymous. Female spikes 4-10 inch long, pendulous flowers 1/8-1/4 long sepals as in male. Capsule 2/3-1 by 1/3-1/2 inch membranous, three winged. Seeds flat or with a broad globose basal wing. It is found commonly throughout India ascending upto 6,000 feet in the Himalayas. Locally it is cultivated on a small scale in gardens for its edible tubers.

MEDICINAL USE : Tubres are used in piles, dysentry, syphilis, and applied to ulecers.

DIOSCOREA ALATA LINN (SYN. D.ATROPURPUREA ROXB)

SANS.- PINDALU, HB CHUPRI ALU., **BO.-** CHOPRIALU., **TEL.-** PENDALAMU., **TAM.-** PERUMVALLI KIZHANGU. Cultivated practically in all the states in India

MEDICINAL USE : Tubers anthelm useful in leprosy, piles, gonorrea. Tox alk, (Meded pituin, Batavies, 1894, 68, 1899, 123)

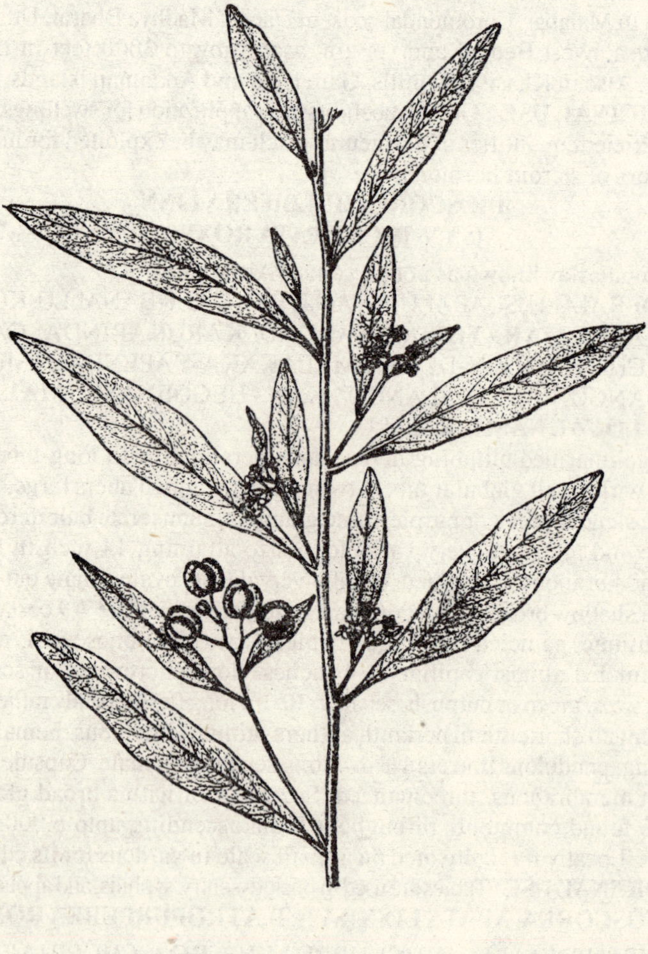

SAPINDACEAE

DODONAEA VISCOSA (LINN) JACQ.)

H.- AHAI, SANADHA., **BO.**- BANDURI., **BOMBAY**- JAKMI., **TAM.**- VALARI., **TEL.**-BANDEDU., **P.**-BENGMENU., **KAN.**-BANDRE, HUNGRIKAAE., **MAL.**-UNATTRUBI., **BIHAR**-MHENDHI., **ORRISA**-MOHRA.

It is an evergreen shrub to 5 m, with leathery bright green shining oblanceolate entire leaves which are commonly sticky with yellow resin, leaves alternate 3-9 cm. long flowers are sexed, 3-5 mm across, greenish yellow in terminal and lateral clusters C. 2.5 cm long; sepals 4-5, blunt, petals absent; stamens usually 8 (5+5 two whorls, 2 stamens are missing). Ovary superior, carpels, with 1-6 chambers each 1-seeded. Fruit is compressed capsule C 1.5 cm. with 2-4 valves, each valve with a broad membraneous wing. It is often gregarious in August - February, fruiting January - June.

It is quick growing shrub often used for hedges. It is reported from Afghanistan to Himachal Pradesh India, Pantropical to 1500 m. open slopes, often gregarious August - February. Almost throughtout India North West Himalayans upto 4500 ft. in South India ascending to 8000 ft. the Nilgiris commonly planted in Northern India, as a hedge plant.

MEDICINAL USE : Leaves - febge sudorific in gout and rheumatism, for wounds swelings and burns. Bark employed in astrin baths and fermentations. Plant fish - poison. The bark and leaves contain crystalised dodogen which resembles sapogenin virtue.

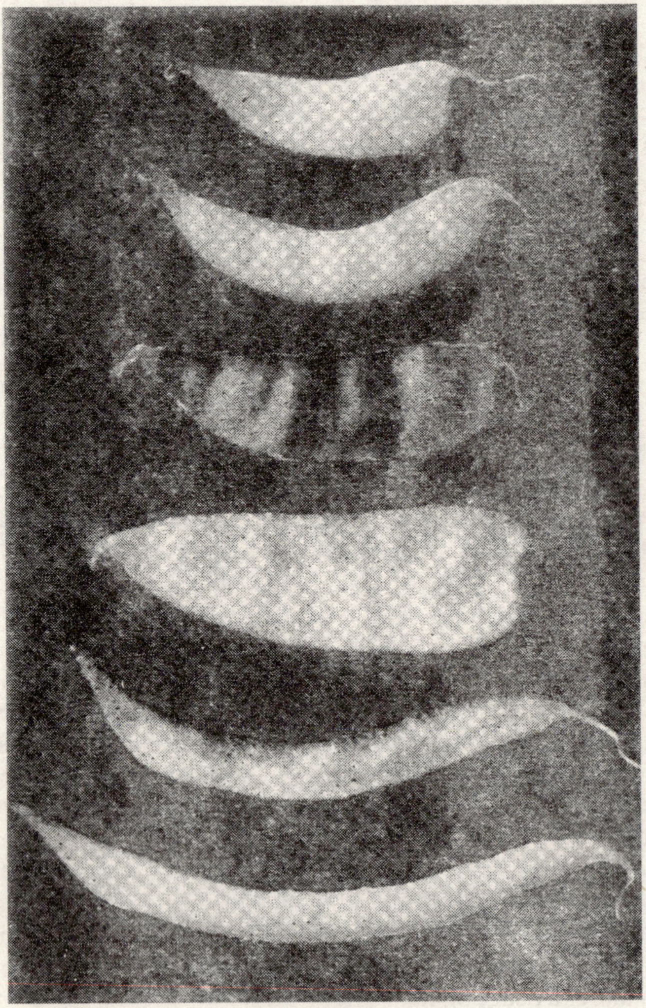

PAPILIONACEAE

DOLICHOS LABLAB LINN
SYN. L. PURPUREUS (L) SWEET)
" L. VALGARIS SAVI
"L. NIGER MEDI.

ENGLISH- LABLAB., **HINDI**- SEM., **LOCAL NAME**- SEM., **SANSKRIT**- SHIMBI., **BENGALI**- MAKHAM- SIM., **BOMBAY**- PANTI., **TAMIL**- AVARAI.

A sub globose perenial wide twining or creeping herb generally 3 foliate. minute subpersistent bracts. Bracteolas and stipules. Stipules lanceolats, basifixed, leaflets as broad as long, always entire, acute 126 inch long, broad ovate or deltoid membranous rarely down before beneath. Flower middle sized white or pink, racamose or axillary. racemes and peduncles each reaching 1/2 - 3/4 ft. long. Pedicels short densely fascicled, 1/8 or finally 1/4 bracteoles oblong, sometimes as long as the calyx 1/8-1/4 " teeth short deltoid, calyx tube companulate, corolla much exerted, petals usually equal in length, keel obtuse or rostrate, not spiral reddish or white 1/2 - 3/4 stamens diadelphous, anthers uniform, ovary nearly sessile, many ovuled. Style filiform or thickned upwards bearded down the interface or round the terminal stigma, style thickned upwards narrowed to the base, bearded down the inner edge. keel narrow rostrate, pod 1.1/2 - 2 by 1/2 - 3/4 tipped with the hooked persistant base of the style. Flowers september - October. Fruits found in cold season.

Wild and universally cultivated throughout India ascending in the Himalayas from 6000 - 7000 feet.

MEDICINAL USE : The roots are poisnous. Seeds are considered fabrifuge, stomachic, anti sposmodic and aphrodis.

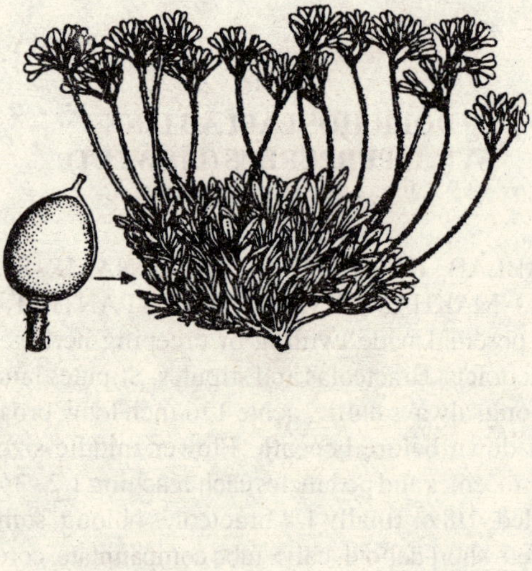

CRUCIFERAE

DRABA MURALLIS LINN
or
DRABA SETOSA ROYLE

A small cushion - forming plant with tiny rosettes about 6-8mm across of densely hairy leaves and erect leafless stems bearing a lax cluster of few yellow flowers. Flowers C 3-5mm across; sepals much shorter than petals, with papery margins, hairless, leaves linear 1-1. 5mm long with bristly margins, flowering stems, slender 3-4cm. Fruit elliptic 4-6mm hairless.

Found in Kashmir upto 6000 ft.

MEDICINAL USE : In spain plant used as antiscorn.

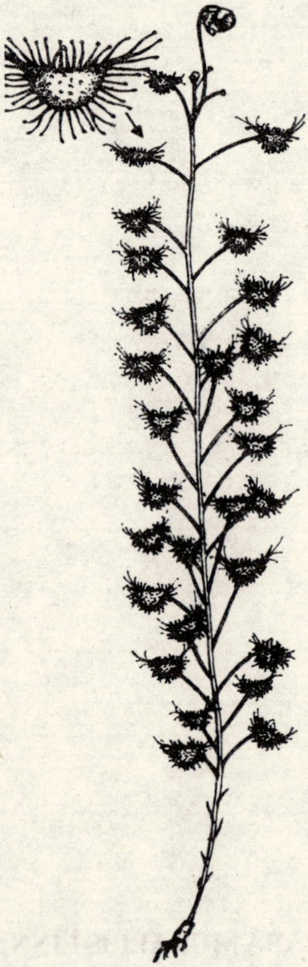

DROSERACEAE

DROSERA PELTATA SM
VARIETY D. LUNATA BUCH - HAERAM- EX. DC

H.- MUKHAJALI., **PUNJABI**- CHIBRA.

It is known as a carnivorous plant. It is distinguished by its half moon shaped - leaf baldes C - 6mm across, with the upper side of the blades cared with long red glistening gland - tipped hairs on their leaves. These attract insects which are trapped in the sticky gum. The leaf blade then folds round the prey and slowly digest it. Flowers white, small C-6mm across, in terminal branched clusters, petals 48 (usually5) stamens many; sepals variable, toothed, slightly fringed, ovary with 3 styles. Leaves stalks, borne alternately on an erect slender stem 10-30 cm (in var. LUNATA). According to C.B. Clarke smaller rosette leaves absent at flowering.

It is found in Uttar pradesh to South West China, India, S.East Asia, Australia, 1500 - 3600 metre grassy slopes, not common July - August. Hilly regions through out India upto 10,000 ft. in the Himalayas and 8000 ft. in the Nilgiris.

MEDICINAL USE : Crushed leaves with or without salt used as blistering agent. Plant used in the preparation of gold bhasm which is used as antisyp. and alter. and tonic. Leaves contain a protolytic enzyme of the pepsin type (whomer, I, 420: Dymock, Warden and Hooper, I, 593, Nadkarni, 314).

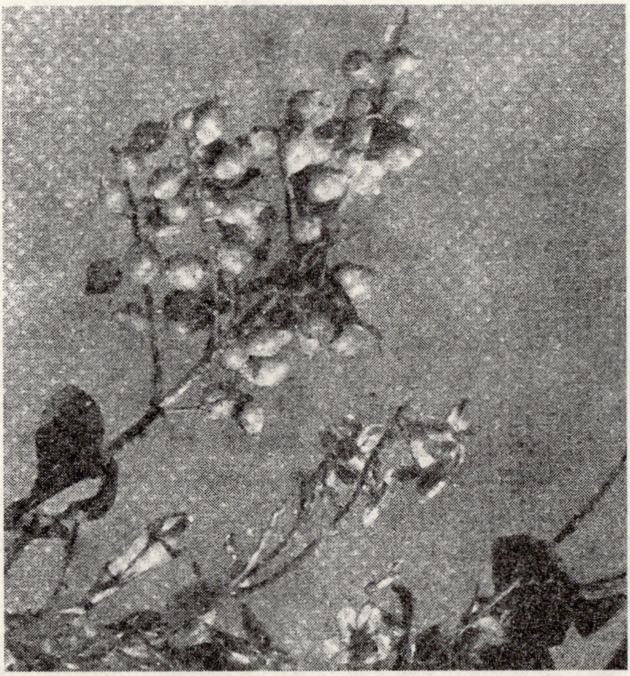

VERBENACEAE

DURANTA REPENS LINN
(SYN. D. PLUMIERI JACQ.)

Popularly known as GOLDEN DEW DROP. creeping skin FLOWERS PIGEON BERRY;

It is a spiny shrub to 3 m. with bright leavender - blue flowers with pale centres, borne in terminal pyramidal branched clusters. The branches are spiny and stem qudriangular. Flowers C 1.5 cm, with corolla tube about twice as long as calyx and with rounded spreading lobes,stamens not exserted, calyx 4mm, lobes tiny, linear. Leaves opposite, broadly elliptic entire, stalked, mostly 3 5 cm, spines stout to 1.5 cm. Ovary eight (8) celled. Ripe fruit orange a drupe globular C. 5 mm with 42 - seeded nutlets.

It is a native of C. America 200 - 1600 m. very common as a hedge plant in the Nepal Valley and many other places in West H imalayas. May - August.

MEDICINAL USE : Plants believed to be poisonous. Leaves contain a saponin and the fruits an alkaloid analogous to narcotine, macereted fruits yield a juice which even in dilations of 1 : 100 parts of waters lethal to mosquito larvae. The action is less marked on culicin larvae, the juice can be used as a larvicide in ponds and swamps.

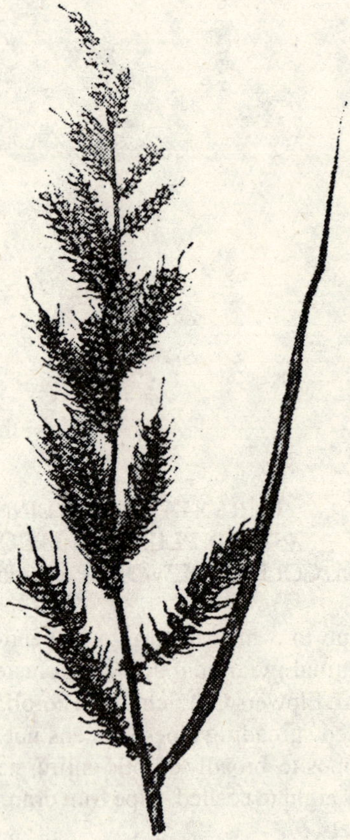

GRAMINAE

ECHINOCHLOA STAGNINE BEAUV.
(SYN. PANICUM STAGNINUM RETZ.
E. CRUSGALI BEAUV)

BENG.- DUL., **BOM.-** BANTI., **KANN.-** KADU DEPHAI HULLU., **TEL.-** BONTHA ODDU., **TAMIL-** BONTHA, UDDUDU., **LOCAL NAME-** SAMA, SAMAK.

It is annual or perennial. Clums 1 metre or so in length, decumbent or shortly creeping below, simple or branched. Leaves 10 20x0.5 - 1 cm linear; margin finely cartilaginous, ligule absent. Panicles erect, 5 - 12 cm long. branches solitary or pinate, suberect or spreading distant except the upper ones or more or less lobed in appearence. Spikelets crowded 3-3.8 x 2 mm ovate elliptic, cuspidate or awned, greenish or tinged with purple. Lower floret barren, floral glumes cuspidate, or produced into a long, flexuous awn. Upper floret. hermaphrodite polished. Grains broadly ellipitic. Flowering and fruits - July to November.

Common in the fields of sugarcane and other rainy season crops grown in Najafgarh and Timarpur. Also met along irrigative channels and canal banks. Found throughout India.

MEDICINAL USE : The decoction of the pith is used as diur.

E. CRUS - GALLI - BEAVU.

(SYN. PANICUM - CRUS - GALLI LINN).

BENGALI- BURASHAMA., **HINDI-** SAMAK, SANWAK., **S.-** JALSAMOKA., **TEL.-** PEDDAWUNDU., **TAMIL-** OOTHUPUL., **P.-** BARASANWAK., **BOM.-** SARVANK, BANTI.

It is common throughtout the grater ports of India specially in wet places and rich soils, and up to elevalions of 6000 ft.

MEDICINAL USE : Plant is used in dieases of spleen and to check hoemor.

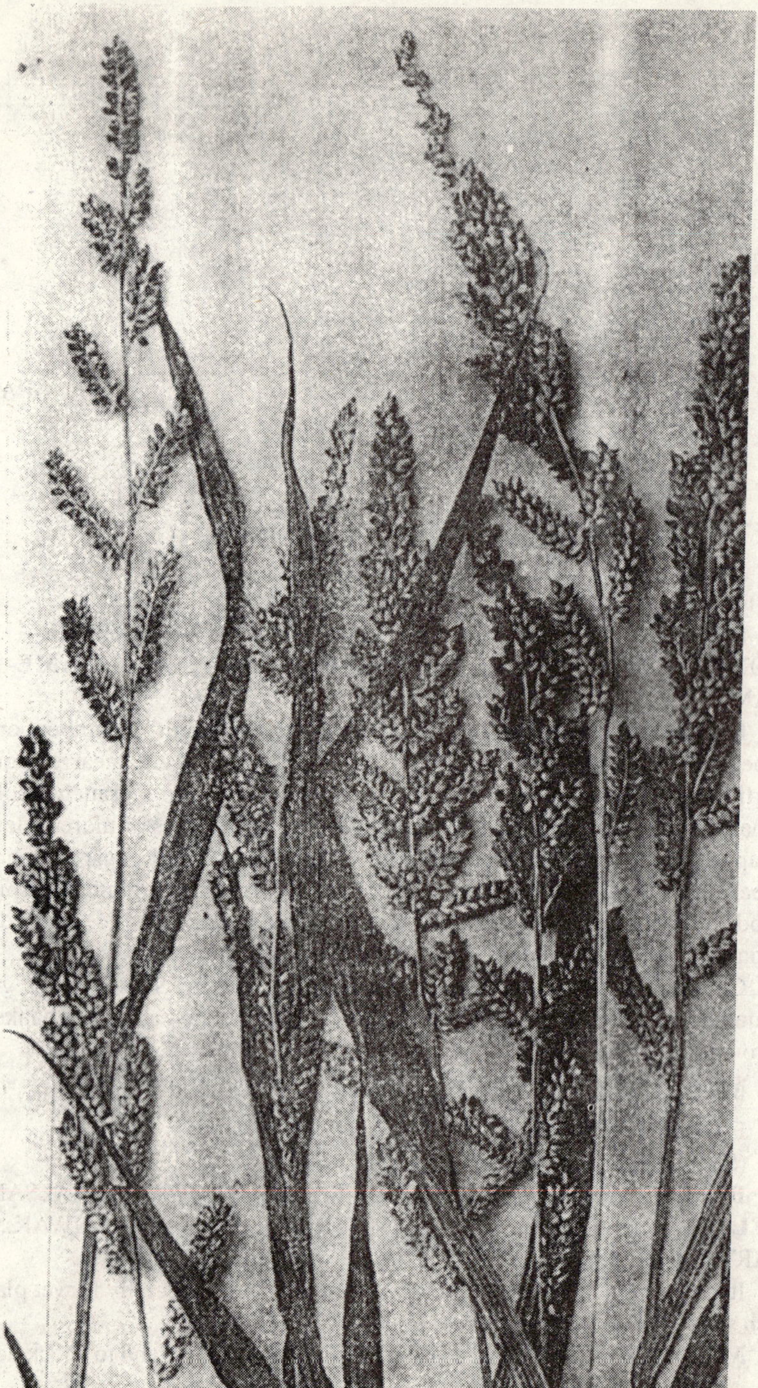

GRAMINAE

ECHINOCHLOA FRUMENTACEA LINK
(SYN. PANICUM FRUMENTACEUM ROXB.)

BO - BAVT; **HINDI & BENG.** - SAMWA, **SANKS** - SHYMA, **TELGUE** - CHAMOL, **PUNJABI**- SEWANK, **TAMIL** - KUDRAVALI PILLU, **MARATHI** - SMAUL.

It is cultivated over the greater part of India and on the Himalayas upto 6,500 ft.

MEDICINAL USE: Plant useful in biliousness and constipation.

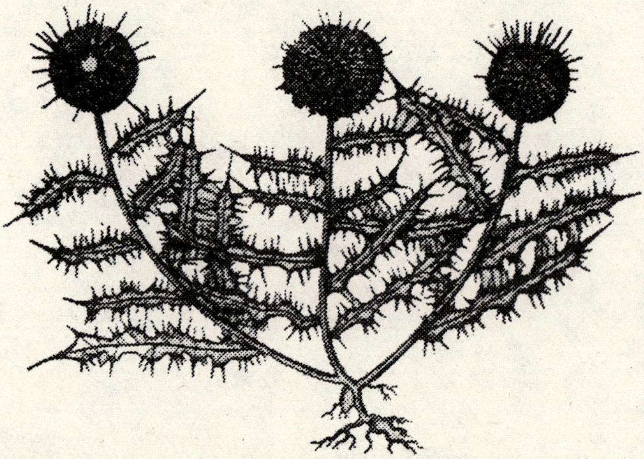

COMPOSITAE

ECHINOPS ECHINATUS ROXB.

HINDI- UTAKANTA, GOKRU., **MARATHI-** UTANTI, KADECHUBUK., **SANSKRIT-** KANTALU, UTATI., **ENGLISH-** CAMELS THISTLE., **GUJARAT-** UTAKANTO, SHULIO, UTKANTO., **LOCAL NAME-** OONTKATELA.

A diffused and erect much branched, white woolly annual. The leaves thistle like lanceolate to oblong, pinnatifid; the triangular lobes ending in long rigid and narrow spines Flower heads grouped together in a compact globose capitula. Uniflowered. Flowers pale blue with long spine tipped in volucral bracts. One or two braets produced into sharp spines exceeding the compound heads. Achenes obconic, silkly.

Commonly found in waste and dry places and open ground. It is also recorded from moist places throughout India, ascending upto 2000 m. on the hills.

MEDICINAL USE : Plant alter, diur. nerve tonic, used in hoarse cough, hysteria, dyspep, scrofula and opthalmia. Powered roots applied for killing maggots in wounds, and with gumacacia applied to the hair to kill lice.

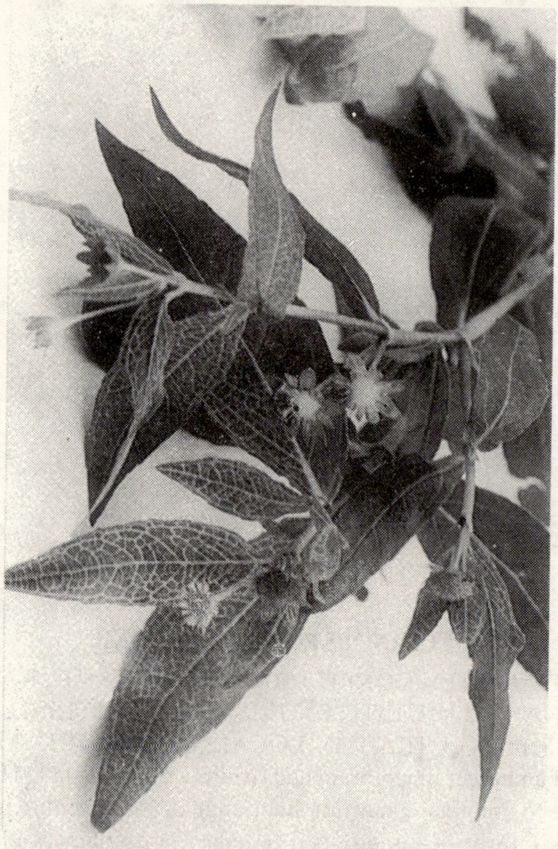

COMPOSITAE

ECLIPTA ALBA (LINN) HASSK.
(SYS. E. PROSTRATA L. VERBESINA PROSTRATA LINN
E. ERECTA LINN

SANS.- BHRINGARAJA, KESARAJA, AJAGARA., **HINDI-** BHANGRA, MOCHKAND, BABRI., **BENGALI-** KESUTI KESHUKTI, KESHORI., **MARATHI-** BHRINGRAJA, MAKA., **GUJ.-** BHANGRA, KALUGANTHI, DODHAK, KALOBHANGRO., **TEL.-** GALAGARA, GUNTAGALI JERU., **TAMIL-** GARUGA, KAYANTHAKARA., **KAN.-** GARAGADASOPPU, BHRINGORAJA GONIGA., **MAL.-** KYONNI., **URIYA-** KESARDA.

It is a rough erect or prostrate annual. Leaves variable, 2.5 - 8 x 0.8 - 1.5 cm; linear or oblong - lanceolate, turning black when dry. Heads white, 7x9 mm, solitary or 2-3 together. Achenes winged on the margin, with warty excresceneces. Pappus absent. It is found common in different habitats. Flowers and fruits are found throughout the year.

It is a common weed growing in moist places throughout India, ascending to 2000 m. on the hills.

MEDICINAL USE : Whole plant is tonic and deobstruent in hepatic and spleen enlargements and is emetic. Plant juice in combination with aromatics is administered for catarrh and jaundice. Leaf juice alongwith honey is used as a remedy for cattarrh in infants. Root is emetic, pergative and is applied externally as an antiseptic to ulcers and wounds in cattle.

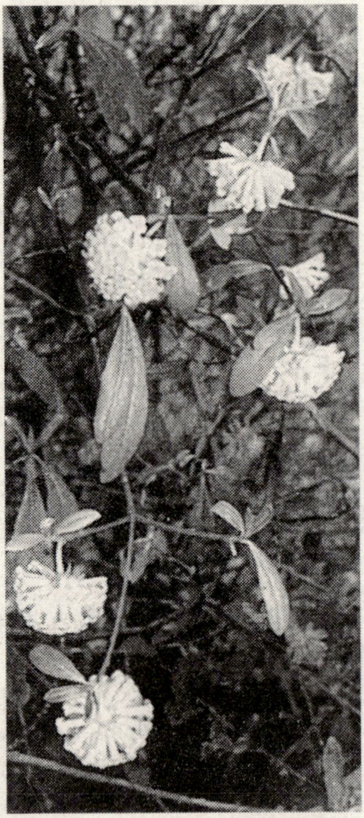

THYMELAEACEAE

EDGEWORTHIA TOMENTOSA (THUNB) NAKAI.
(SYN. E. GARDNERI (WALL) MEISSN)
NEPALI - ARYILI.

A large densely branched shrub with long and profuse. branches, with elliptic - lanceolate long - pointed leaves and with dense pendulous globular clusters of numerous small golden - yellow, sweet, scented, tubular flowers fading to white. Flower clusters are 2.5 - 5 cm across, very hairy, receptacal tube cylindrical, lobes four blunt. Style long, stigma linear; nectar disk a ring or lobed. 1-2 cm long, densely silky haired lobes short rounded, spreading to 1 cm braets linear - oblong, conspicuous in bud. Leaves 7.5 - 12.5 cm hairless above, hairy or silky - haired beneath, narrowed to a short stalk, stems brownish 10 cm. or more.

It is reported from central and eastern Himalayas, Assam - Nepal, Bhutan and Sikkim, 5000-7000 ft.

MEDICINAL USE-Plant fish - poison, rootstock and stem, used in China as remedy for buboes.

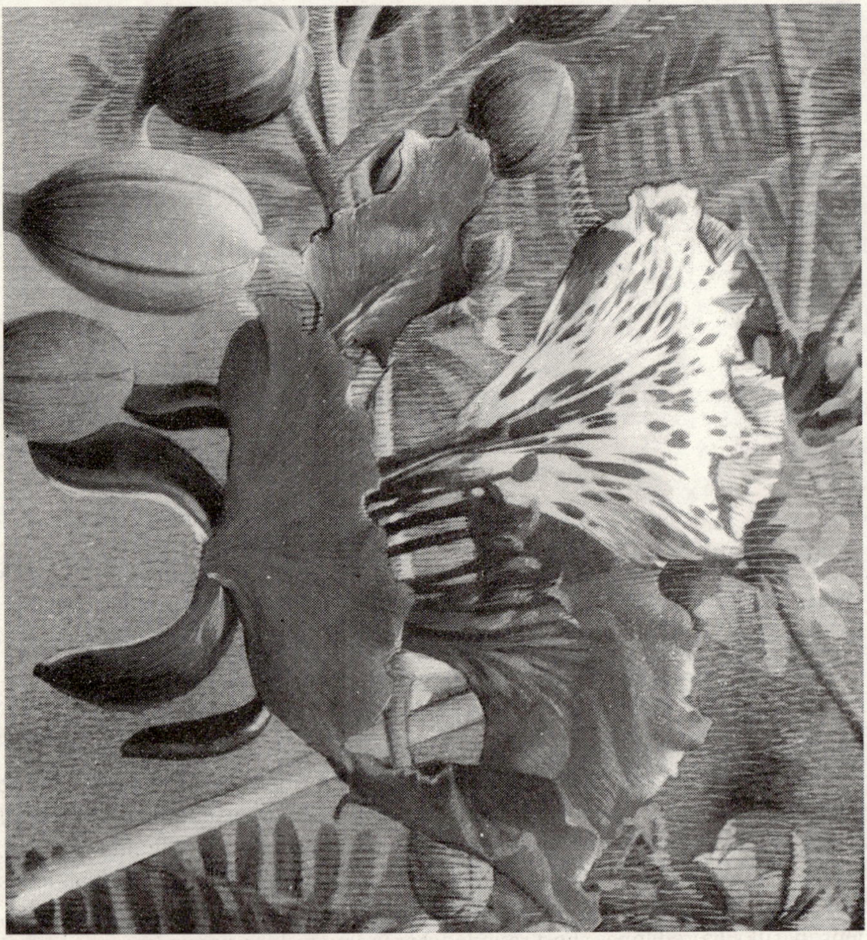

PAPILIONACEAE

EDLONIX REGIA (RON)RAF (SYN. POINCIANA REGIA NOJ. EX. HOOK.)

BO.- VAYNI., **TEL.**- VATANARAYANA., **TAM.**- VADANARAYANS., **LOCAL NAME** : GUL-MOHAR.

A magificent tree with an umbrella shaped crown leaves bipinnate, feathery, 60 cm long, leaflets about 1.2 x 0.5cm Flowers red or orange red. Pods 30x60x5 cm flat, seeds numrous, oblong. Flowers : April. September and fruit Nov-April. Commonly planted in gardens, squares and avenues for ornamental purposes and for the shade given by its dense foliage. The flowring period is irregular, almost throughout the year. The tree often produces vegetative buds after the 1st few showers. very likely introducd in India. Reported to ocean in some parts of Kathiawar & South India and frequently planted as an avenue tree.

MEDICINAL USE : Laves used in rheumatism and flatulense. Bark-in Indochina considered antiper and febge.

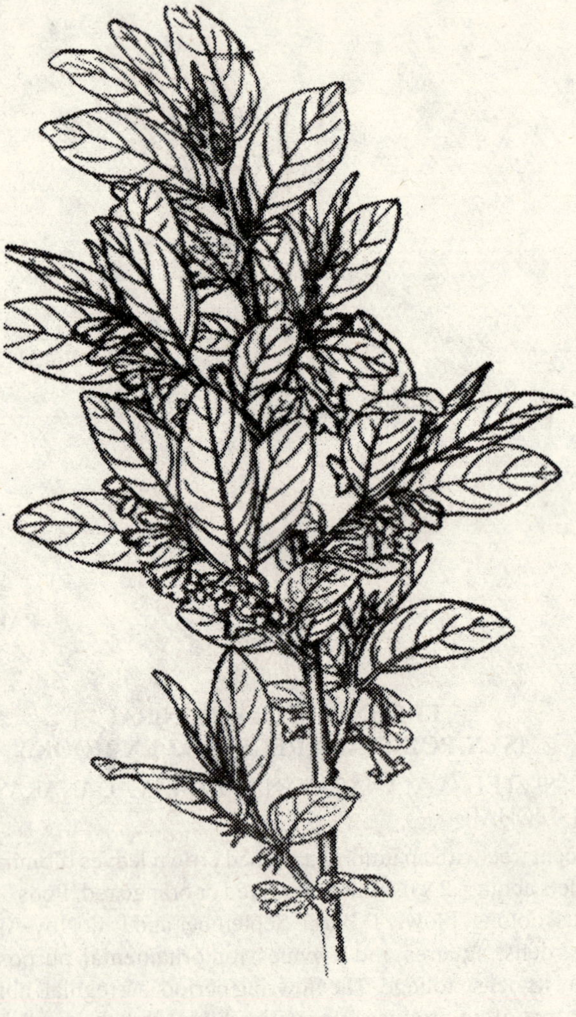

ELAEAGNACEAE

ELAEAGNUS LATIFOLIA LINN

BENGALI- GUARA., **MARATHI-** AMBGUL, NEELDUCK, NURANGI., **HINDI-** GHIWAIN., **TAMIL-** KULARI KOLUNGAI., **MAL.-** KAYOLAMPUVALLI, KAPALAMPUVALLI., **ENGLISH-** BASTARD OLEASTER., **KAN.-** HITTELY, HUNSABALLI.

It is a deciduous big shrub or small tree somewhat spiny. The shape of this plant keeps on changing. The leaves are oblong elliptic which are silvery scaly beneath. The leaves are leathery, entire without stipules. The flowers are dull yellowish - white with small tubes with fragrance appearing with the young leaves. Flowers are few in axillary clusters; perianth tube 8 mm with four triangular acute to oval lobes, silvery scaly outside; Stamens 4 slightly exserted; leaves alternate, 2.5 - 5 cm, stalked; shoots and young branches are covered with silvery scales, lateral shoots ending in a straight thorn; shrub to 2 m or more. The fruits are ovoid red to orange red 18-38 mm long fleshy, edible nut is bony.

It is widely distributed in all the hilly parts of India particularly reported from Kashmir to Nepal, temperate Himalayas and also in Manipur.

MEDICINAL USE : The flowers are cardiac, astring. the fruits are astringent.

Its another species E. UMBELLATA is also used medicinally The flowers are stim. cardiac and astrin. seeds used as stim. in coughs the oil extracted out of the plant is used in pulmonary infections.

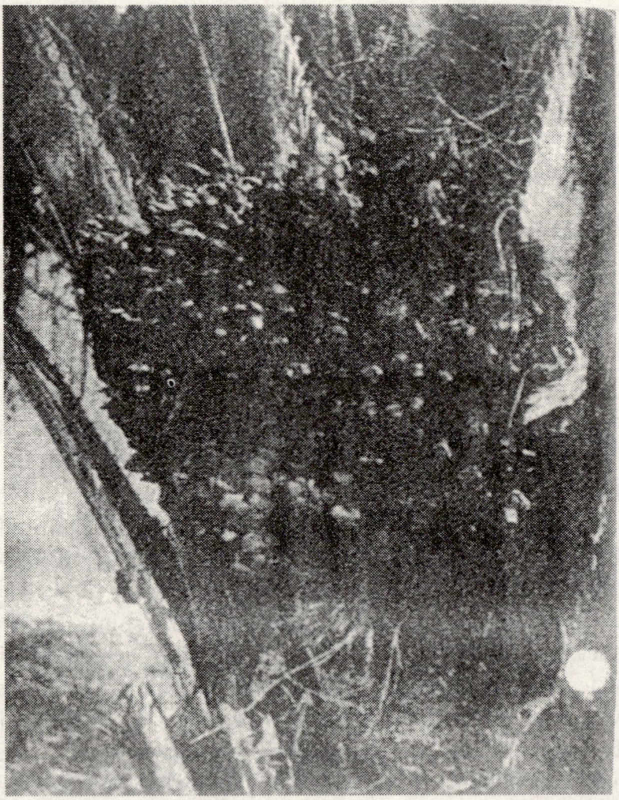

PALMAE

ELAEIS GUINEENSIS JACQ

ENGLISH- OIL PALM, AFRICAN OIL PALM.

It is an erect elegant tree reaching a height of 6-24 metres In appearance it resembles a coconut tree. The stem is thick bearing a series of ring like feathery leaf fronds. As the tree grows up, the trunk becomes narrower systematically. The lower leaves dropping off but leaving behind their bases encircling the stem in the form of indistinct ring streaks and the upper leaves are found in the form of tuft or crown which bear flowers and fruits. A single tree bears male and female flowers separately (Monoecious). Normally a series of upto 10-12 consecutive inflorences which are compound spikes) are of the same sex followed by a similar sequence of the opposite sex. The flowers appear afer 4-6 years. The adult tree yield on an average 6 to 8 (spadix) simultaneously. Male spadix always appear a few weeks earlier than female spadix. The fruits are sessile, oval drupes with pointed ends 2.5 - 5 cm. long and 18 - 36 mm. broad. They are in clusters of yellow, orange, red or shiny black-colours and in nature one fruit contains 1-3 seeds. The seed coat is hard and the cotyledons are white in colour.

It is known as a native of tropical Africa, but cultivated in botanical gradens and in Travancore. It has been introduced in Maharashtra, karnataka and Kerala recently.

MEDICINAL USE : Guinea oil applied to wounds as volume vary used as liniment for rheumatism and courbature. oil is a rich source of carotene, can be used in place of codliver oil, for correting vitamis A deficineycy.

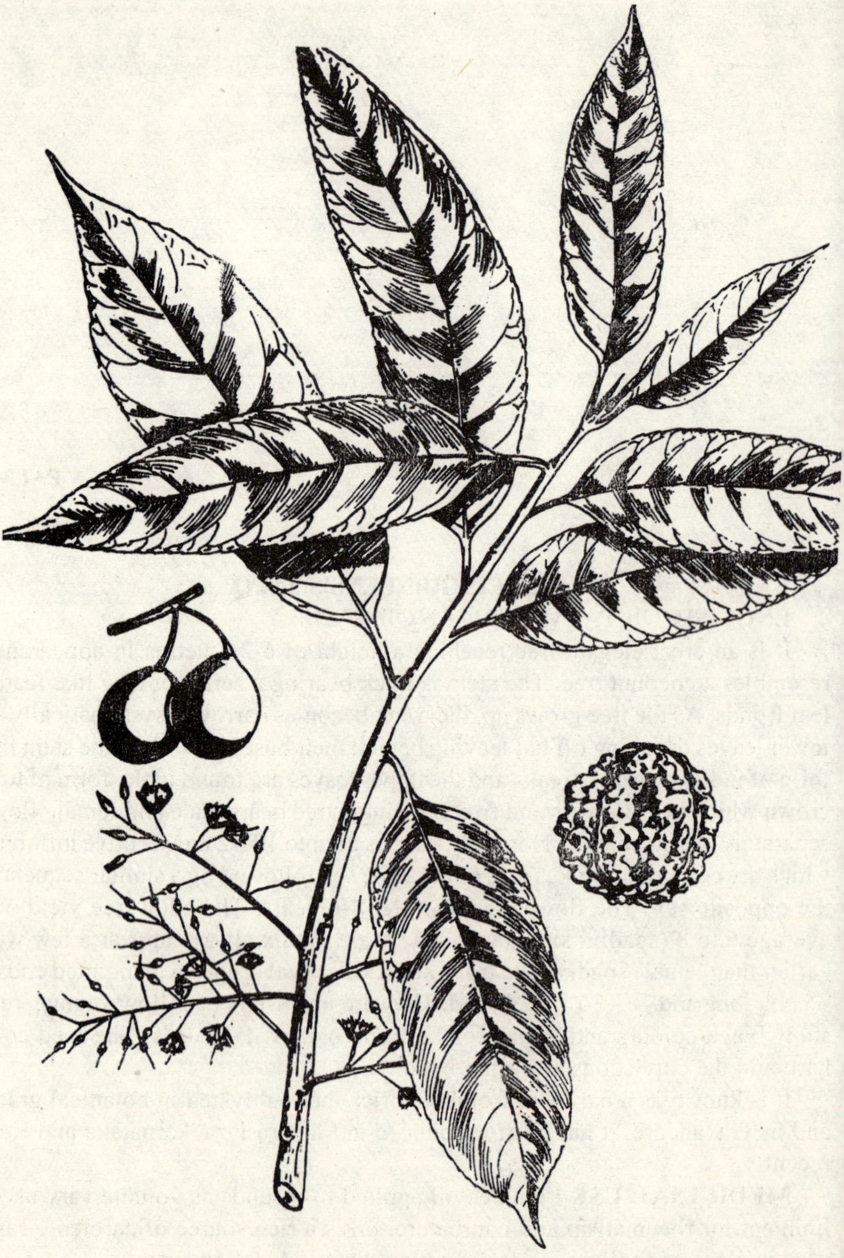

ELAEOCARPACEAE.

ELAEOCARPUS GANITRUS ROXB.
(SYN. E. SPHAERICUS (GAERTN.) K. SCHUM

ENGLISH- UTRASUM., **HINDI-** RUDRAK, RUDRAKI., **SANS., TAMIL, TEL. & MAL.-** RUDRAKSHA., **BENGALI-** RUDRAKYA., **KAN.-** RUDRAKSHA., **MARATHI-** RDUROKSH., **URIYA-** RUDRAKYO., **ASSAME-** RUDRAI, SOHALANGKAYI, LADROK, UDROKK.

This tree is very tall like mango tree and the top portion is occupying the position of an umbrella. The leaves are elliptic to orbicular, non-hairy, margine is serrate arranged in a circle around the stem. The flowers are white occuring in dense non-terminal spikes on the droping branches in the axil of old leaves. When dirty white flowers drop off than dark mouve or green coloured fruits appear which are pulpy in nature and sour in taste. The stone of these fruits forms Rudraksh. These fruits are round and sometimes half in shape appear the radius varies from 1.25 - 2.5 cm. The stone of the fruit is marked by lines. It is believed that these lines vary from one to 38, though only from 1 to 14 line rudrakshs are available in general. It is said that no. of lines on a rudraksh determine the quality and importance of these beads. It is found in Bihar, Bengal, Assam, Madhya Pradesh, Bombay, Nepal and occasionally cultivated as an ornamental plant.

MEDICINAL USE : The fruits used in the diseases of the head and epileptic fits, It is helpful in curing paralysis, blood purifier, it increases the virility, vermiform, cough, and diseases of throat and diseases after child birth. Four line rudraksha is responsible for good health and in general, and eyes in particular.

Five line head is responsible for heart diseases including blood pressure and also as a blood purifier. Seven lined beads is responsible and extremely useful for cancer, heart attacks, skin infection, piles, toxic. effect, delivery without pain; gas trouble, meditation, diseases connected with legs.

Eight lined bead helps in preventing accidental death and early death.

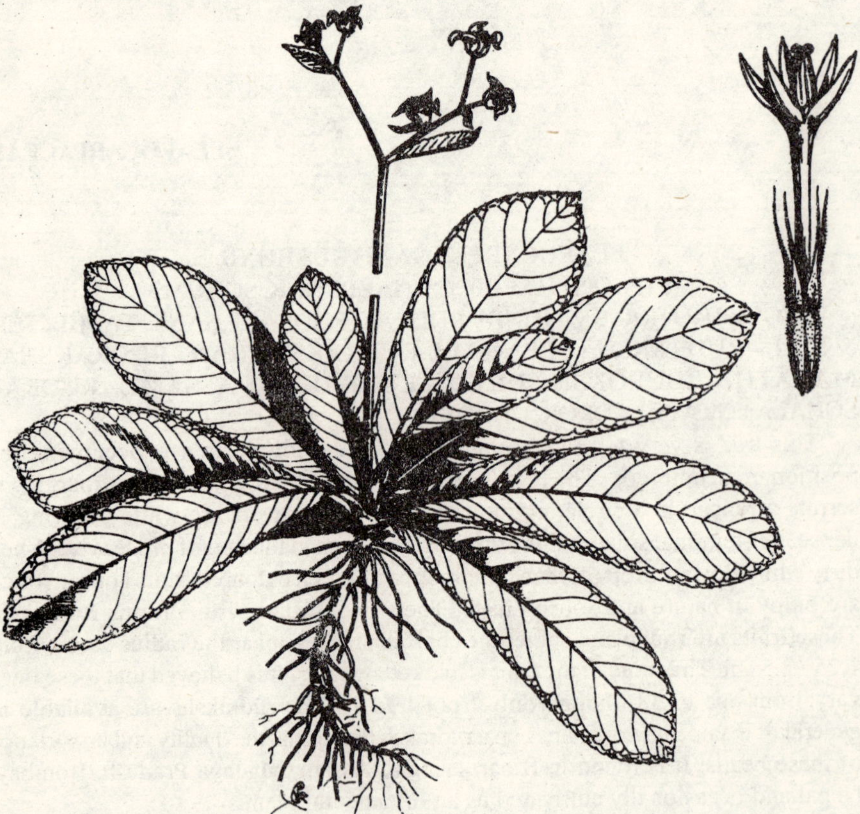

COMPOSITAE

ELEPHANTOPUS SCABER L.

HINDI- JUNGLI GOBHI, GAOJBAS GOJIA., **BENGALI-** GOJIALOTO, NAKDSHAKA, **ENGLISH-** PREKLY LEAVES, ELEPHANTS FOOT., **KAN.-** HAKKARIKE., **MARATHI-** GOJIBHA, PATHRI., **TAMIL-** ANSHAVADI, AANAICHCHU VADI., **TELEGU-** HUSTIKASAKA., **SANS.-** GOJIBA., **GUJARAT-** GULJIBI, MOPATHREE., **FARSI-** KALAMRUMI.

It is a small herb. Leaves are lamceolate ;and glabrous. In the center one round flower (yellow eoloured) appears. In the centre of the flower the axis elongates which bear many yellow coloured flowers. These flowers bear small beans. It is cultivated infields, and found throughout India in shady places specially in Bengal.

MEDICINAL USE : The plant is musilaginous and is used as cardiac tonic, astringent, altrative and fabrifuge. Decoction of the root and leaves with cumin and buttermilk is given in dysurea and other urethral complaints. Also given in diarrhoea and dysentery. The drug is also used in snake bite.

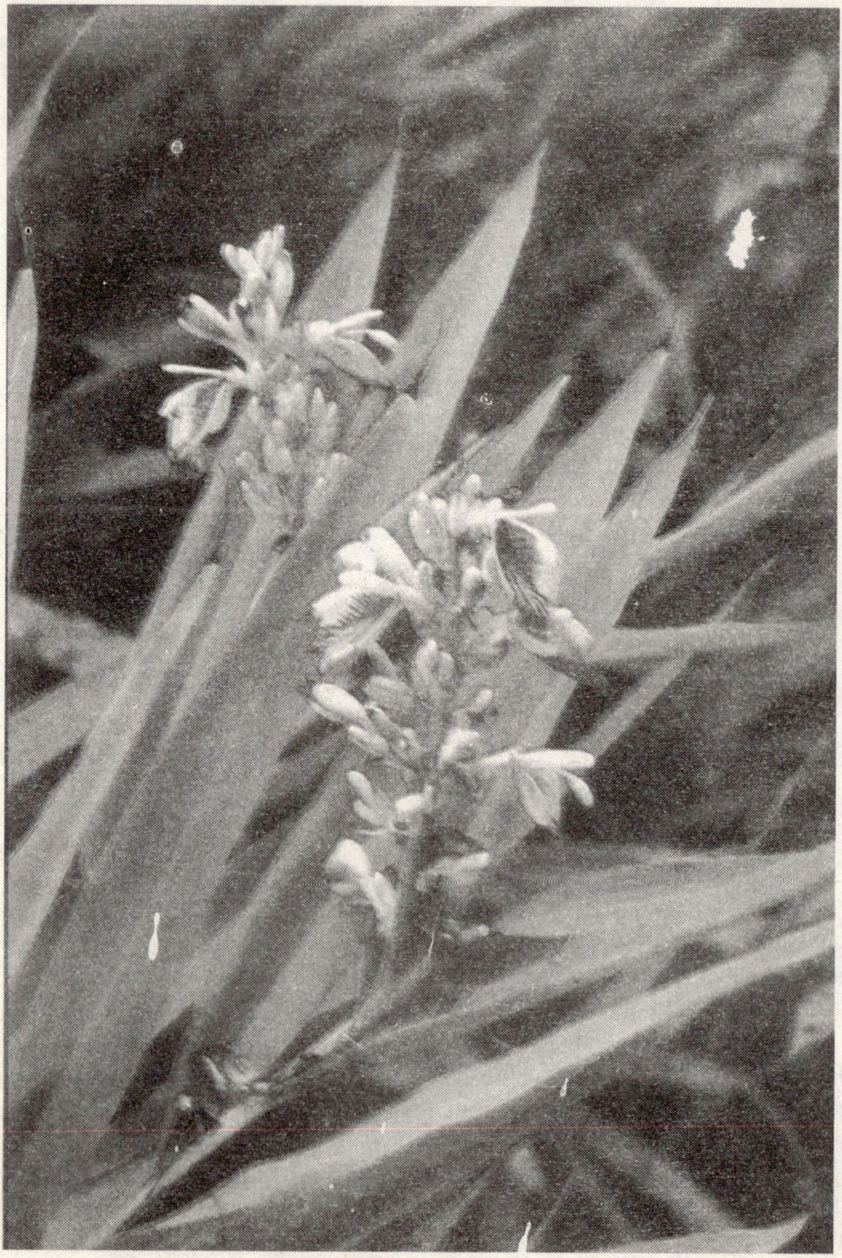

ZINGIBERACEAE

ELETTARIA CARDAMOMUM MATON
(SYN. CARDAMOMUM OFFICINALE SALISB
" AMMOMUM CARDAMOMUM L.

SANS.- ELA., **H&B.**- CHOTI ELAICHI., **BOMBAY**- ELACHI., **TAMIL**- YELAKKAI., **TEL.**- YELAK-KAYALA., **ENG.**- CARDOMOM.

The plant is tall perennial and herbaceous with underground branched rhizomes from which arise many aerial erect leafy shoots or decumbent panicles. Rhizome is somewhat woody and stout and gives horizontal roots. Leafy shoots in clusters of 10-20 enclosed in leaf sheath, 2-5 m tall, leaves distichous dark green, glabrous and petiolate. Inflorescence arising from rootstalk at the base of leaf shoot, erect, decumbent slender panicle. Flowers white, tinged with rosy or purplish, fragrant 3x1.5 cm, in 15-30 cm long terminal thyrses, at length moddling. Bracts large white, calyx cylinderical, 3 toothed. Fruit is a capsule, trilocular varying in size fusiform to globose yellow to pale green. Seeds 15-30 per fruit dark brown angled, round, aromatic with thin mucilaginous aril.

It grows wild in evergreen rain forests in the western ghats in India between 750-1600 m and in Sri Lnaka above 10,000 m. Reported from Malabar on the Western Ghats between 2,500 - 5000 ft. wild or cultivated. India is the biggest producer of this spice with cultivation mainly confined to the southern states of Kerala Mysore and Tamil Nadu.

MEDICINAL USE : Cardamoms are used as an aeromatic stimulant and carminative; seeds arom. stim. stomach, carmin. diurnal.

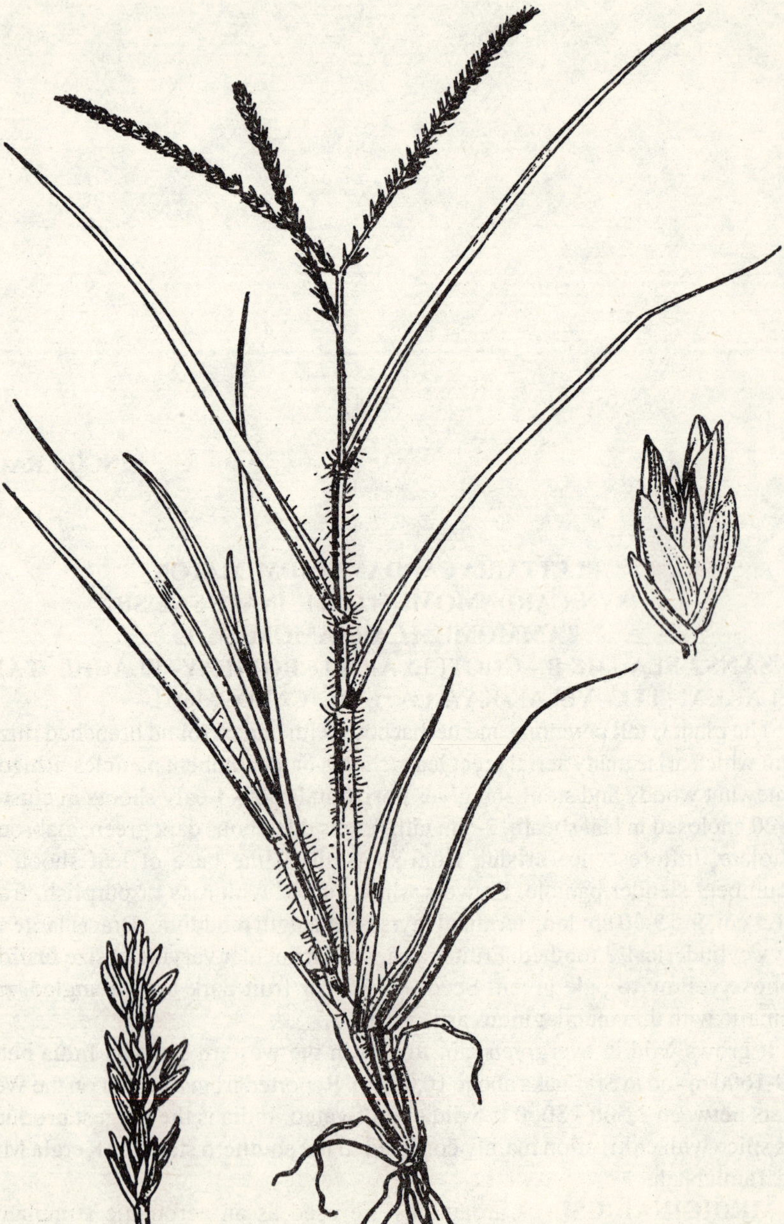

GRAMINAE

ELEUSINE CORACANA (L) A. GOERTN
(SYN. CYNOSURUS CORACANUS L.
" E. INDICA GAERTN.)
SYN. DACTYLOCTENIUM AEGYPTIUM (LINN) BEAUV).

BENGALI- MORUA., **KON.-** NAVCHAUO., **MARATHI-** NACHNI., **GUJARATI-** BAVTO., **PUNJABI-** CHALODRA., **HINDI-** HAKRA MANDUA, MANDAL., **TELGU-** RAGULU, KANN., **MAL. & TAMIL-** RAGI., **LOCAL NAME-** MAKRA., **ENGLISH-** FINGER MILLET, AFRICAN MILLET, RAGI: INDIAN MILLET.

An erect or decumbent annual, variable in habit. culms rooting at the base and from branched nodes; Leaves disticous, narrowly linear, flat. Spikes 2-6 (1.3 - 3.8 cm. Long) digitately radiating; rachis keeled, Spikelets, densely crowded spreading at right angles to the rachis, 3.5 x 3 mm Lower involucral glume cuspidate; upper awned. Floral glumes mucronate or awned. Grains obovoid-globose, rugose. Flowers and fruits - May - October.

Common during monsoon period on waste land and as a weed in cultivated fields. it is an important grain crop of karnataka also grown in large scale in Tamilnadu, Andhra Pradesh and Maharashtra. It is practically grown all over India.

MEDICINAL USE: Seeds are tonic, cooling, useful in biliousness and are also astringent.

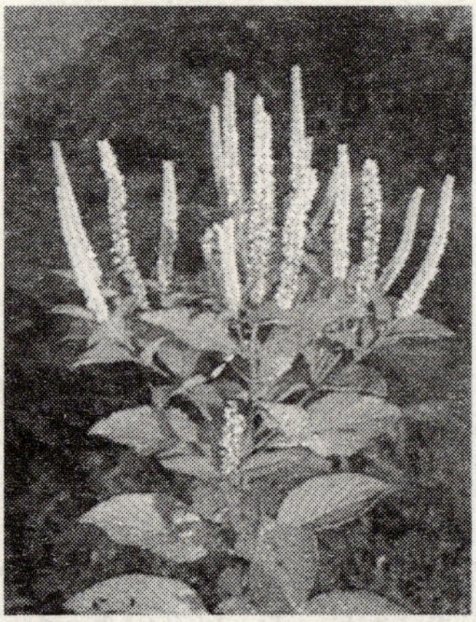

LABIATAE

ELSHOLTZIA CRISTATA WILLD
(SYN. E. PETRINI (LEP) GARCKE)

It is a tender herb with stems to 2m, branches rough, four angled. Leaves glandular opposite 10-20 cm. with heart shaped bases with conspicuously impressed lateral veins above. long stalked. Ovate pointed toothed. Inflorecence in dense slender terminal and axillary spikes of numerous tiny yellow flowers. Spikes strongly aromatic 8-20 cm. long with lanceolate bracts. Calyx 5-toothed, enlarging in fruit, corolla 4-lobed the upper lobe erect the others spreading, tubular 5mm long twice as long as the calyx. Stamens exerted.

It is found in temperate and sub-tropical Himalayas from Kashmir to Mussoorie at 1200 m. It is also recorded from Assam hills upto 9,000 ft. Introduced in Nilgiris.

MEDICINAL USE : In Assam flowering tops given as diur. In China the drug regarded as carmin., stomach and astrin. Dried leaves and flower tops are a source of an aromatic oil (with presence of thimol, which is used in medicine.

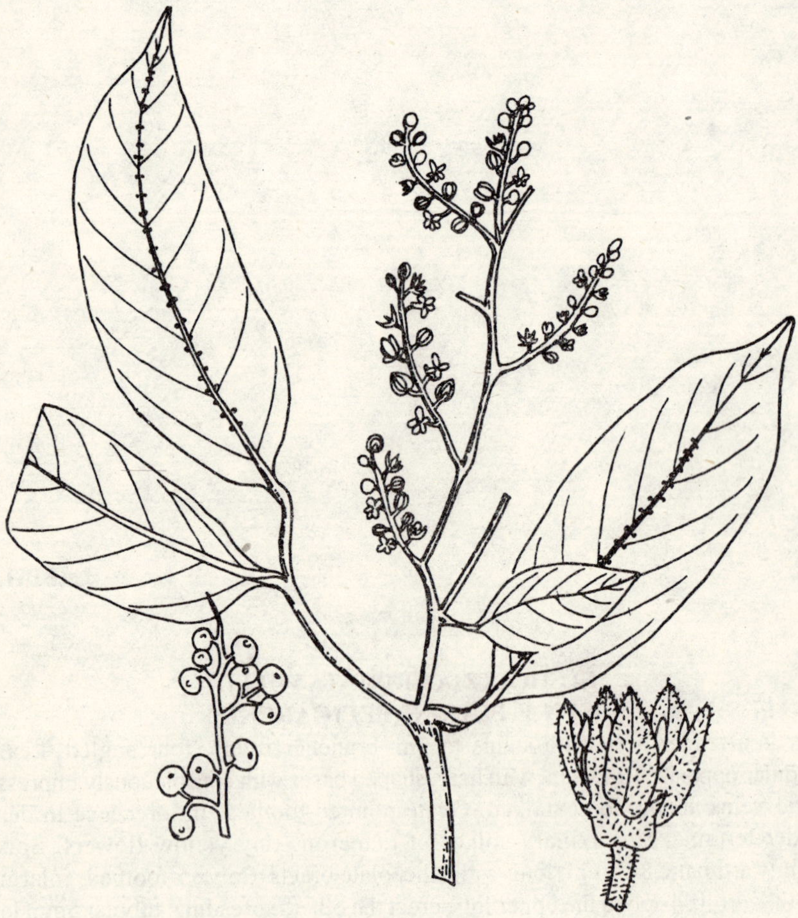

MYRSINACEAE

EMBELIA RIBES BURM F.
(SYN. E. GLANDULIFERA WIGHT)

ENG.- ACEITIPET ALUM CLAM, EXFLASSK ALMECDA & ALMEIDA., **HINDI-** BAIBIRANG, BHUNGI, GAIYA., **BENGALI-** BIRANGA DHADKI, JHANTI., **MARATHI-** AMBATI, VAIVARUNG, VAVADINGA., **ORIYA-** NUNUNIYA., **SANTALI NAME-** BHABRI., **SANS.-** VIDAHGA., **GUJARATI-** KARKANNIE., **PUNJABI-** BABRUNG., **TAMIL, TELUGU & KANNADA-** VAYRI VILANGA.

It is a shrub or small tree, the new branches are covered with brown hairs while mature branches are smooth and glabrous. Speacked with white glands. The leaves are upto 12 cm. long lanceolate dotted all over with glands. Margins of the leaves are simpler or toothed, leaves sometime reddish on lower surface, hairy on veins. Flowers minute, pale green, in short, axillary, densely hairy clusters. Fruits small - globose oval red when ripe.

It is found in the hilly parts of India from Central and lower Himalayas down to Ceylon and Singapore. It occurs also in Eastern India and Deccan peninsula. In general it is recorded throughout India upto 5000 ft.

MEDICINAL USE : Dried fruits - anthelmic, astrin. alter. tonic in scorpion sting and snake bite. Decoction of dried fruit used for fevers and diseases of chest and skin. Infusion of roots given for coughs and diar. Embelic acid contains drug embelin - which has no effect on hook worms and tape worms but effective in the treatment of ascariasis. (Ind. Med. Gaz. 1947-66) aqueous extracts of fruit show anti bacterial activity against STAPHYLOCOCCUS AUREUS and ESCHERICHIA COLI (Ind. J.med. Researsh. 1949-169)

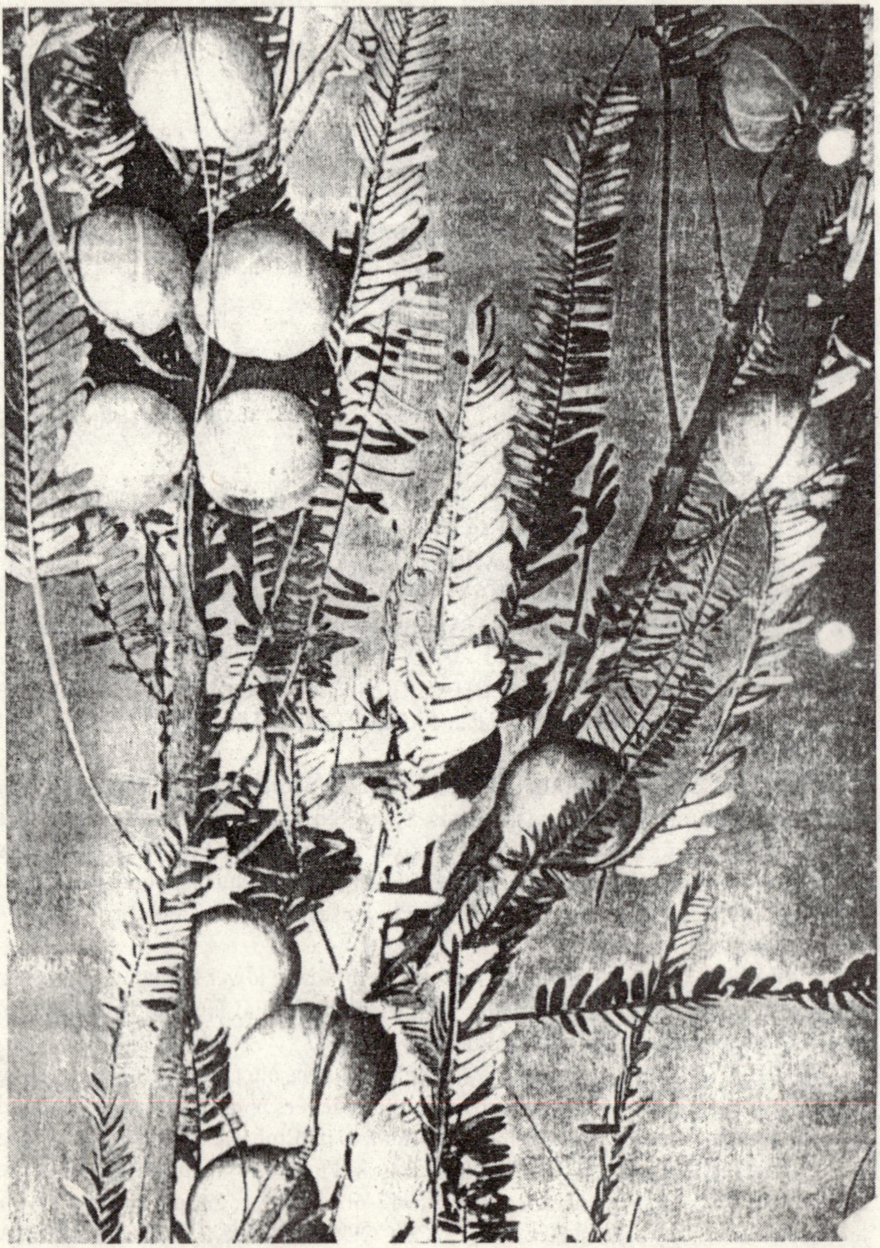

EUPHORBIACEAE

EMBLICA OFFICINALIS GAERTN
(SYN. PHYLLANTHUS EMBLICA LINN.)

ENG.- EMBLIC, INDIAN GOOSEBERRY, EMBLIC MYROBALAN., **HINDI**- AMLA, AONLA AMLIKA., **BENG.**- AMLA, AMLAKI., **KAN.**- AMALAKA, NEELI, NEELIKAYI., **MAL.**- NEELI, NEELI KAYI., **SANS.**- ADIPHALA, AMALAKA, DHATRI., **TAM.**- NEELI., **TEL.**- AMALA-KAMU, USIRAKAI, NEELI., **GUJ.**- AMALI, AMBALA, AMBLA, AMLA., **KASH.**- AONLA., **MAR.**- AMLA., **LOCAL NAME.**- AMAL, AONHLA, AOLA.

A small or medium sized deciduous tree with smooth, greenish grey, exfoliating bark. (Bark peeling off in flakes). Leaves feathery with small narrowly oblong, pinnately arranged leaflets; distichous, alternate, quite entire. Flowers small, monoceious, usually in axillary clusters, pale yellow, apetalous. Disk-various, rarely o. Male flower.- no disk; sepals 5-6, imbricate in two series. Stamens.- three (3) in the centre of the flower; filaments united in a short or long column; anthers two celled oblong or didymous, rarely reniform, cells parallal or diverging, slits extrose vertical. pistillode o or very minute, Female flower: sepals 5-6; ovary 3-or more-celled; styles 3 free or connate below, 2 fid with slender arms; rarely united; ovules 2 in each cell. Fruit: a capsule of three crustaceous 2-valved cocei, depressed, globose 1/2-1 in diameter, fleshy and obseurely 6 lobed containing 6 trigonous seeds. Seeds estrophiolate. testa crustaceous, albumen fleshy; cotyledons flat or flexuous. Flowering period is March to May and fruiting season is winter.

Common in the mixed deciduous forest of India, ascending to 4,500 ft on the hills. It is considered a native to tropical South Cast Asia and is now distributed throughout India. Locally it is planted in public parks, lawns and squares.

MEDICINAL USE: Amla has been held in high esteem in indigenous medicine. It is acrid, cooling, refrigerant, diuretic and laxative. It is the richest known natural source of vitimin 'C' and the raw fruit is eaten as an aperient. Dried fruit is useful in haemorrhage, diarrhoea and dysentery. In combination with iron, it is used as a remedy for anaemia, jaundice and dyspepsia and cough. It form an essential constituent of commercial chavan prash which is the richest source of nutrition since last one century. With lemon Juice, the amla juice is a good remedy for bacillary dysentory. Triphala consisting of equal parts of powered emblic myrobalan, chebulic, myrobalan and belleric myrobalan is used as a laxative and in headache, billiousness, dyspepsia, constipation, piles, enlarged liver and ascites. The exudation from incisions on the fruit is used as an external application for inflamation of the eye. The flowers are cooling, refrigerant and aperent. The root and bark are astringent (kirt and Basu, III, 2220; Nadkarni, 19114, 151, koman, 1918, 6; Das Indian for; 1949;75;293). A fixed oil extracted from the fruits is reported to have the property of promoting hair growth. (Das, Loc. cit. Nadkaeni, Loc, cit.

The seeds are used in the treatment of asthma, bronchitis and biliousness. It is considered as a rich source of natural vit C. and hence ingredient of Bonnisan, septelin, styplon & Geriforte. The fruit has been used successfully in the treatment of human scurvy.

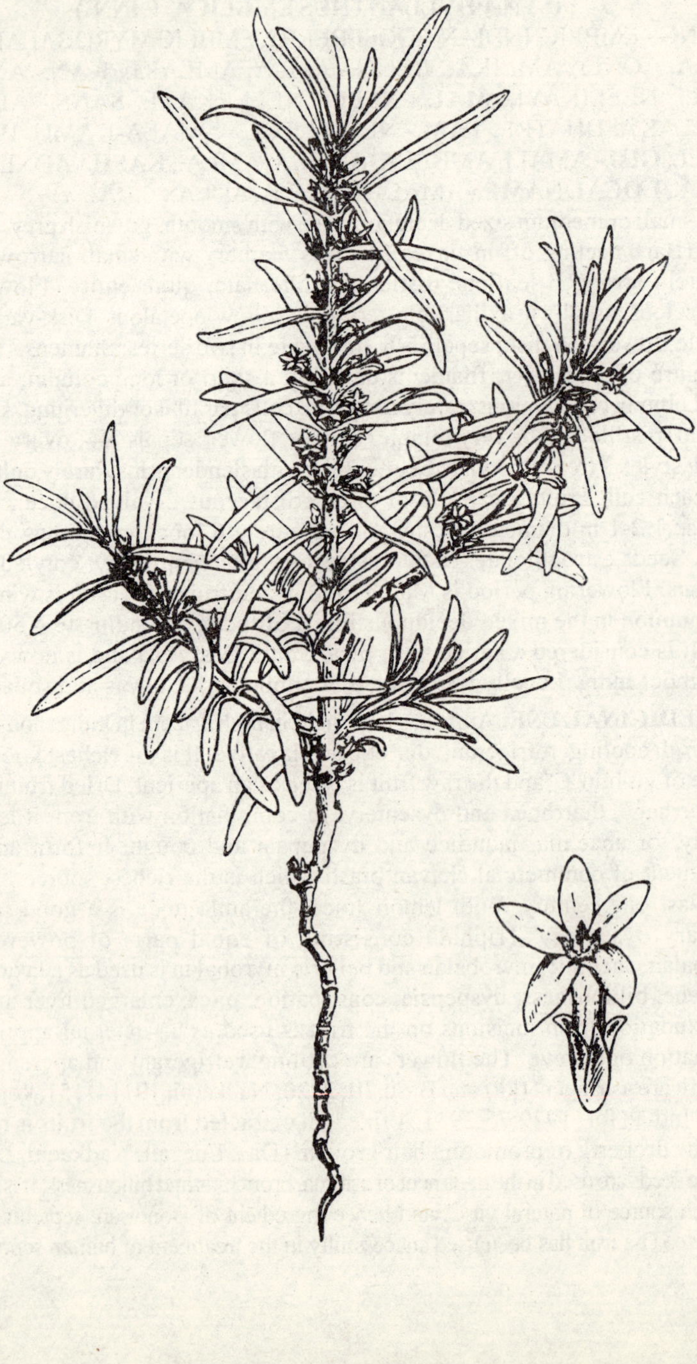

GENTIANACEAE

ENICOSTEMA HYSSOPIFOLIUM (WILD) VERDOORN
(SYN. E. VERTICILLATUM ENGL.)
E. LITTORALE BLUME,
GENTIANA VERTICILLATA L. F. NON L.)

ENGLISH- INDIAN GENTINA., **BOMBAY STATE-** KADAVINAYI., **SANSKRIT & BENGALI-** NEGAJIBHA., **HINDI-** CHHOTA - CHIRAYATA., **TELGU-** NELA GULI., **TAMIL & MAL.-** VALLARI., **MARATHI-** KADA VINAYE.

An errect procumbent, glabrous herb 10-30 cm tall. Leaves decussate, 2.5 - 6x0.5 - 1. cm, ovate lanceolate to linear. Flower white, in sessile, whorled, axillary clusters, usually 3 in the axil. Stigmas bilobed large, capsule subglobose, about 6x9 mm. Seeds minute brown, faveolate. Flowers and fruits June - September.

It is not very common. Few samples collected in pathches from moist and sandy places and crevices. It is also reported from hilly tracts. It grows throughout India upto 5,000 m from Punjab and Gangetic plain to ceylon.

MEDICINAL USE : Whole plant is stomachie, bitter tonic, laxative and carminative. Dried powder is given with honey as a blood purifier and in dropsy, rheumatism, abdominal ulcers, hernia, swellings itches and insect poisoning.

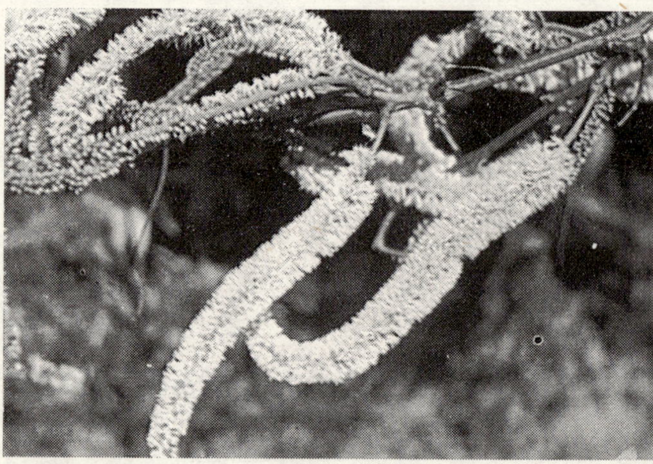

LEGUMINOSAE
(MIMOSACEAE)

ENTADA PHASEOLOIDES (L.) MERR.
(SYN. E. SCANDENS (L.) BENTH.
E. PURSAETHAOLDC.
LENSPHASEDOIDES L.
MIMOSA SCANDENS L.

HINDI- CHIAN, GILAN., **TEM.-** CHILLU, SILLU., **BENGALI-** GILAGACT, BARABI - CHAIN., **ASSAM-** GILA LEWA., **BOM.-** GARDAL., **ENGLISH-** NICKERBEEAR., **TEL.-** GILATIGE.

A very large woody climber with twice pinnate leaves, with paired woody tendrils and with tiny pale yellow flowers either born in long slender axillary spikes or in terminal branched clusters. Flower spikes 25 cm long or more, flowers 2-3 mm across, petals 5, equal, stamens longer, leaves with 2 pairs of pinnae each with 3-4 pairs of oblong to obovate shining leaflets 3-8 cm. long. Pod enormous, 60- 170 cm. by 8 - 10 cm broad with 10 - 30 rounded or square flattended joints, seeds flat shining brown.

It is distributed in C&E Himalayas, Bengal, Orissa, Bihar. U.P. and Western Ghats, forests of the Bombay State, hill forests of Northern Circars, The Deccan and western ghats from S. Kanara to Travancore.

MEDICINAL USE - Seeds, stem and bark - poisonous. Seeds - fish poison, considered tonic emetic, antiper and anthelm. Paste prepared from seeds, applied locally for inflammatory glandular swellings. Stems - emetic juice of wood and bark- external application for ulcers. Seeds contain saponins.

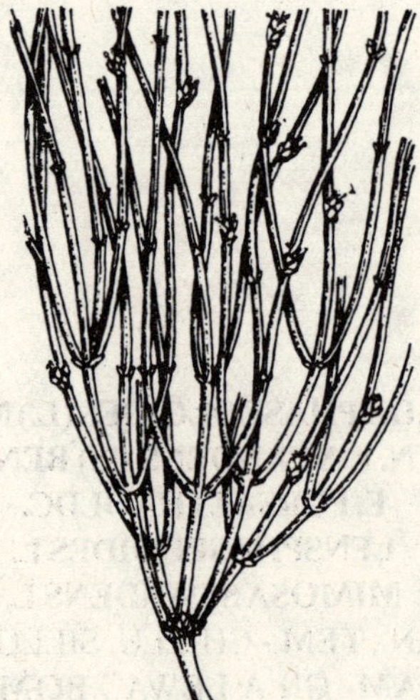

EPHEDRACEAE

EPHEDRA GERARDIANA WALL. EXSTAPF
Syn. E. VULGARIS HOOK. F. NON A. RICH)

PUNJAB- ASMANIA, BUDAGUR, CHEWA, BUTSHUBR., **LADDKH**-TSETEAPAT, TRANO., **BUSHAHR**- RACHI, KHANDA PHAG., **ENG.**- EPHEDRA., **MAR.**- HUMA., **HINDI**- KHANDA, PHOK., **ENG.**- EPHEDRINE.

The plant is dioecious, green, woody and xerophytic. It is a low-growing rigid tufted shrub with usually a gnarled stem and erect green densely clustered branches, 6-4 ft; the branches are fascicled, rather slender, striate nearly smooth and jointed from a branched woody base. Branches with scales at the joints. The stem perform the function of assimilation. The leaves are opposite and connate, reduced to deciduous brown scales present at the nodes of the stem. Spikelets 1/4-1/3"; subsessile, often whorled; fruiting with often fleshy red suculent bracts, 1-2. seeded. Flowers dictinous, with no trace of carpels in male, or of stamens in female; male in spikes, female in pairs or solitary, usually bracteate. The male has a perianth of two antero-post united petals; beyond which the axis is prolonged and bears 2-8 sessile 2-10 c-anthers. The female has a tubular perianth and one erect orthotropic ovule with a long micropy projecting at the top of the flower; the flowers are enclosed by bracts which become red and fleshy after fertilization and enclose the fruit. The seed is biconvex or planoconvex enclosed in the perianth which becomes woody, and the fleshy bracts cover this again. There are two cotyledons in the embryo. Seed albuminous.

A small family with sporadic distribution in regions of the tropics and subtropics of both hemisphers. Temperate and Alpine Himalaya and WesternTibet in the drier regions, alt. 7-12,000 ft; 12-16,000 ft. in Sikkim. Distribution Europe, W. and Central Asia. Afghanistan to Bhutan, 2400-5000 m. Stony slopes, gravel terraces, in drier areas, May-June.

MEDICINAL USE : Dried stems constitute the drug which is used to cure asthma, cold, hay fever and rashes of allergic origin. Drug is also considered to be an effective cardiac stimulant, and nasal spray, prepared of drug, is used in asthamatic attacks and inflammation of mueous membrane.

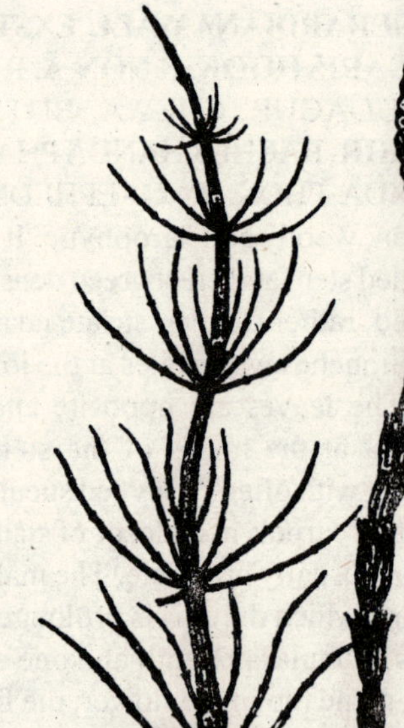

EOUISETACEAE

EQUISETUM AREVENSE LINN
(SYN. E. DEBILE)
ENG. FIELD, HORSETAIL

Horsetails are rush-like perennials with deep creeping (Sym-podial) rhizomes from which arise erecte or scrambling, hollow, jointed aerial branches each year. The plants inhabit swampy ground and sandy banks of streams and rivers. The aerial shoots may be of one or two kinds; in some spp the ordinary green shoot bears the reproductive spike at the end, while in the others there is a special reproductive shoot usually appearing early in the year and often without chlorophyll, the ordinary shoots performing assimilation work only. The stem is very distinctly jointed and at the nodes are borne whorls of small leaves which are reduced to scales and are united to form a sheath closely pressed against the stem, and of little or no use in assimilation. The branches emerge through the leafsheath and thus appear at first sight endogenous; in reality they are exogenous, but formed so much later than the leaves that their points of origin are already covered by the leaf sheath, and so they are complled to burrow through it. Stages in this process may easily be observed. The surface of the stem is grooved; the ridges are occupied by mechanical tissue, whilst the green tissue and stomota are at the base of the furrows. This is a marked xero structure. In many spp. the internodes of the rhizomes are swollen into tubers, which serve for hibernation and vegetative reporduction.

The spike is very like the 8' flowers of a conifer, and has as much (or as little) right to the title of "flower". It is a terminal axis with short internodes, bearing a dense strobilus of peltate sporengiophores. Each of these bears a number of sporoangia upon the underside of the head (i.e. towards the stem) arranged like the horses of a (merry-go-round). The spores are of one kind only, each has, running round it, two spiral cuticularised bands of membrane, formed from the outer wall and termed claters. These are hygroscopic, unfolding in damp air. In the rolling up again on drying, the elaters of one spore become entangled with those of others and cause them to adhere together, so that several prothalli may be formed near one antother when they germinate. This is advantageous, for the prothalli are dioceous, through so far as we can tell the spores are all alike. The prothallus is fairly large, the male being smaller than the female.

It is a genous of vascular cryptogams, known as Horse-Tails, found practically all over the world. Four apecies occur in India. E. ARVENSE; E. DEBILE ROXB.

MEDICINAL USE : The entire plant has been recognized by the German pharmacopeia under the name Herba Equiseti and used as a dimetic. It has haemostatic and harmopoietic properties and its oral adminstration produces a decided increase in corpuscles followed by an increase in physical energy on the part on the patient. It is considered useful in dropsy, gravel and kidney affections. The ashes of the plant are beneficial in aeidity of the stomach and in dyspepsia (U.S.D., 1443 Chem. Abstr; 1937, 31. 3149; 1939, 33, 3966, 4672; 1935, 29, 1981; Wren, 179).

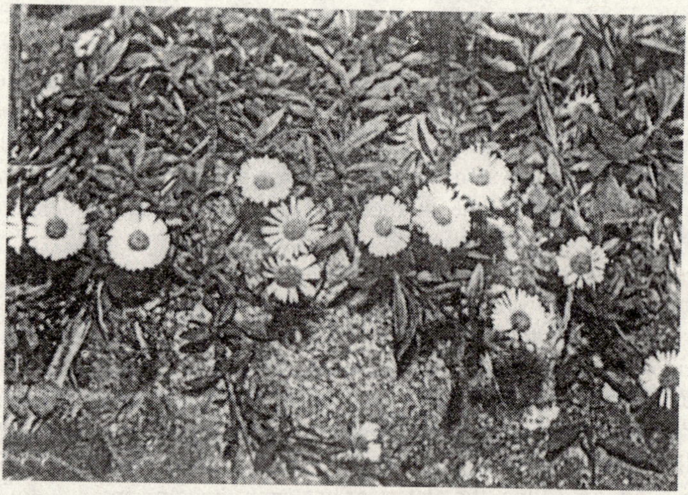

COMPOSITAE

ERIGERON CANADENSIS LINN

SANS.- PALITA, JARAYUPRIYA., **MAKSHIKA**- VISHA., **CAN.**- ADAFLEABANE.

An erect, much branched, stout, hairy herb upto 1 m. tall. Leaves simple 3-8x0.3-0.5 cm. narrowly linear, entire or coarsely toothed; the upper stalkless.

Heads heterogamous, 3.4x4-6 mm, in branched panicles, yellowish. Ray florets usually in two or more rows thread like ligulate not yellow. Pappus-hairs is in one row; stamens blunt at base. Achenes flat, glabrous. Flowers and fruits May-July.

Occurs in moist shady places and waste grounds near fruit orchards and fields. It is reported from West Himalayas, Punjab and upper Gangetic plain upto 3000 ft.

Kashmir Valleys, Assam, Western Ghats and the Nilgiris, uto 7000 ft.

MEDICINAL USE : The whole herb is astrin, stim; haemostatic and diur, used in diarr. dysentry and uterine haemor.

Steam distilation of dry plants yields Erigeron oil of commerce which is used in dysentry, diarhoea, bronachial caterrh and cystitis.

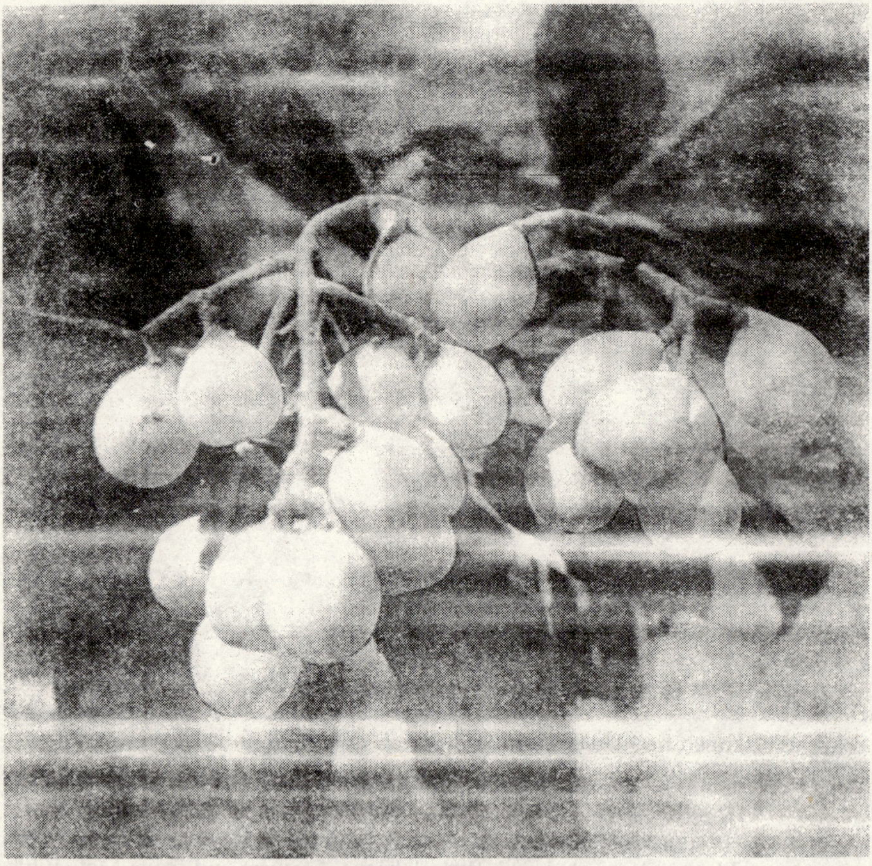

ROSACEAE

**ERIOBOTRYA JAPONICA THUNB.) LINDL.
(SYN. MESPILUS JAPONICUS THUNB.
PHOTINIA JAPONICA GRAY).**

ENGLISH- LOGUAT, JAPAN MEDLAER., **HINDI-** LOKAT, LOGAT., **KANS.-** LOKKATE., **TAMIL-** NOKKOTTA, ILAKKOTTA., **LOCAL NAME-** LOKAT, LUKAT.

It is an erect or suberect evergreen, small or medium sized tree 6 - 7.5 m. tall. Bark is dull black branches and branchlets spreading terminally. Leaves are large clusters at the ends. Leathery 30 x 10 cm or more tappering at the ends, prominently veined. They are dark green and bright and beautiful and look ornamental in apperance. Flowers dull white, fragrant in terminal panicles. The fruit is a pome pyriform or globose baccate, yellow or orange 2.5 - 3.75 cm in loose bunches. Each fruit contains 1-10 seeds (and each seed is 3-5 angled). The flowering season is November - December. Fruits - March - April.

It is cultivated locally in fruit orchards and is reported from Sharanpur, Dehradun, Mujaffarnagar, Meerut, Kanpur, Bareilly Districts of Punjab, U.P. Amristar, Gurdaspur and Hoshiarpur, District of Punjab. Also reported from Assam, Maharastra the Nilgiris and Karnataka.

It is grown all over India upto the height of 5000 ft.

MEDICINAL USE : Fruit considered sedative, used in allaying vomitting and thirst. Flowers expect., infusion of leaves in diar. Chief constituents of ripe fruit are laevolose, sucrose and malie acid, amygdalin in pericarp of unripe fruit. Leaves contain d-sorbitol, and ascorbic acid oxidase and vitamin B.

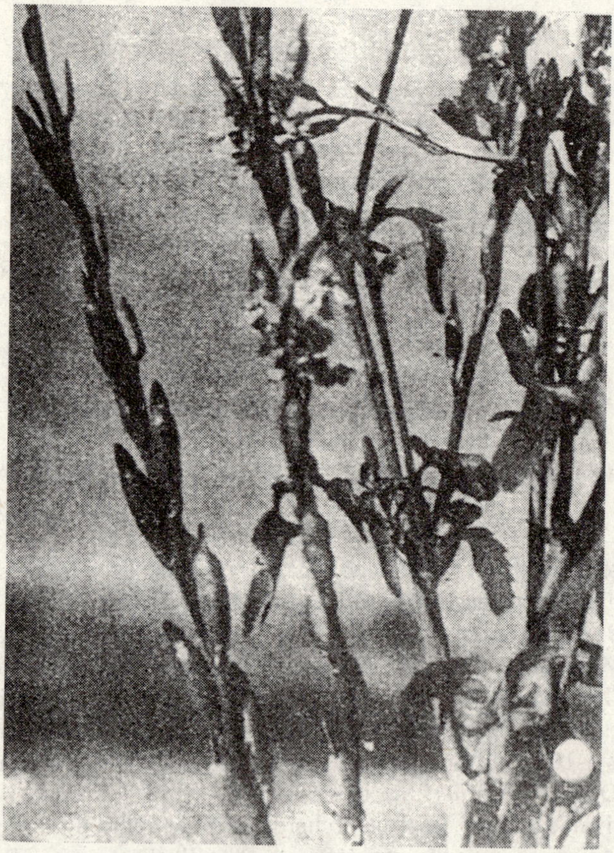

CRUCIFERAE

ERUCA SATIVA MILL

Syn. E. VESICARIA (L.) CAV. SUBSP. SATIVA (MILL.) THELL POPULARLY KNOWN AS ROCKET-SALAD OR ROQUETTE, TARAMIRA.

SANS.- BHUTAGHNA, DARADHARSHA, SIDDARTHA., **HINDI**-TARAMIRA, SEOHA, SAFED SARSON., **BENG**.- SHWETSURSHA., **PUNJAB.**-ASSU, JAMBA, TARA, USAN., **MAR.**- JAMBHO., **ENG.**- ROQUETTE, ROCKET-SALAD., **LOCAL NAME**- TARA, TARAMIRA.

Glaucocus, glabrous, or subhispid, errect branching herb. rarely undershrub; juice watery, often pungent, stem 6-18'. Leaves variously toothed, rarely obovate and subentire, lyrate pinnatifid; alternate; exsitipulate. Flowers large, yellow, or lilae or white, veined with voilet; recemed, rarely solitary on scapes, or axillary. Sepals 4, free, 2 lateral (opposite the placentas) sepals often tipped with hairs; errect, lateral saceate at the base; imbricate; petals-viened, and clawed 4, free, hypogynous, placed crosswise imbricate. Stamens:- 6 rarely 1,2 or many; 2 outer opposite the lateral sepals; 4 inner longer in opposite pairs; Disk with usually 4 glands opposite the sepals. Ovary- 2-celled by a placental membrane, or 1-celled, or with superimposed cellules; style short or 0, stigma simple or with 2 lobes opposite the placenta; ovules 1-2 or indefinite 2-serriate on two parietal placentas rarely solitary and errect Fruit a 2-celled, 2-valved pod, the valves deciduous and leaving the seeds on the persistent placentas (replum) or indehiscent or transversely jointed. Pods-closely adpressed to the axis, ovoid-oblong, turgid. terete, with a large ensiform seedless beak; valves concave, 3-nerved; stigma simple, seeds numerous, 2 serriate, globose; cotyledons conduplicate. Fruiting and flowering season is April and March of every year.

It is reported from cultivated places in Northern and Central India, the Western Himalaya, ascending to 10,000 ft. and upper Gangetic Valley. Distribution Westward to the canaries. Locally it is cultivated as a cold season crop in the fields of Timarpur, Najafgarh, Shahdara and Ghaziabad with BRASSICA COMPASTRIS VAR, sarson Preeni, CICER ARIETINUM LINN, and HORDEUM VULAGARE LINN.

MEDICINAL USE : Seeds are aerid and used like mustard. Leaves are stimulant, stomachic, dimetic and antiscorbutic.

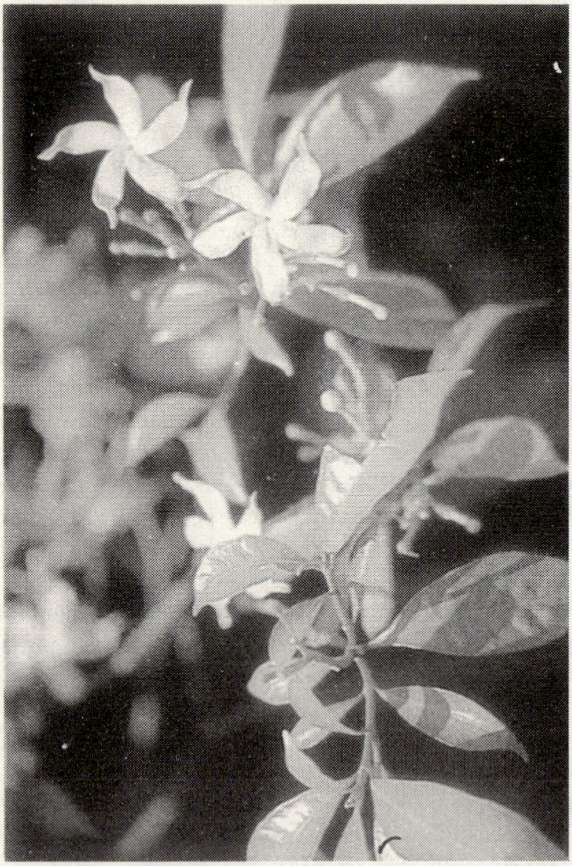

APOCYNACEAE.

ERVATAMIA CORONARIA STAPF. (SYN. E. DIVRICATE (LINN) ALSTON. TABER NAEMONTANA CORONARIA RBR.)

BENGALI & HINDI- TAGAR., **TAMIL-** KARUDUUPLAI, NANDIYAVATUNA, NANDIYAAVATTAI., **TEL.-** GANDHI TAGARAPU & NANDIVARDHNUM). **SANS.-** NANDIPLANT, TAGAR., **GUJARATI-** SAGAR, TAGAR., **MARATHI-** ANANTH, GONDETAGAR, SAGAR, TAGAR., **KAN.-** KOTTATHA NANDIBATALOO., **MAL.-** KUTTUMPALAE, NATTYAVATTUM, TAKRUM., **LOCAL NAME-** CHEMELA, CHANDNI.

It is an ever green shrub, 2.5 m or more in height. The bark is buff coloured and the top of the plant is rosette like. The leaves are oblong to lanceolate, 7.5 - 15 cm long, dark green glabrous and shiny. The stipules are cuplike. The flowers are pure white and bloom throughout the year. They bcome odourless. Flowers occur in few flowered eymes. Follicles 2.5 -5 x 1.1.5 cm. with recurved beats. The seeds are 3-6, embededed in a red, pulpy aril. The flowering period is May-October and fruits are available in winter.

It is cultivated in gardens and is reported from upper Gangetic plain, Garhwal, East Bengal, Khasia hills, Assam, Northern circars and hills of Vizagapatnam.

MEDICINAL USE: Wood is refrigerant. The root is aerid and bitter, used as local anodyne and chewed for relief of tooth ache. Milky juice used for various diseases of eye such as Caruai and cattract. It is also used for skin diseases. It is also used to prevent swellings and burning of ulcers.

Bark of stem and root contains a crystalline substance and alkas tabernaemontanine and coronarine the alks are Pharmacologically active.

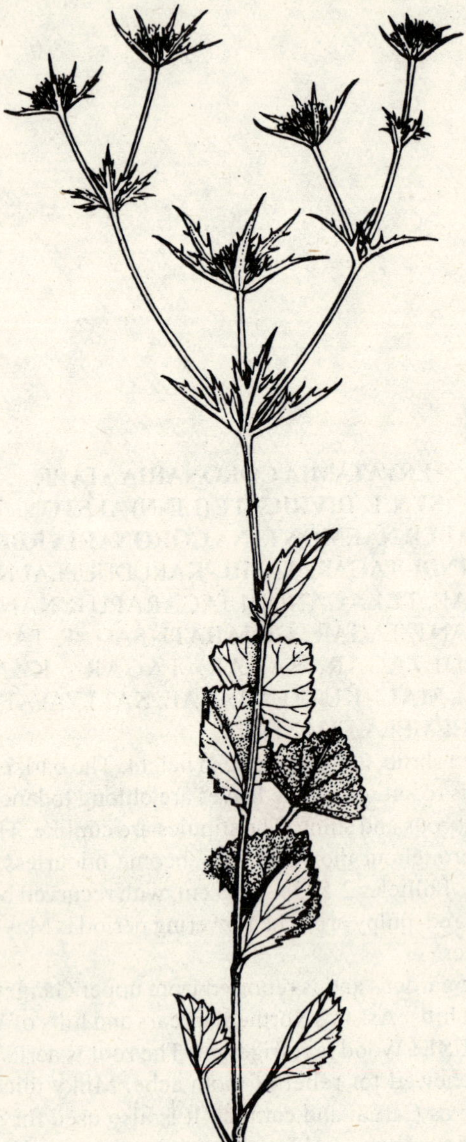

UMBELLIFERAE

ERYNGIUM CAERULEUM BIEB
(SYN. E. BIEBERSTEINIANUM NEVSKIEX BOBROV.

HINDI- DUDHALI., **URDU-** SALELIMICRI, KANDU, DUDHALL., **PUNJABI-** PAHARI GAJAR., **ENGLISH-** ERYNGO SPRINYPERENNIALS.

It is distinguished by its bluish stems and undivided (radical and caline) leaves and its small blue globular flower - heads with 5-8 much longer spine - tipped involucral braets. Flowers globular head C. 1.5 cm. spiny involucral brects to 2.5 cm or more; calyx with lanceolate scales and spiny tipped lobes, petals notched; bracteoles longer basal leaves stalked, oblong to heart - shaped, coarsely toothed; stem leaves stalkes; deeply spiny lobed, fruit ovoid, flattened, scaly.

It is reported from Pakistan to Kashmir, West Asia, 1500-1800 m. Wasteland; common in valley of Kashmir. July - grows in western Himalayas at 2,000 m.

MEDICINAL USE : The ashes of the plant are useful in haemorrhoids, Roots are expactorant, diuretic and diaphoretic and are considered to be haematinie. Roots are also used as nervine tonic and as aphrodisiae. In the unani system of medicine, the plant is used as tonic and stimulant.

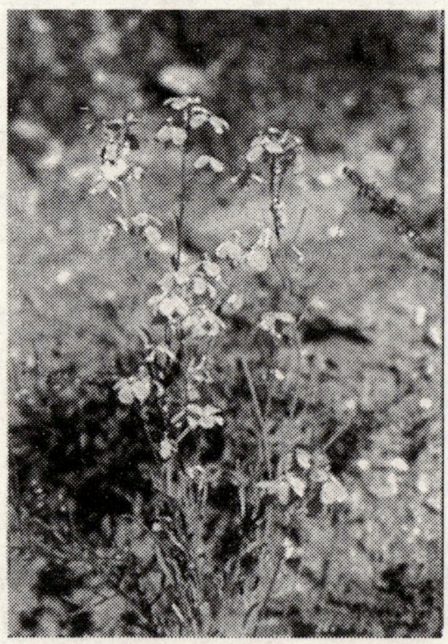

CRUCIFERAE

ERYSIMUM ASPERUM DC
(SYN. E. ARKANSANUM NUTT)

A tall leafy plant 30-80 cm. very variable biennial or perinnial clusters of numerous bright larger yellow flowers 1 - 1.5 cm with longer and broader petals 12-18 mm by 6 - 9 mm. Hairs adpressed, mostly with 2 branches. Style distinct, stigma, usually two lobed. Leaves linear acute, with or without few widely spaced teeth. Fruit long narrow four angled, with valves conspicuously one veined. Seeds in one row.

It is reported from Pakistan to Kashmir 1800-3000 m. Rocks open slope May - August.

Grown in Indian Gardens.

MEDICINAL USE: Seeds contain cheiroline, resembling quinine in Pharmacological action.

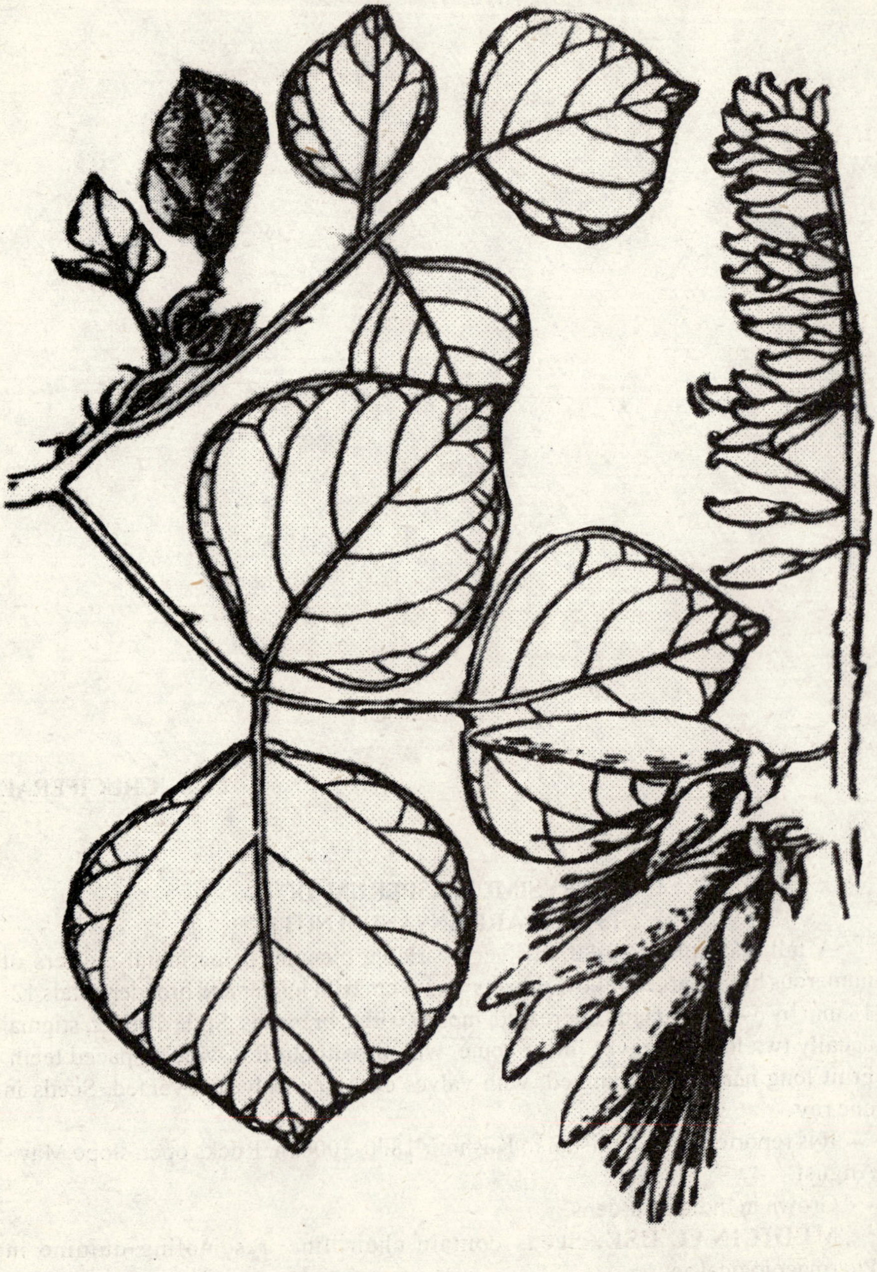

LEGUMINOSAE.

ERYTHRINA STRICTA ROXB.
(SYN. E. INDICA LAMK.
(SYN. E. CORALLODENDRON LINN)

ASSAM BENGALI - PALITA MADAR., **KON.**- PANGIRO., **ENGLISH, INDIAN**- CORAL TREE., **GUJARATI PANARAWAS, HINDI**- FERRUD, MANDAR., **KAN.**- HAARAWAANA., **MAL.**- MOOLOOMOGRIKAH, MULLUMURUKKU., **MARATHI**- PANGARA., **TAMIL MULLO**- MURUKOO, KALIYANMURUNGAI., **TEL.**- BARIJAMY + MULLAMODUGOO., **K.**- KEECHAGA, HEMURUKOO., **SANSKRIT**- MURA.

A large tree with trunk and branches covered with sharp conical whitish prickles. Trunk is corky, crooked, prickly or smooth. Leaflets rhmboid, entire or lobed. Each leaflet is 18 cm., verybroadly ovate, broder than long. Flowers appearing with leaves in dense one sided spike like clusters 10-13 cm long occuring at the ends of stout branches in spring. Flowers are scarlet; calyx companulate spathe - like and split to the base; standard oblong - lanceolate, 4-5 cm. twice as long as keel. Pod is hairless, lanceolate 5-10 cm. Flowering season is summer.

It is cultivated in private and public gardens as hedge plant. It is commonly found in Bengal, deciduous forests of Konkan, north Kanara, Malabar and travancore, Assam and Manipur, extending west wards to Nepal. In many parts of South India it is grown in gardens as a support for black - appear vines.

MEDICINAL USE : Bark is febrifuge, anthel, expectorant and antibilious juice is vermufuge and cathartic. Leaves are diuretic, laxative, emmengogue and galactogogue. In its action erythrine, the alkaloid, is antagonistic to strychnine and may be used as an antidote to strychnine poisoning.

ERYTHRINA SUBEROSA ROXB. (Coral tree)

BO. & HINDI- DOLLDHAK, MADAR, MANDAR, PANGRA, NASUT PAUGRA., **TAMIL**- MALLUMURUNGAI, MULLUMUROOKU., **KAN.**- KADDUPARIVAL MULLOHARIVAN KADU AARIBAANA., **TEL.** - BARIYAMA BARIDAPU, BARJAMA; BARIJAPU., **PUNJAB**- THAB., **GUJARAT**- JAGGARI, VOKHA KHARO, JANGARIYA., **MARATHI**- PANGARA: ASSAM, MANDAL., **BIHAR & ORISSA**- PEERI.

A medium sized tree with spiny. corky, deeply fissured bark, and with scarlet flowers appearing before or with the young leaves in small short crowded clusters at the ends of branches. Flower clusters 5 - 10 cm. standard 4-5 cm. Oblong, keel scarcely half as long, wings, minute, leaflets 3, broadly, ovate, the terminal largest, 8-12, cm all densely hairy beneath often with reddish-brown hairs. Corolla companulate. Pod hairless, cylindrical long - pointed somewhat constricted between seeds, 13-15 cm leaflets rhomboid entire or lobed. Flowers summer season.

Cultivated in public and private gardens. Grows in Punjab plains, upper gangetic plain, central and south India.

MEDICINAL USE - Bark used in medicine.

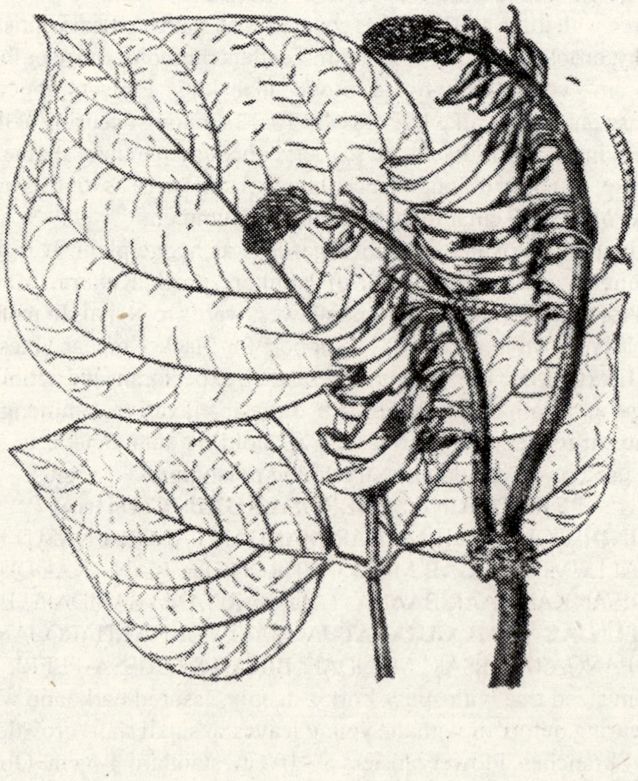

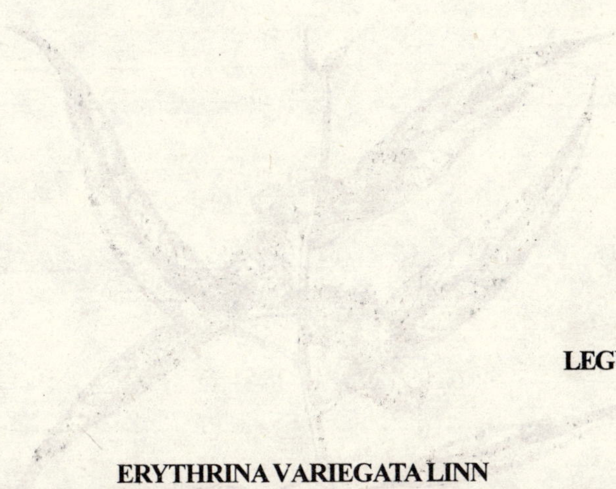

LEGUMINOSAE

ERYTHRINA VARIEGATA LINN
(VAR. ORIENTALIS (LINN) (MERRILL SYN. E. INDICA LAM)

SANSKRIT- MANDAR., **HINDI**- DADAP., **BENGALI**- PALITAMANDAR., **MARATHI**- PANGARA., **TAMIL**- KALIYANAMURUKKU., **TEL.**- BADISA., **LOCAL NAME**- RAKTA MADAR.

It is a medium sized tree; stem is covered with numerous prickles. The leaves are trifoliate and the leaftlets are broad ovate to rhombic ovate, nearly as long as broad. Flowers appear (before the leaves) on leafless branches with one bright scarlet showy in numerous bunches. Calyx spathaceous. The flowering season is from March - April.

These plants are grown in gardens and bungalows. It is found throughout India in deciduous forests and in Andaman and Nicobar Islands.

MEDICINAL USE : Bark astrin. febge, in liver troubles, anthelm. as a collyrium in opthalamia, antid to snake bite. Leaves laxt, diur., anthelm, galaet, emmen, applied externally for dispersing veneral buboes and for relieving pain in joints.

Juice of leaves - vermifuge, cath.

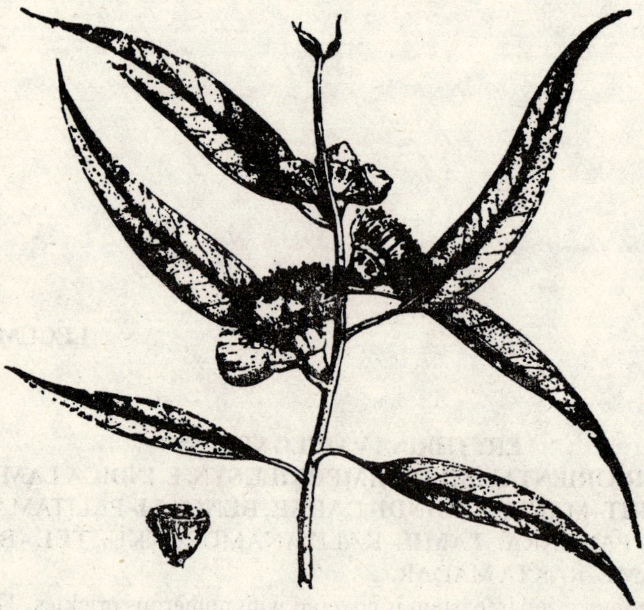

MYRTACEAE.

EUCALYPTUS CITRIODORA HOOK
(SYN. E. MACULATA HOOK)
VARIETY - CITRIODORA BAILEY:

TEL.- TALANOPPI., **ENGLISH-** LEMON SCENTED EUCALYPTUS., **MAL.-** KARPURUM ARAM., **TAMIL-** KARPOORAMARAM.

A tall handsome tree; Bark shining, whitish or reddish grey. leaves 15-20 cm long lanceolate, bright green, usually falcate. Flowers white found in three (3) flowered unbels arranged in panicals on short leafless branches. Calyx lobes and petals united to form an operculum of cap. Operculum double, inner transparent; outer hemispheric pointed. Stamens opening by slits; fruit a dehiscent capsule large 1.5 cm long by 1 cm diameter ovoid, valves deeply enclosed.

It is planted in the plains of North India and in the mountain traets. Also grown in Malabar, the Nilgiris and Coorg. In recent years extensive plantation of this species has been undertaken in Punjab, U.P. and Andhra Pradesh.

MEDICINAL USE : An essentail oil is obtained from leaves and terminal branchlets is a source of citronellal for manufacture of citronellol and menthol which is used in medicine. A small portion of the oil is also used as germicides and disinfectants.

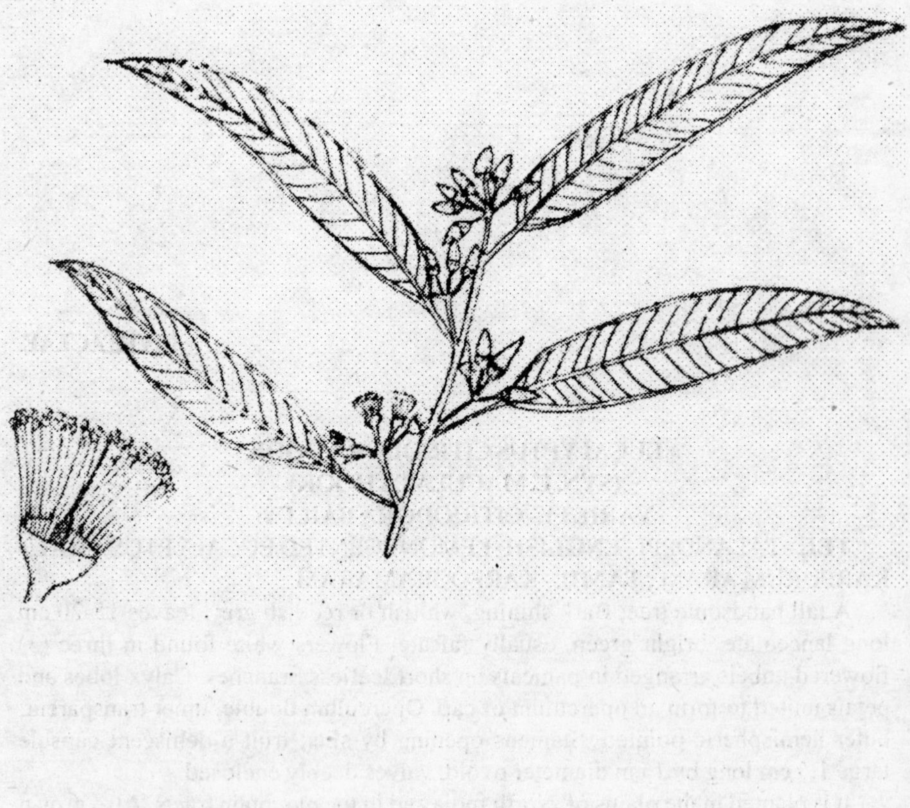

MYRTACEAE.

EUCALYPTUS GLOBULUS LABILL

MADRAS STATE- KARPURA MARAM., **ENG.-** THE AUSTRALIAN GUM TREE, BLUE GUM., **TAMIL-** KARPOORAMARAM, **MAL & KANNADA-** PURAMARAMTALIA., **TELGU-** TALANOPPI-AKU.

A tall tree, bark peeling in long strips or sheets and thus exhibits discrimination and forms an identifying character. Leaves are bifacial, lanceolate, scytheshaped, glabrous, sessile, thin and wax coated; a few round internal oil glands are present and calciumoxalate crystals of prismatic and rosett type are also found. Infloresence an umble which by lengthening of the axis passes to a panicle or corymb. The floral receptacle is hollow and woody in the front (fr). The Calyx is thrown off as a lid when the flower opens. Flowers large white, 1-3 together in axils. Operculum depressed hemispheric, abruptly pointed.

Cosmopolitan, it is reported from all over the country, the mountains as well as plains. Also grown in Malabar, Nilgiris and Coorg. It is known as a native of Australia. Anamalai and Palni Hills in south India, Simla Hills (4,000 - 7000 ft.) and at Shillong in Assam.

MEDICINAL USE : Leaves are fabrifuge and carminative, stimulant, expectorant, diaphoretic and antiseptic, Anti malarial properties are attributed to the volatile oil. Eucalyptus oil is a powerful antiseptic and disinfectant.

There are many other species of this plant, out of which E. ROSTRATA; E. VIMINALIS and E. POLYANTHEMOS Are used more or less for the same purpose.

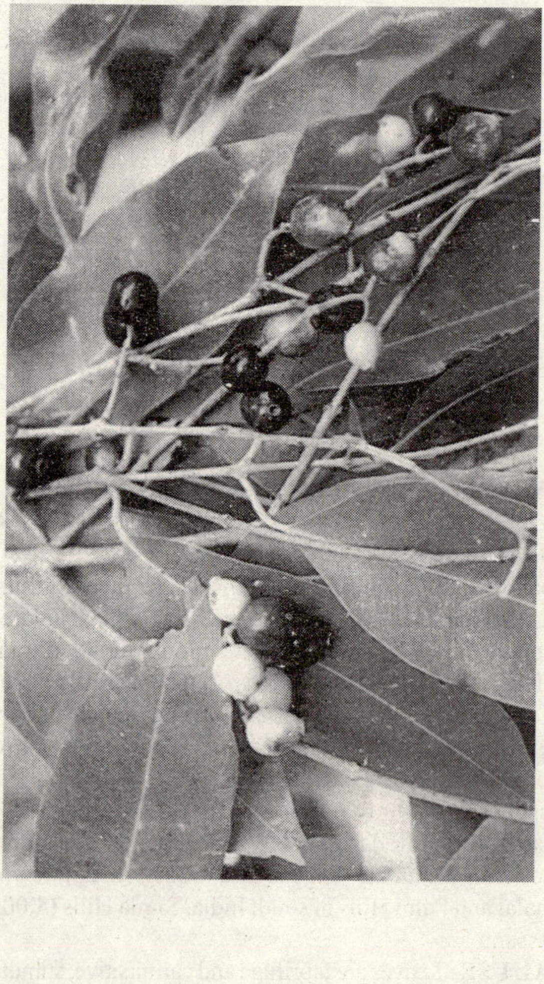

MYRTACEAE

EUGENIA JAMBOLANA LAMK
SYN. MYRTUS CUMINI L.
(SYN. SYZYGIUM JAMBOLAUM DC.)
SYN.S. CUMINI (LINN) SKEELS
(SYN. E. CAYOPHYLLIFOKIA)
"S.AROMATICUM
"E. AROMATIICUM

BENG., KALA-JAM ENG.- JAMBUL. BLACK PLUM, BLACK BERRY; JAVA PLUM, JAMBOLANA., **GUJ.**- JAMBUDO., **HINDI**- JAMAN, PHALINDA, JAMUN, JAMBU, JAMBAVA., **KAN.**- NEARLY., **KON.**- JAMBUL., **MAR.**- JAMBUL., **MAL.**- NAVAL., **TAM.**- NAGUM, NAAGAMA RA, NEREDAM., **TEL.**- NALRAEDU, JAMBUV., **SANS.**- JAMBU., **BOMB.**- JAMBU., **LOCAL NAME.**- JAMUN.

A tree, usually of considerable size with a thick and rather crooked trunk. Bark smooth gray. Leaves :- 3-6 inches; extremely variable in shape and opposite smooth and shining, the numrous nerves uniting within the margin; ovate or oblong obtuse or more or less acuminte coriaceous closely nerved. Petiole 1"2-1 panicles lateral below the leaves rarely axillary or terminal. Inlorescence : cyme short and compact or laxly paniculate panicles lateral from the scars of fallen leaves bracts usually small and deciduous. Flowers greenish white calyx shortly turbinate limb truncate or obscurely 4-lobed, petals 4; calyptrate; stamens in many rows, free or slightly combined into four bundles, filaments filiform; anthers small, versatile, bursting longitudinally, ovary 2, rarely3 celled style filiform stigma small; ovules in each cell. Berry : Drupe like often obliquely oblong olive shaped to globse purple from size of a pea to a pigeons egg; rarely dry and fibrous, crwoned, with the prsistent calyx dark purple and juicy seeds few globose, variously compressed, testa one seeded membranous or cartilaginous, embryo thick and fleshy, radicle short, cotyledons thick; distinct. The floweing period April-June and fruiting period is June-July every year.

It is Common wild or cultivated and generally distributed throughout India in both peninsulas and in Ceylon; from the planes to 4-5000 ft. Distribution . Malay archipelago to Australia. Locally it is commonly cultivated in the Subzimandi, sarai Rohilla, Kingsway Camp and Karnal Road. Gardens for its fruits which are eaten raw and sold in the market has been planted as a road-side tree in New Delhi.

MEDICINAL USE : (1) Blossoms are an important source of honey. Bark is used in dyeing and fanning and is also asstringent and used in preparation of gargles and mouth washes. A decoction of bark and seeds is said to be useful in diarroea and dysentery. Alcoholic extraet of seeds has been reported to reduce level of blood-sugar in diabetic patients. The cotyledons dried in shade and ground to a fine powder for effective medicine in reducing blood sugar in body.

Its related species used in geriforte syrup and tablets.

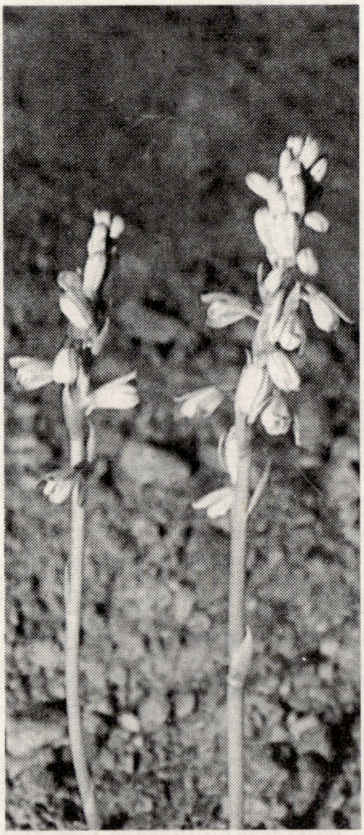

ORCHIDACEAE

EULOPHIA DABIA (D.DON) HOCHR.
(SYN. E. CAPESTRIS WALLICH EX LIND LEY)

BENGALI- SALIBMISRI., **SUNG.-** MISRIE., **PUNJABI & HINDI-** SALIBISRI., **BOMBAY-** SALUM., **SANS.-** AMRITA, PRANADA.

It is a terrestrial plant with bleshy tuber or rhizome. Stem 15-40 cm. sheethed with papery braets. Leaves appear after flowering spikes, leaves 2, linear pointed, 25-40 cm. long by 1 cm broad. Flowers appearing before the leaves, pale pink with darker lines, many in a one-sided spike 6-9 cm long. Flowers 1 to 2 cm long; petals blunt, shorter than the acute sepals, lip short, three lobed, with short side lobes and with transersely oblong, orange, toothed mid-lobe, which is three ridged at base and with a patch of densely crowded short bristles at apex. spur short, conical.

It is reported from Himachal Pradesh to C. Nepal 1500-2400 m dry hill sides, pine forests. April-May. Throughout the greater part of India mostly in the plains.

MEDICINAL USE : Rhizome valuable as tonic and aphrodis, used in stomatitis, purulant cough and heart troubles.

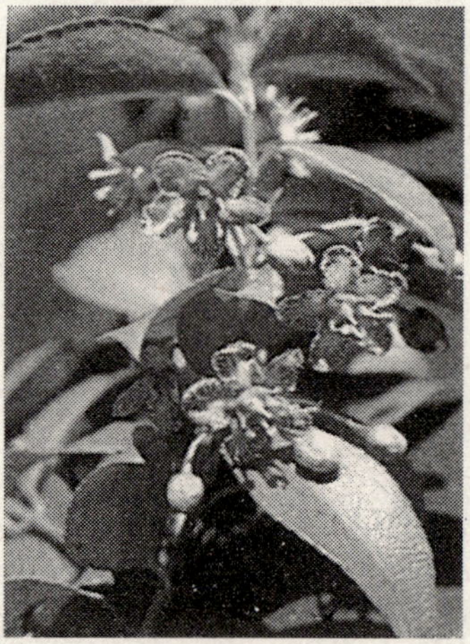

CELASTRACEAE

EUONYMUS TINGENS WALLICH

HINDI- KUNGKU., **SIMLA-** CHOPRA.

It is ever green shrub or tree with dark ash grey corky bark and with thick dull green leathery wrinkled elliptic to ovate - lanceoate leaves, which are closely toothed and paler beneath. Flowers in long - stalked axillary clusters, often at base or apex of branches; flowers yellowish white and strongly veined with purple c. 1-3 cm across. Petals usually 5, toothed; anthers red. Leaves 2 - 5 cm. Fruit top shaped C. 1-5 cm across, 3-5 angled, not winged, seed half encircled in orange aril.

It is reported from temperate Himalayas from the Sutlej to Nepal, 6,500 - 10,000 ft. Himachal Pradesh to S.W. China, Burma, 2100-3300 m Forests April - June.

MEDICINAL USE : Bark considered usful in eye diseases and used in cases of chronic constipation and dyspep.

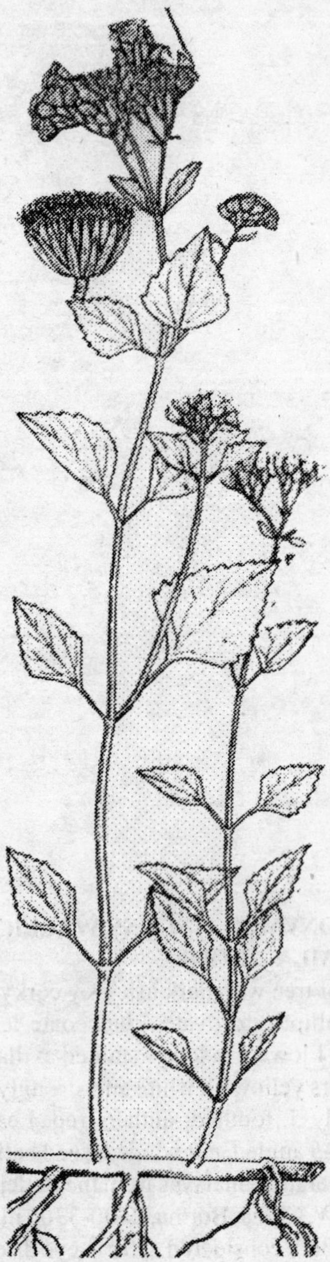

COMPOSITAE

EUPATORIUM TRIPLINERVE VAHL
(SYN. E. AYAPANA VENT)

MARATHI, HINDI & BENGALI - AYAPANA., **TAM. & TEL.**- AAYAPANNAI., **ENGLISH**- AYAPANA TEA., **GUJ.**- ALLIPA., **KAN.**- AYAPNUM.

An aeromatic, erect shrubby perennial to 1 m or more. Stem herbaceious with simple and slippery leaves glandular - hairy beneath. Flowers head white, slightly larger to 8 mm long usually in dense domed or flat - topped clusters, and with opposite, lanceolate to ovate, acutely - toothed leaves. Flower heads C. 6 mm across; florets all tubular, dilated upwards; involueral bracts lanceolate and mostly spiny. Leaves C. 7 cm, stalked; stem 30-90 cm; fruit black, angled with a pappus of slender hairs.

It is a native of Brazil, cultivated in various parts of India in damp places, meadows and river banks. It is also distributed in the temperate Himalayas and Khasi hills.

MEDICINAL USE : It is used as diaphoretic, diuretic emetic and in Jaundice, thermogenic for fomenting sores and ulcers. Juice of the fresh leaves is used as haemostatic agent particularly for checking internal haemorrhage. In higher doses it is an aperent given in derangement of the stomach and bowls, dyspepsia, & cough. In small doses it is a tonic and stimulant. Fresh bruised leaves are applied to foul ulcers, sores and to bites of venomous reptiles. It is also used in sanke bite internally and in Cholera.

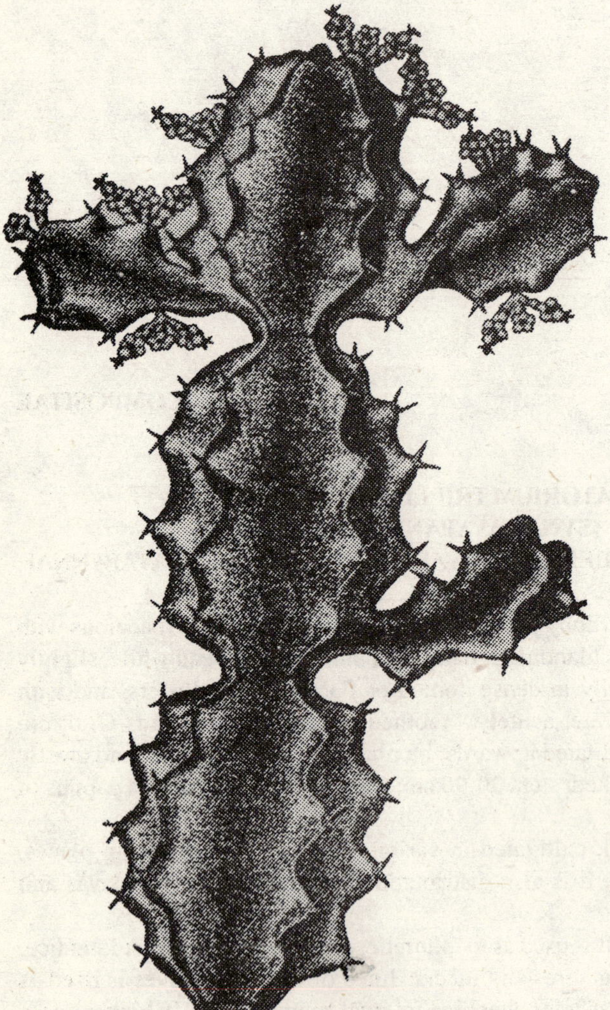

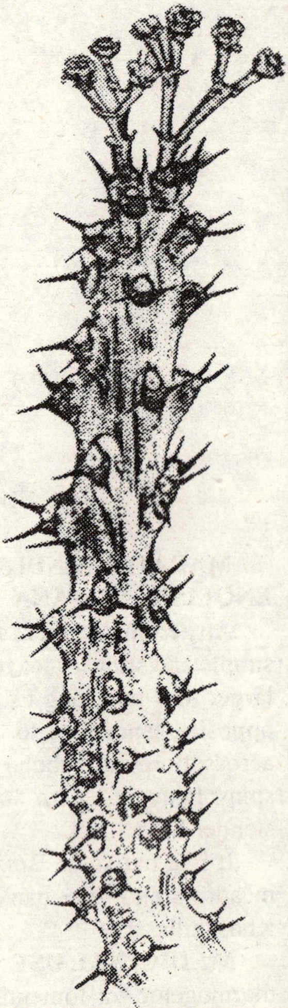

EUPHORBIACEAE

EUPHORBIA ANTIQUORUM LINN

SANSKRIT- VAJRAKANTAKA, SNUHI, VAJR., **HINDI-** TREDHERA SEHUND., **BENGALI-** TIKATA, SIJ: BAJWARAN., **MARATHI-** NARASYA, NARASEJA., **GUJ.-** TANSHARISE HUND., **TEL.-** BOMAJEMUDU., **TAMIL-** VACHIROM., **KAN.-** MULAJEMUDU, KEDARAVALLI., **MAL.-** CHADURAKALLI.

It is a shrub perennial, erect upto a height of 50 cm - 2 m. Branches are 3-5 angled. It grows throughout India in warmer regions, in dry plates assending to 2000 ft. on hills.

MEDICINAL USE : Plant purg. digest. pungent. Root bark - purg. decoction of stem in gout. Juice of plant purg. irrit, in rheumatism and toothache, used in nervine diseases dropsy, palsy, deafness to kill maggots in wounds and application for warts and other cutaneous affection.

EUPHORBIA NERIIFOLIA AUCT. PL. NON. LINN

SANS.- SNUHI., **HINDI-** SCHAND, THUAR, THOR, SEHUND., **MARATHI-** MINGUTA., **TAM.-** ILAIKALLI., **TEL.-** AKUJEMUDU., **PUNJ.-** GANGICHU., **BENGALI-** DUDHIAPHUL.

A seculent shrub or small tree. It has got five angled branches.

It grows wild in Orissa Deccan peninsula but is cultivated in hedges throughout India.

MEDICINAL USE : JUICE of the plant is used in earach and asthma. Milky juice used as purg; rubft; and expect. to remove warts and cutaneous eruptions. Root is used in scorpion sting and snake bite; antisep. fish poison.

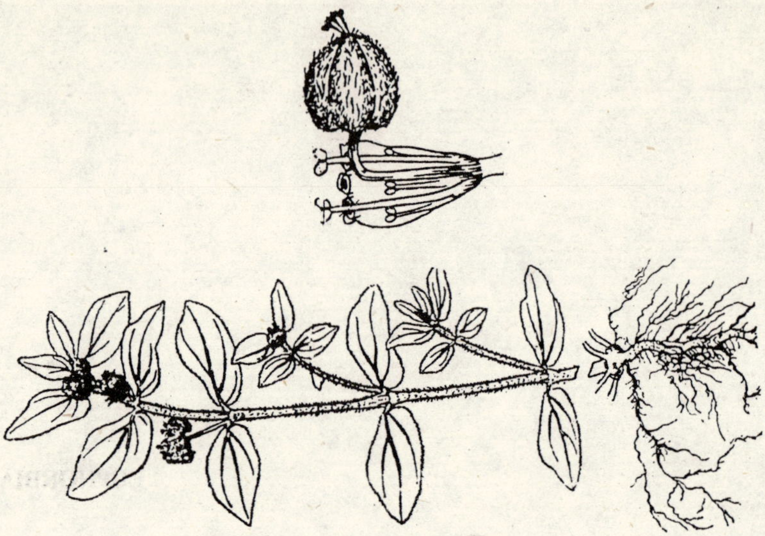

EUPHORBIACEAE

EUPHORBIA DRACUNCULOIDES LAM

BENG. - CHHAGUL - PUPTI., **HINDI**- CHEAGULPULPUTI., **PUNJAB**- KANGI., **TEL.**- TILLA - KADA., **LOCAL NAME**- JAIEHI.

It is an erect smooth dichotmously branched, deep rooted herb. Branches many leafy. Leaves 3-5.5x0.3-0.4 cm. linear to linear-lanceolate, alternate to opposite, 2-3 at each node. Involucers nearly sessile, solitary, glabrous; lobes tanceolate glands moon - shaped; flowers pale yellow. Capsules glabrous, about 5x4 mm. seeds ellipsoid, strophiolate. Flowers and fruits - April to August.

Commonly in cultivated and fallow fields on sandy and clayey, dry soils. Throughout India in the plains and low hills.

MEDICINAL USE : Fruits used to remove warts in the skin.

EUPHORBIACEAE

EUPHORBIA HIRTA LINN.
(SYN. E. PILULIFERA AUCT. NON L.)

HINDI-LALDUDHI DUIHI., **BENG.**- BARO-KHERUIE., **MAR.**- DUDHI, MOTHIDUDHI, DUALI, NAYETI., **GUJ.**- DUDELI., **TEL.**- REDDINANABROLU, BIDARIE., **TAM.**- AMAMPATCHAIARISI, PATCHAIYARISSI., **MAL.**- NELAPALAI., **BOMB.**- NAYETI., **SANS.**- PUSITOA, AMAMPATCHAIARISI., **LOCAL NAME**- DUDHI, DUDHIBEL.

An annual, erect prostrate or ascending hispid herb, branching from the root stock. Stem is with copious crisped hairs, 6-20 inch high. Leaves-dark green or reddish above, white-villous beneath, 2.5-1.5 cm; elliptic or ovate-oblong lanceolate with obligue bases, opposite, acute toothed or serrulate, nerves distnict; very shortly petioled, 3/4-1-1/2 inch long, base usually narrow and obliquely cordate. Inflorescence of many male and one female flower in a small 4-5 lobed turbinate or campanulate perianth-like involucre. Involucres about 1/30; glands small, globos, without a perceptible limb. Floral minute, involucres numerous in axillary and terminal dense-floweres. Sessile or peduneled eymes minute pubescent, limb of glands very narrow or obsolete, coeci compressed keeled pubescent, seed pale brown acutely angled transversly shallowly rugose. Capsule. 1/24 inch in diameter. Patently hairy breaking into 3 cocei seeds trigonous and reddish to brown. The acute leaves, hispid, hairiness, and small fruit render this species easily recognizable.

Common throughout the hotter parts of India from the Punjab eastwards and Southwards to Ceylon and Singapore. Distribution-all tropical and sub tropical countries; Locally it is common and abundant weed throughout on the ridge, in cultivated and waste ground. Also met in the crevices of wall and unused land near habitations; after ascending along the walls. Flowering and fruiting continues for the greater part of the year.

MEDICINAL USE : Entire plant is used in diseases of children i.e., in worms, bowel complaints, cough etc., Juice of plant is used in dysentery and colic. Decoction of plant is beneficial in bronchial affections and asthma. Latex of plant is used as application for warts.

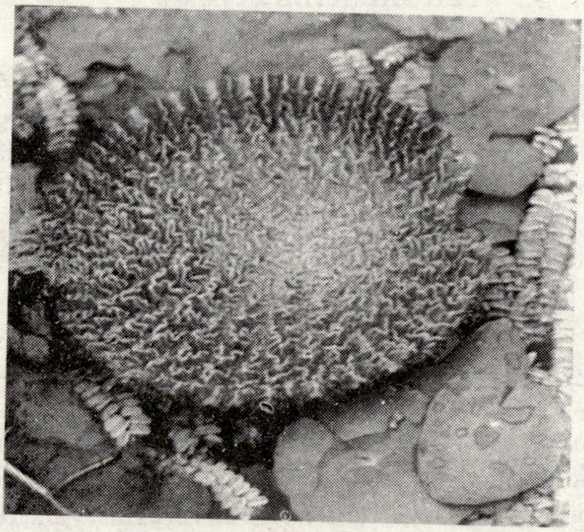

NYMPHAEACEAE

EURYALE FEROX SALISB.

SANS., HINDI & BENGALI- MAKHANA., **PUNJABI-** JAWAR., **TEL.-** MELLUNIPADMAMU.

It is an aquatic plant with large underwater rhizome. Stems and leaf stalks - prickly. Leaves floating, rounded or elliptic 30 - 120 cm. across, green and corrugated above, red or purple with thick spiny veins beneath. Flowers solitary, partially submerged, bright red within shining green outside, petals many; stamen numerous; fruit 5-10 cm across; spongy berry crowned with persistent sepals, seeds 8-20, black imbeded in pulp.

It is common in fresh water tanks and Jheels of northern, central and western India.

MEDICINAL USE : Seeds in spermatophorea, tonic, astrin, deobstruent. Seeds are also a rich source of protein.

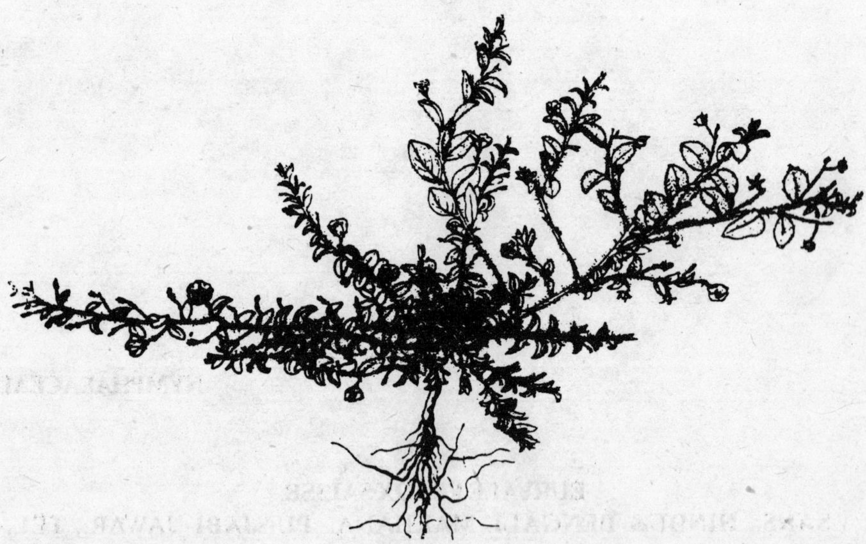

CONVOLVULACEAE

EVOLVU LUS ALSINOIDES LINN
Syn. CONVOLVULUS ALSINOIDES LINN.

HINDI.- SANKHAPUSHPI, SHYAMAXRANTA., **KAN.**- VISHNUKRANTI., **MAL.**- VISTNAUCLANDI., **MAR.**- SHANKHA VALLI, VISHNUKAANTA., **SANS.**- VISNUKRANTI, VISHNUGANDHI., **TAM.**- VISNUKARANDI., **TEL.**- VISHNUKARAANTA., **GUJ.**- KALISANKHAVLI., **BOMB.**- SHANKHA WALLI.

A genus of small herbs or under shrubs distributed in the warm regions of the world. Two species occur in India.

(1) E. ALSINOIDES LINN

(2) E. NUMMULARIUS LINN

A densely hairy perennial herb with spreading, prostrate annual branches numerous, wiry arising from a small woody rootstock. leaves linear, oblong or wide - elliptic, nearly sessile 1/4-1; rarely 11/2 by 1/2", very variable distichous clothed with appressed pubescence or moderately silky with white or fulvous hairs. Petiole 0-1/8". Flowers light blue or blue, in 1 to 3 flowered, axillary, filiform peduncles. Peduncles 1/8-1 1/2"' bracts small, linear, hairy, persistent; pedicels 0-1/2", sepals; subequal, unaltered in fruit; corolla funnel-shaped; limb 5-plaited, subentire. Stamens included or exserted, filaments filiform ovary 2-1 celled, 4 ovuled; styles 2, seperate from the base, each cleft into 2 linear or subclavate stigmas.

Capsule: 1/8-1/6" globose, 4-valved, normally 4-seeded. Seeds glabrous; cotyledons doubly folded radicle incumbent. Flowering and fruiting seasons is July to Novermber ever year.

Found throughout India and Ceylon, very common; rare in very damp regions. The tropical and subtropical area of the globe. Locally it is common throughout on moist or dry sandy soils ascending to 6,000 ft in Himalayas occurs on the Ridge in gravelly soil or in the crevices of stones.

MEDICINAL USE : The plant is bitter and is reported to be used as tonic and febrifuge, and vermifuge, in dysentry. The plant with oil is used for promoting growth of hair (Koman, 1919, 15; Kirt and Basu, III, 1738; Brown, III,225). Leaves are made into cigrettes and smoke in chronic bronchitis and asthma. It is also used as anthelminitic and anti-phlogistic.

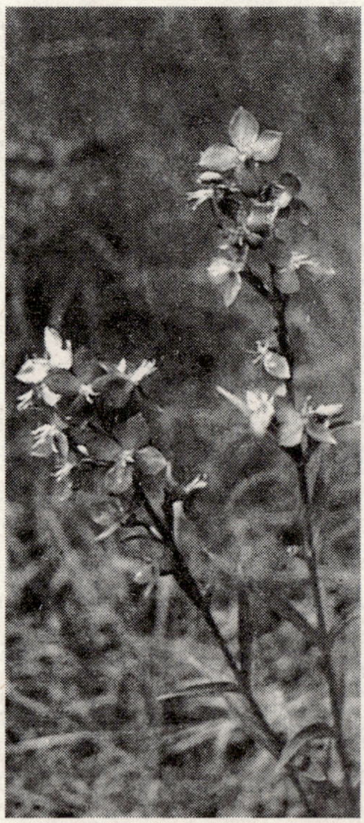

GENTIANACEAE

EXACUM TETRAGONUM ROXB.

HINDI- AVE CHIRETTA., **BENG.-** KOOCHURI., **ASSAM-** SHER - RI - TAKTI.

It is a herbaceous plant. stem is profusely branching four angled erect 30- 120 cm. leaves 3.5- 12.5cm. opposite clapsing at base and broadly Ianceolate; usually con>spicuously 3-veined; Flowers blue, in terminal spike like clusters borne on branching stems; Flowers 3 cm across,with four spreading ovate acute lobes much larger than corolla tube and with long exserted anthers and style. Calyx with 4 ovate long pointed Keeled lobes,braets lanceolate;the lower larger ovary two chambered;stigma is entire capsule globular with persistent calyx and corolla.

It is reported from Uttar Pradesh to Bhutan, India, S. China, S.E. Asia, 1000 - 1800 mm. open slopes damp places. August to October; Also from Himalaya from Simla to Bhutan upto 5000 ft. upper Gangetic plain from Bengal to Chhota Nagar, Madhya Pradesh, N. Circars and khasia Hills to Burma.

MEDICINAL USE : Tonic in fevers, stomach, bitter.

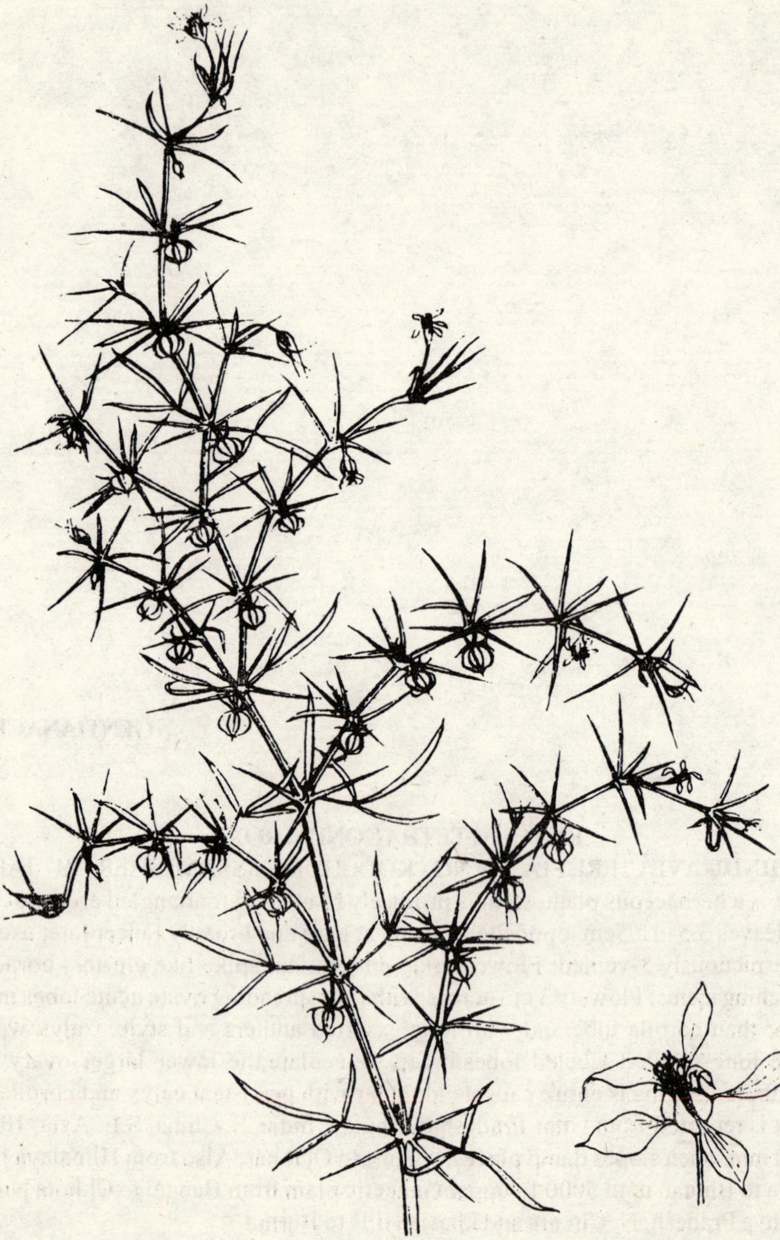

ZYGOPHYLLACEAE

FAGONIA CRETICA LINN
(SYN. F. ARABICA LINN)
"F. HRUGUIERI D.C.
"F. MYSORENSIS ROTH.

HINDI- DAMAHAN USTARKHAN., **MARATHI-** DHAMASO., **PUNJABI-** DAMA SAMADA., **SANSKRIT-** DUSPARSHA., **TEL-** CHITTIGARA., **LOCAL NAME-** DHUANSA.

It is a small diffused spiny shrub with crrect branches. It reaches a height of 60-70 cm. Branches are glandular, nodes swollen. Leaves are 1-3 foliate. Leaflet is linear or elliptic. Stipular spines in 3-4 at each node. Flowers pink or sometimes whitish. Nutlets 1 seeded - seeds brown. Flowers and fruits July - october.

Locally it is found on hilly tracts of Delhi on dry yellowish brown soil. Recently it is located from other parts of Delhi also. It is also reported from Deccan/W Khandesh, Kutch, Sind, Baluchistan Wazirstan, W. Rajputana Upper Gangetic plain, Punjab and Westwords to Afghanistan.

MEDICINAL USE : Locally the extract of plant is used for spermatorrhoea, the ash is given to children, suffering from anaemia. Plant bitter, astrin. tonic febge, prophylaetic against small pox, in dropsy, delirium and any disorder arising from poisoning. Leaves and twigs are cooling.

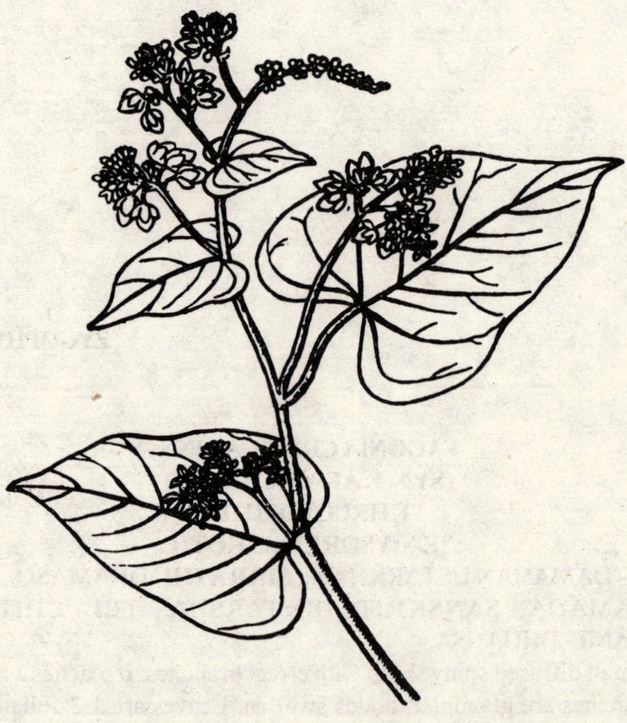

POLYGONACEAE

FAGOPYRUM ESCULENTUM MOENCH

HINDI- KOTU., **PUNJABI-** OGAL, DERAN, OBUL PHAPHAR, PHAPHRA., **ASSAMESE-** DORON., **KUMAON-** OGUL., **SIMLA-** PHAPHRA., **DARJEELING-** TILAPHAPUR., **ENGLISH-** BUCK WHEAT.

A slender erect annual glaborous unbranched 30 - 100 cm. tall. often tinged red at maturity to 60 cm. Stem angular, hollow with swollen nodes Leaves 4-8 x 3.5 - 5 cm ovate - cordate alternate. Leaves with a triangular heart shaped blade (hastate or cordate) mostly as long as broad, 2-5 cm. and with rounded or triangular basal lobes the lower leaves stalked, the upper stalkless stipules ochraceous, inflorence axillary and terminal sub-capitate cyme with densely clustered flowers often in white, red or pink colours, perianth five partite, stamens eight (8) with alternating eight glands at the base, ovary one chambered with one ovule. Superior, ovules erect, style tripartite each with a capitate stigma. The fruit is not an achene, distinctly triangular c-6 mm. with smooth faces and angles.

Flowering and fruiting in cold season. It is reported from Pakistan to Bhutan 2000-4400 m.Grown for grain throughout temperate Eurasia, widely cultivated in the Himalaya - June - September.

MEDICINAL USE : Grains recommended at a diet in colic, choleric diarr. fluxes and abdominal obstructions in China. Seed flour used in Spain as an emol. and resolv. Plant yields glued. rutin, which is used in medicine in the treatment of capillary frazility with associated hypertension. It is found useful in other kinds of haemorrages such as bleeding from kidney; hereditary haemorrhages Bleeding from kidney is such hereditary haemorrhagic telamgiectasia.

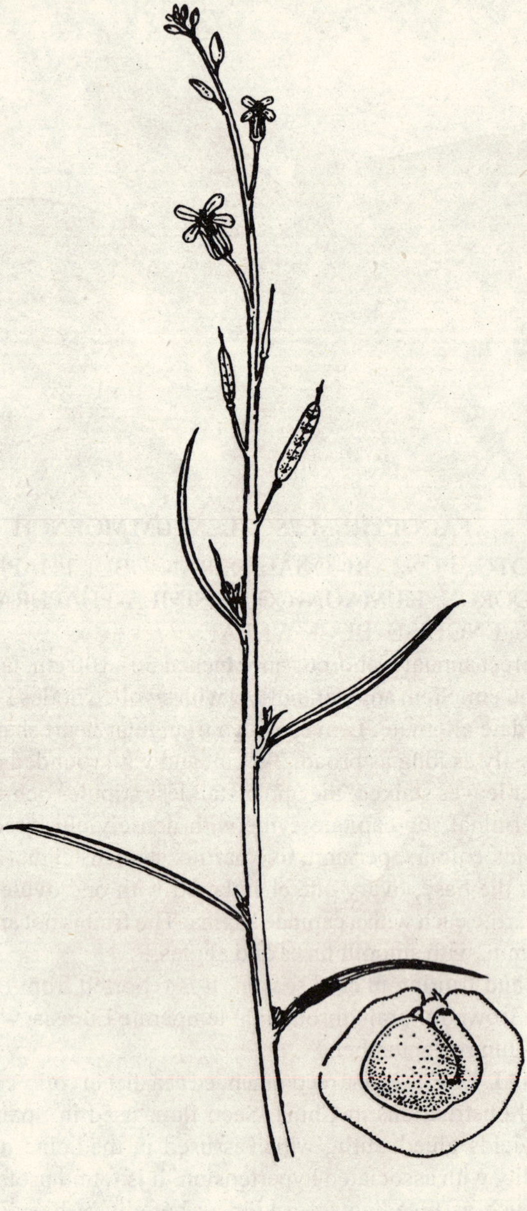

CRUCIFERAE

FARSETIA HAMILTONII ROYLE

PUNJABI- FARID BULT., **FARID-** MULI, LATHIA MULEI., **LOCAL NAME-** BUI.

It is an erect branching hoary herb. Leaves narrowly linear opposite Margin is entire. Axilary stipules present. Flowers whitish small. Pods 1-2 x 0.4 0.5 cm, short and broad linear oblong pointed. Seeds one or two serriate; winged; deep brown orbicular. flowers and fruits April - October.

Found in dry sandy or clayey soil as a local weed . It is distributed in punjab, sind, baluchistan, west Rajputana and North India.

MEDICINAL USE : Plant is specific for rheumatism, and taken as cooling medicine after pounding.

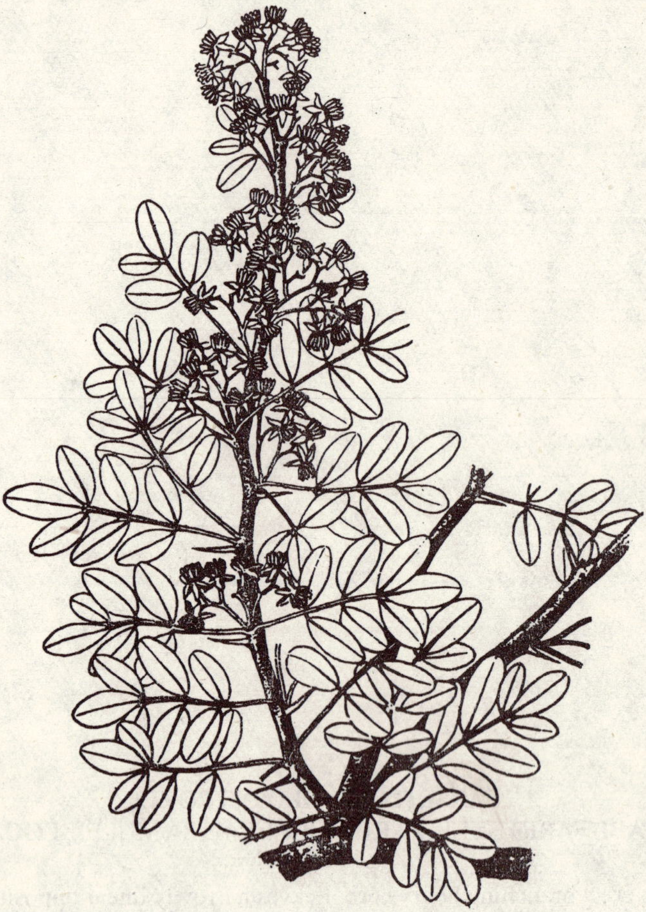

RUTACEAE

FERONIA LIMONIA (LINN) SWINGLE.
(SYN. F. ELEPHANTUM CORREA.
CRATAEVA VALLANGA KOEM.
LIMONIA ACIDISSIMA L.
SCHINUS LIMONIA LINN.

SANS.- KAPITTHA., **HINDI**- KAVITHA, KAVA, KAITHA., **BENGALI**- KATHBEL., **BOMBAY**- KAVIT., **TAMIL**- NARIVILA., + VILAAMBAZHAM., **TEL.**- VELEGA., **ENGLISH**- ELEPHANT or WOOD APPLE., **LOCAL NAME**- KAITH., **GUJARAT**- KOTHA., **KANN.**- BELADA - HANNU.

It is a small to medium sized tree, bark grey - brown thorns 2 - 3 0.1 - 0.15 cm long. Branches spreading horizontally. Leaves aromatic sweet smelling 3-7 foliate petiole and rachises often winged. Flowers pale green anthers dark red. Fruits large and globose; rind woody. Flowers - March to may. Fruits; October.

it was located in Semi wild condition in the Delhi ridge since then it has been planted in other parts of Delhi such as Chauburayha and Rajpur Road. It is often seen in gardens. It is indegenous in S. India, cultivated throughout India.

MEDICINAL USE : The fruit is aromatic, antiscorbatic, astringent and refrigerant. Gum from the stem is demulcent. Leaves are aromatic carminative and astringent, Bark is prescribed for biliouness.

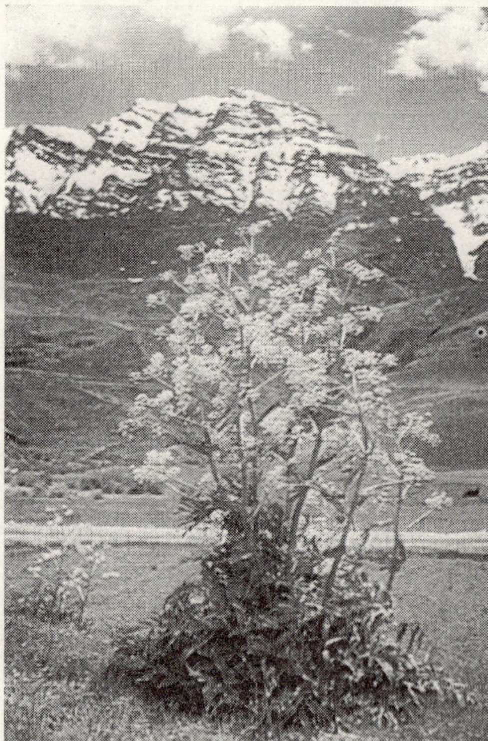

APIACEAE
(UMBELLIFERAE)

FERULA JAESCHKEANA VATKE

It is a tall perennial plant reaching to an height of 3m. Stem is hollow, Leaves large compound with 2-3 pinnate leaves with broad, oblong and toothed segments being 40 cm,ultimate segment to 10 cm by 1-2 cm broad with margins finely toothed,upper leaves reduced to large sheathes often with umbels in their axils.flowers yellow found in long compound umbles secondary umbles globular c.1 cm across bracts and bracteoles absent.

Fruiting umble to 20 cm. across fruit 1 - 1.5 cm long by 1 cm broad flattened with lateral wings, dorsally compressed with very slender dorsal ribs and somewhat smooth and swollen winged lateral ribs,resin canals numerous.it blooms in May - June.

It is reported from Pakistan to Himachal Pradesh C. Asia open slopes, common around Dras in Ladakh and in the chenab valley. 2400 - 3600 m, Kashmir.

MEDICINAL USE : Gum resin applied to wounds and bruises.

Several other species of this genus such as F. ALLIACEA Boiss F. FEETIDA Regel, F. GALBANIFLUA Boiss and F. SUMBUL Hook F. are used more or less for the same purpose AS F. NARTHEX. Boiss

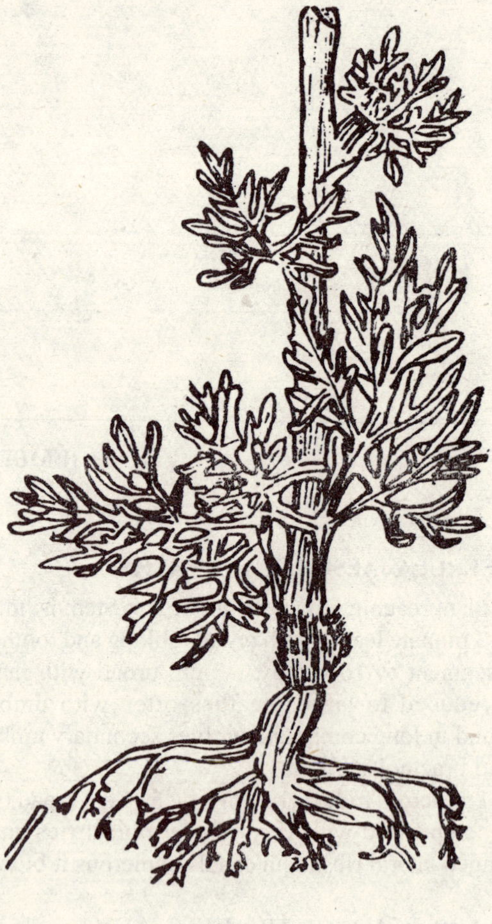

APIACEAE

FERULA NARTHEX BOISS
(FERULA ASSAFOETIDA L)

HINDI, BENGALI & MARATHI- HING., **GUJARATI-** HING., **KAN.-** HING., **SANS.-** HINGUKA, AGUDAGAUDHA, BALHIKA, KASHMIRI ANJUDAN SAP, YONG., **MAL.-** PERUNGAYAM., **ORIYA-** HENGU., **TAMIL-** PERUNGAYAM., **TELGU-** INGUVA., **PERSIAN-** ANGAJAD, ANGOJ., **ARAB.-** HILLATIT., **ENG.-** ASAFOETIDA.

It is a tall perennial herb or plant reaching a height of 2 metres. The root is a rhizome which is carrot shaped. Leaves are of two kinds. The upper leaves are much divided into numerous segments. Looking like the leaf of castor oil plant. The lower leaves are simple, 30 - 60 cm. long. ovate; young leaves are densely hairy. flowers are small, in terminal bunches of bright yellow colour. Fruit is 8 mm long, about half as broad or broader. Morphologically it resembles F. JAESCHKEANA to a greater extent, anatomically there is resemblance to a certain extent.

It is mainly grown in Punjab and Kashmir.

MEDICINAL USE : Asafoetida is the resinous and scented substance obtained by incision in the living rhizomes or roots of this plant and its allied species. Gum resin thus obtained is used in medicine in treatment of asthma, whooping cough and flatulent colie, as an antispasmodic, expecorant and nervine stimulant. It is known to produce remarkable effects in advanced stages of pneumonia and bronchitis in children. It is also used in dentrifice (carrious teeth), dyspepsia, hysteria and tympainetics, infantile convulsion, indigestion and worms. It is applied externally on stomach to stimulate intestine.

Commercially it is used in the prcparation of hingavaty rosanvati, hing goli; Karen jadiyog, yograj - guggulu; hingastak - churna, hing karpm. Vatika, raja - parvartani-vati modern medicine are pilula asafoetida, tincture asofoetida and plaster of asafoetida.

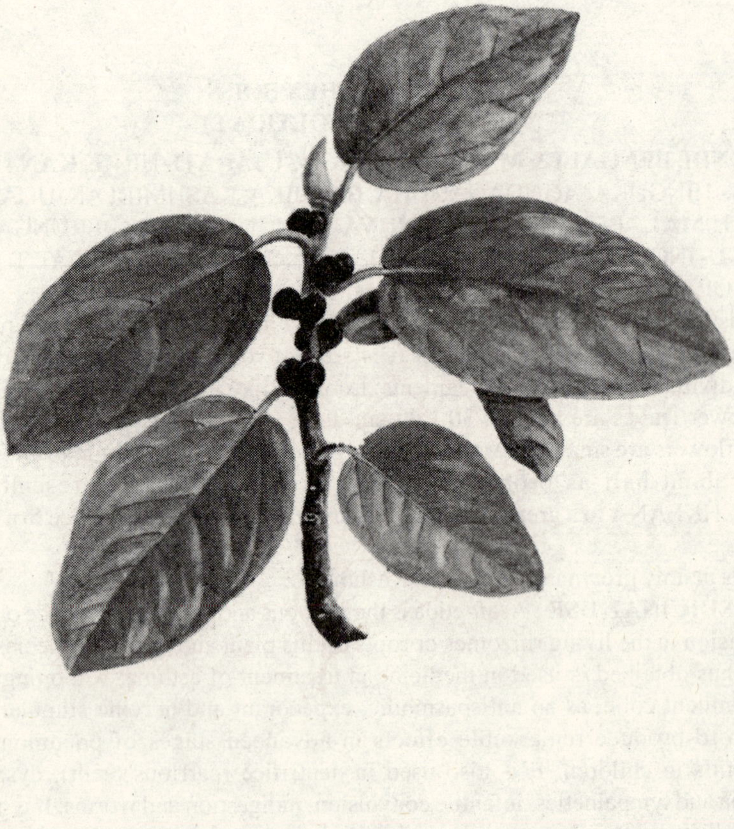

MORACEAE

FICUS - BENGALENSIS LINN.
(SYN. FICUS INDICA.)

SANSKRIT- VATA, BAUPAD., **HINDI & PUNJABI**- BOR, VAD, BIGAD, BENG BAR., **BOMBAY**- VAD, BAAT., **MARATHI**- VADA., **P.**- BOR., **TAMIL**- PUDAVAM., **TEL.**- PEDDAMATH., **ENGLISH**- BANYANTREE., **KAN.**- AALADAMARA, AALA, ALAD, NARR, VAD., **KON.**- GOEHIRUKU., **GUJARATI**- VAD, VADLOO., **MAL., PAERAL**- BARR, VAD, VATSU., **MARATHI**- VADA., **TAMIL**- AALAMARAM, AAL, PADAVAM., **TEL.**- MARICHETTU, PEDAMATTI, PATTI., **LOCAL NAME** : BARGAD, BARH, BAROTA.

A large evergreen spreading tree, with aerial roots decending from the spreading branches which root in the ground and thicken and become trunklike; thus enlarging the girth of tree. Trees become massive, sometimes spreading to 80-100 mtr. Bark is greyish white, smooth, young trees epiphytic. It is recognised by its leathery (coriacous) ovate, blunt leaves with entire margins, with blades 8 - 20 cms and with thick leaf-stalks 1-5 cm. Receptacles (fruit) axillary, sessile, paired, globular, hairy 1.3 - 2 cm red when ripe. Flowers June - September. Fruit ripening Oct-November also in April.

It is commonly planted along road sides, in lawns and gardens. Young seedlings often met in the crevices of the boundary walls of bunglows. It is commonly planted as a shade tree at wayside resting places. It is found all over India and grows wild in the Himalayas.

MEDICINAL USE: Milky juice applied externally for pains, in rehumatism and lumbago. Infusion of bark-tonic, astring. used in dysen, diarr. diabetes. Seeds are cooling, and tonic, leaves applied as poultice to abseesses. Root fibres - in gonour. (Hoope, Sey1. Z., 1929, 93).

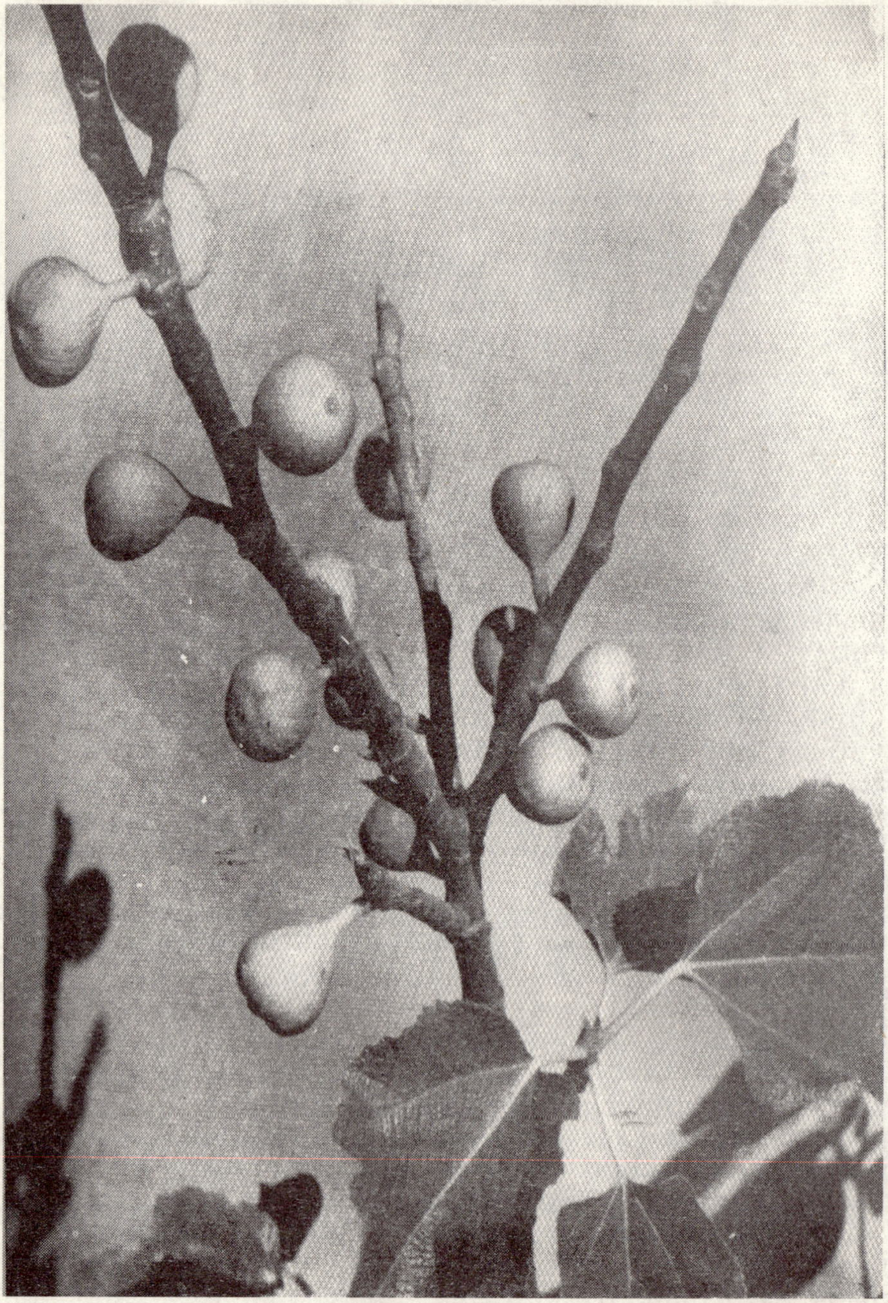

MORACEAE.

FICUS CARICA LINN

SANSKRIT- ANJIRA., **HINDI & BENGALI-** ANJIR., **DAMBUR, JAGYADUNUR + KURALI BO-** ANJRA., **TEL.-** ANJURU ATTI, MANJIMADYY, SIMAYDILI., **TAMIL-** SIMAIYATTI, TENALI (VILAYATIAL)., **PUNJABI-** FAGAIR., **GUJARATI, MARATHI-** ANJIR., **KAN.-** ANJURA., **MAL.-** SIMATTI., **ENGLISH-** FIG., **LOCAL NAME-** PHAKWADA, ANJIR., **HINDI-** JAHARPHALE, KHAIN, KHENAN., **BENGALI-** DAMBUR, JAGGADUMUR KURALI., **TELGU-** BOMMAMANI., **TAMIL-** TARAGADI., **KANNADA-** GARAGASA., **MALAYALAM-** PERINA POROH, TEREGAM.

It is a small tree reaching a height of 4.5 - 9 meters. The trunk is with a distant horizontal wrinkles and branching starts from base. Bark is smooth, grey or dull white. The leaves are broad, ovate to nearly orbicular or 3-5 lobed, chordate crenate - serrate. In size they vary from 20x18 cm. The upper surface of the leaf is rough white lower surface is hairy. Receptacles are solitary or paired, axillary, about 2.5x2.2 cm. globose or pear shaped, yellowish, purple when ripe. Receptacles January - April, ripe figs. June-October.

It is a native to Meditenranean region and is now cultivated in U.P. Rajasthan, Punjab, Andhra Pradesh and Maharashtra. It is reported fron Baluchistan cultivated in North West India and the deccan.

MEDICINAL USE : Fruit - demule, aper, emol, nutri, milky juice from the fresh green fruit known as Ficus rennet is acrid, used to destroy warts.

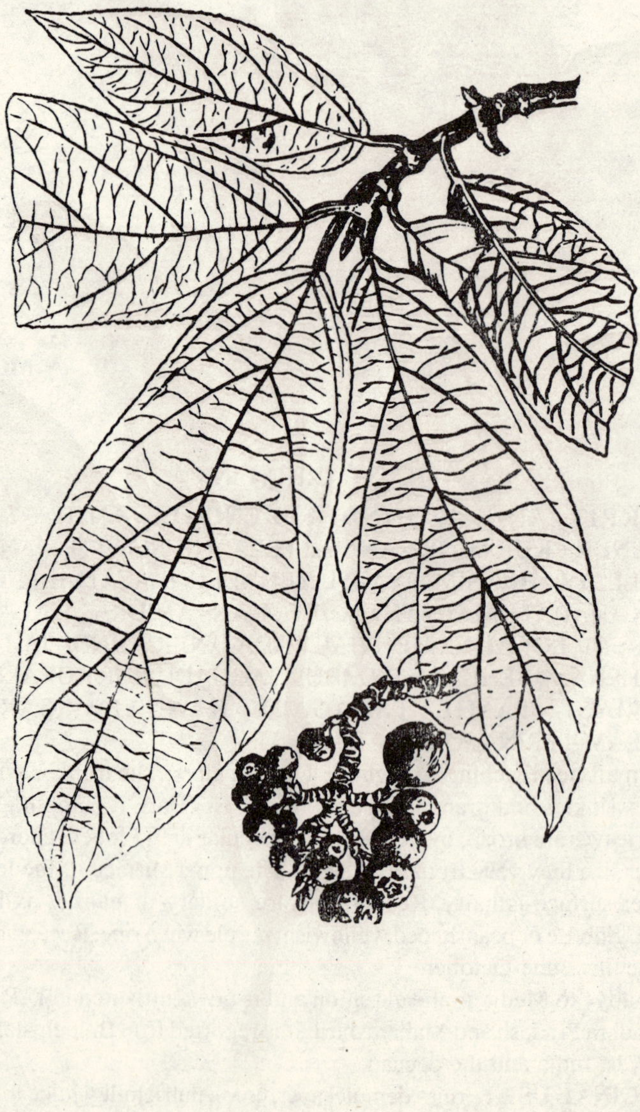

MORACEAE

FICUS HISPIDA LINN. F
(SYN. F. OPPOSITIFOLIA WILLD)

SANSKRIT- KAKADUMBURA., **HINDI-** DABRI, DAGURIN, GOBLA, KATHUMBAR, KAGSHA, KATGULARIA., **BENGALI-** KOKDUMUR, DUMOOR., **B.O.-** RAMBAL., **P.** - RAMBAL., **ASSAM-** KHOSKADUMAR., **TAMIL & MAL.-** PEYATTI, SONATTI, SONATTI., **TEL.-** VETTIYATI, BODAMAMIDI, BRAMNADI., **MARATHI-** BHOKODA, BOKRAI, KALAUMBAI, KHAROTI., **GUJARATI-** DHEDAUMARO, JANGLI ANGIR., **KANNADA-** ADAVI ATTI, KADATTI., **MALAYALAM-** ERUMANKKU, PEYATTI.

It is a small tree or shrub. The leaves are large 10 to 30 cm. long ovate to lanceolate, fruit is ovate to acute being 2.5 cm long. They appear in pairs or clusters on leafless branches. Fruiting season is through out the year. Fruit is greenish and yellowish when ripe and edible.

It is a shade loving plant and is found throughout India; from Himalaya to Andeman; including Bengal, middle and South India.

MEDICINAL USE : Fruits seeds and bark - purg. emetic, and the leaves are used as poultice for wounds and ulcers.

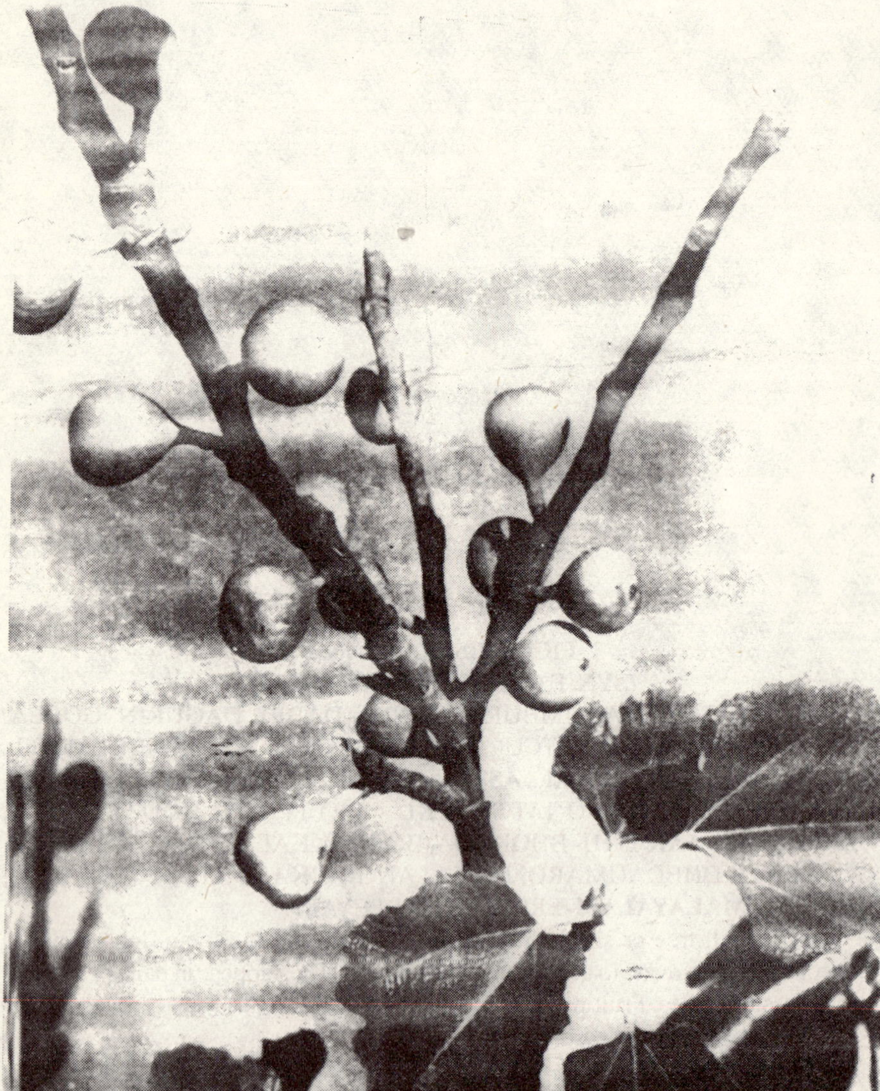

MORACEAE

FICUS PALMATA FORSK
(SYN, F. CARICOIDIS ROXB.
F. VIRGATA ROXB.

HINDI- ANJIRI, BADU, KHAMRI., **PUNJABI-** JAMIR, PHAGPARA., **GUJARATI-** PEPRI., **TEL.-** MEDI MANGIMEDI, PAPPERY., **LOCAL NAME-** ANJIRI, KAIMBAR, KHAT GULERI, PATGULERI.

An erect woody shrub or small tree. Bark dull grey. Young parts tomentose. Leaves 10-15 x 8x11 cm. orbicular or broad ovate, usually dentate or serrate; base 3 - nerved, receptacles axillary, solitary, and pubescent, about 2x1.5 cm subglobose or pyriform, yellow, receptacles February - July.

Common in open places, fruit orchards and waste places near gardens etc. N.W. India from the Indus east Worlds to Oudh, ascending to 3000 ft. in the Himalayas, Mount Abu.

MEDICINAL USE : Fruit demulc. laxt. used as a diet in cases of constipation and in diseases of the lungs and bladder.

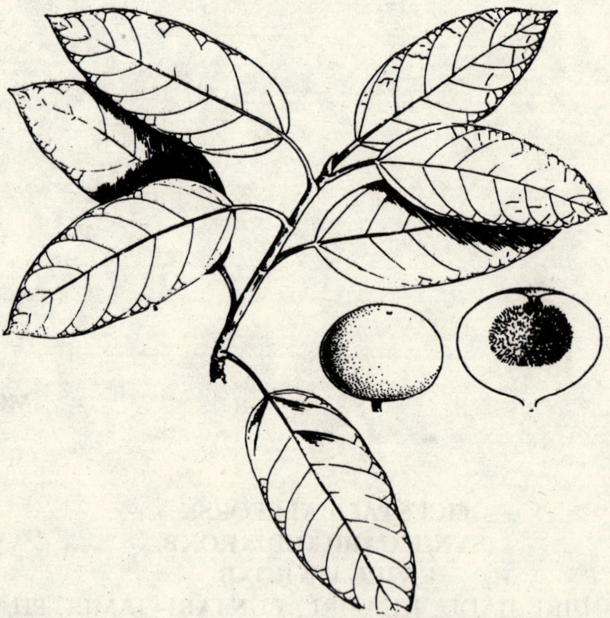

MORACEAE.

FICUS RACEMOSA LINN
(SYN. F. GLOMERATA ROXB.
F. GOOLERERA ROXB.
F. COVLLIA.

SANSKRIT- UDUMBARA., **PUNJABI-** KUMBAL, KATH GULAR., **HINDI-** GULAR UMAR., **BENGALI-** JAGNA DUMAR., **BOMBAY-** UMBAR, DUMAR, JAGYADUMBAR., **TAMIL & MAL.-** ATTIMARAM., **TEL.** -ATTIMANU BODDA PAIDI & UDHUMBARAMU., **ENGLISH-** CLUSTER FIG. GUJARATI UMBARO GULAR., **KAN.-** ATTI MARA., **KAN.-** RUMDI, ROOKU., **MARATHI-** UMBAR., **ORIYA-** DIMYA., **LOCAL NAME-** GULAR.

The tree is small or medium sized sometimes large also, deciduous. Trunk with horizontal lines nearly circular. inner surface of the bark is smooth dull white or reddish brown. The outer surface of the bark has easily remarkble translucent flakes of whitish tissue, greyish to rusty brown, 6-18 mm thick, uniformly hard and non brittle. Leaves 7-15x6-8 cm. ovate oblong to elliptic, glabrous thickly nerved beneath. Stipules ovate, lanceolate, scarious receptacles appear in bunches on short leaf less branches. The top, globular, reddish with sweet fragrance being 2.4 x 2.5 cm.

It is a cultivated plant found in gardens and villages and along the western Jamuna canal locally. Fruiting season is April - July. It is found through out India.

MEDICINAL USE : Bark is astrin. root in dysen. sap of root in diabetes; leaves powdered and mixed with honey given in bileous infections; fruit astrin. stomachi, carmin. given in menor, and haemoptysis. Milky juice in piles and diarroea and haemophilia. It also gives protection against ill effects of atomic radiation and prevents weakening of capillaries due to certain drugs such as, salicylates, arsenicals and thiocyanate sulphadaizaine and gold salts.

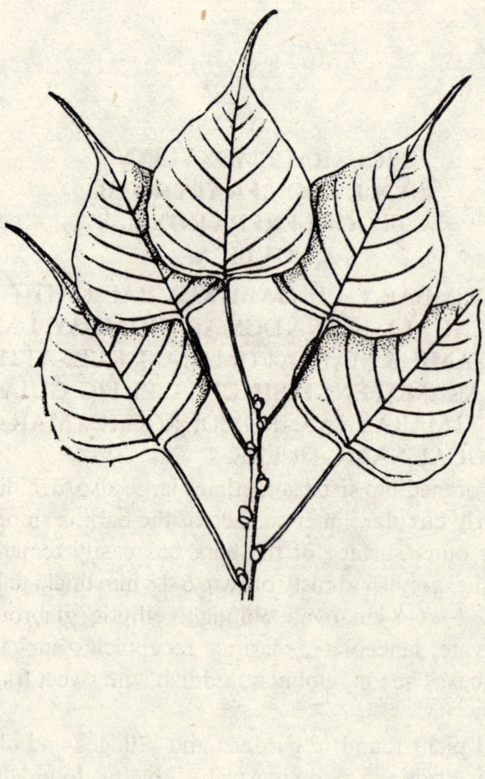

MORACEAE

FICUS RELIGIOSA LINN
(SYN. UROSTIGMA RELIGIOSUM GASP)

BENGALI- AGVATTHO ASUDH., **H. & PUNJAB-** PIPAL ASVATTHA, PIPALI., **BOMBAY-** PIPAL., **TAMIL-** ARASH, ASVATTUM., **TEL.-** PIPPALI, ASVATTHAMMU, BODHI RAVIS., **GUJARATI-** JASI, PIPLO, PIPAL., **MARATHI-** ARASH, ASVATBUM., **KAN.-** ARLI, ASVATTI, RANGI, BASIRI ARALIMARA **MAL.-** ARCH, ARAYAL, ASVATTUTUM., **LOCAL NAME-** PIPAL.

It is a large and glabrous tree found wild as well as cultivated. It is known as an avenue tree but sacred to Hindus and Buddhists. Bark is grey and branches without aerial roots. The leaves are 10 - 15 x 10 - 12 cm, ovate, round, entire, coraceious and apex of the leaf is long tail like point one third to half as long as the blade shining above, reddish when young beneath and with white swelling when mature. Leaf blade including apex 11-18 cm long with undulate margin and rounded or shallow heart shaped base, and with 6 - 8 pairs of lateral veins, leaf stalk 7 - 10 cm. The fruit is a recepticle in stalkless pairs smooth 1-3 cm; depressed globose dark purple when ripe. The tree becomes leafless or so for a short time during the hot weather. Receptacles - April to June and October - November.

It is commonly found as a shade tree in temples road side and open places. It is found all over India. It is also recorded from Pakistan to Bhutan, India widely cultivated in the Himalayas to 1400 m.

MEDICINAL USE: Seeds and fruits are cooling, laxative refrigerant and alterative. Fruits in powder form with honey used for cough and asthma, leaves and young shoots are purgative, bark is cooling astringent, sweet. Infusion of bark is astringent. Fruit is laxative and digestive and with honey is given to baby for cough and cold.

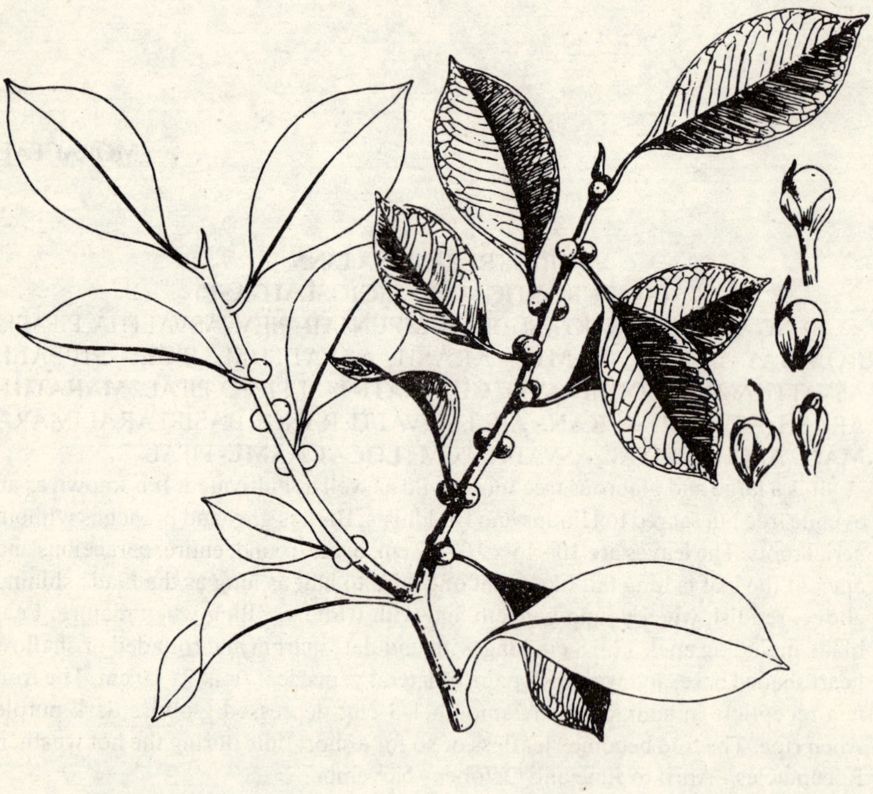

MORACEAE

FICUS RETUSA AUCT (NONLINN)
(SYN. FICUS MICRO CARPA LINN. F.
F. BENZAMINA (NON-L) AUCT.

HINDI & BENGALI- KAMRUP, CHILKAN., **TAMIL-** KALLICHI., **MARATHI-** PILALA., **TELEGU-** YERRAJUVVI.

It is a medium sized, evergreen tree with a dense crown of leaves. Bark is dark grey. Leaves polished, glossy having various sizes and shapes. Size vary from7-9 x 3.5 - 5 cm. The shapes are elliptic, ovate, obovate, obovate, rounded or bluntly accuminate. Venation is not prominent. Fruits (receptacles vary from 6-9x6-9 mm, paired depressed globose, sessile smooth, yellowish reddish, supported by 3 (Three) persistent bracts. Fruiting is from March - October.

It is commonly planted as an avenue tree along streets also in lawns and gardens.

Found in Chhota Nagpur, Bihar, Madhya Pradesh, Western Peninsula South India to Ceylon, Sunderbans and Andamans.

MEDICINAL USE : Juice of bark in liver diseases. Powdered leaves and bark in rheumatic headache. Root bark and leaves boiled in oil application for wounds and bruises.

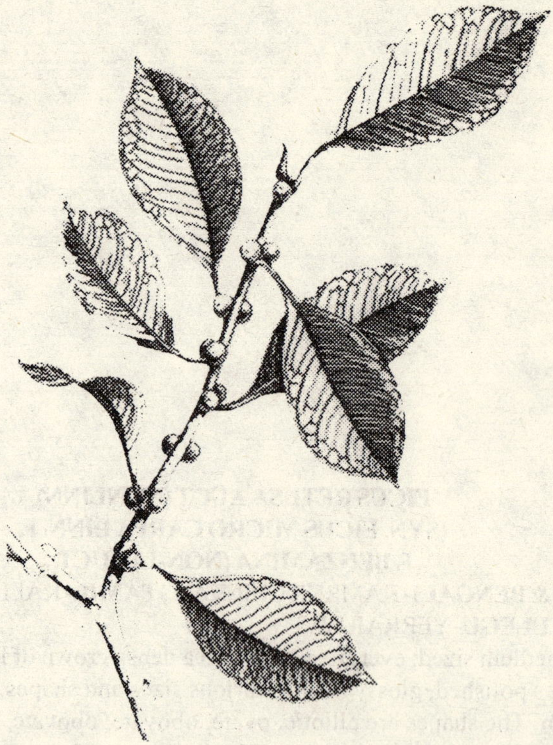

MORACEAE

FICUS TSIELA ROXB.

HINDI- JARI., **TAMIL-** ICHI., **MAL.-** KOYALI., **TEL.-** PEDDJAVVI., **MARATHI-** PIMPRI., **SANSKRIT-** KANINIKA.

A glabrous short (stunted) branched tree having no aerial roots. Bark is greenish grey and rough, due to numerous cracks, wrinkles and lenticels. The inner surface is smooth, longitudinally striated and reddish brown in colour. Leaves leathery (coriacous) 8 - 14 x 6.5 - 8 cm. broad, ovate, entire, smooth with a thick marginal vein, Petiole 2 - 4 cm. Receptacles (fruits) crowded at the top of the branches 13x10 mm sessile, paired smooth. Male flowers sessile, gall flowers pedicellate. Fruit reniform. Fruiting in October. Planted in gardens, lawns and squares.

Found in Madhya Pradesh and Western Peninsula.

MEDICINAL USE : Bark used in colic.

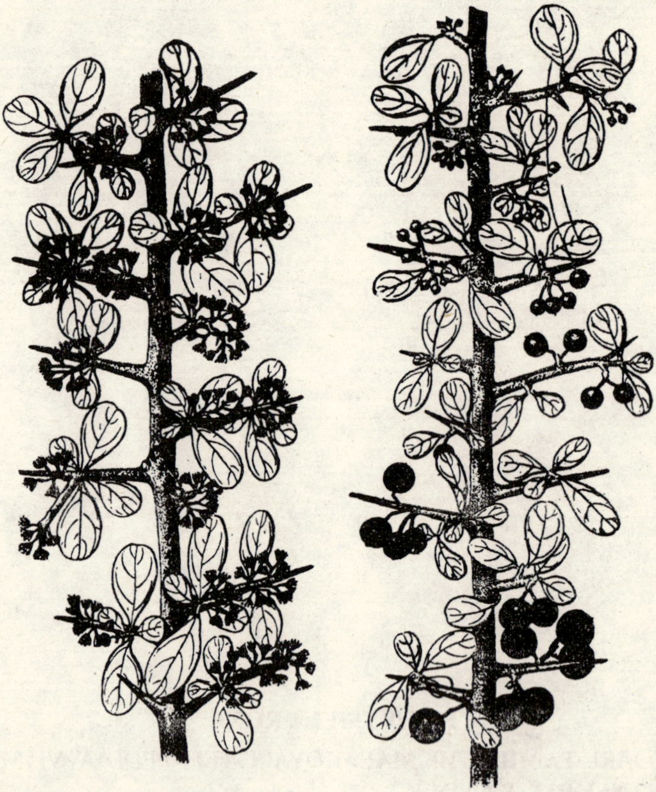

FLACOURTIACEAE

FLACOURTIA SEPIARIA ROXB.
(SYN. F. INDICA. (BURM.F.) MERR
GMELINA INDICA - F.
F. RAMONTCHI L. HERIT.
F. LATIFOLIA COOKE

HINDI- KONDEI, BILANGRE, BAICHI., **BOMBAY-** ATRUNA., **MAL-** KURUMULI., **PUNJ.-** KINGRO., **TAM.-** KODUMUNDI., **TEL.-** KANDREGU., **LOCAL NAME-** KHATAI., **ENGLISH-** GOVERNOR'S PLUM, MADGASCAR PLUM., **BENGALI-** BARCHI, BAICHI, BINGA, KATAI., **GUJARATI-** KANKID., **MARATHI-** BHEKAL, KAKER, PAKER., **TELUGU-** KANDREGU., **TAMIL-** KATUKALA, SOTTAI KALA., **KANNADA-** HATTARINULLU, MUNNUUKI.

It is a small tree or densely branched horny bush. The branchelets ending in sharp rigid needle like long spines 4-6 cm, leaves are glabrous - ovoid - ovate or suborbicular, Pubarulous particularly on the veins, often crenate to serrate; cuneate at base. Style short 4-5. Fruit a drupe, round or globose, purple, 5-7 mm in diameter. Fruiting season is in summer.

Locally it is found on open places growing as wild. Reported from Kumaon, dry jungles throughout Bengal, Orissa, the Andamans, the West Penninsula, Scrub forests in all districts of the Madras State, especially on the commondal coast and in the Deccan.

MEDICINAL USE : Infusion of leaves and roots in snake bite. Bark - trituated in Sesamum oil is used as a liniment in rheumetism and joint pains. Fruit is given in jaundice and enlarged spleen, gum of the plant is used for cholera.

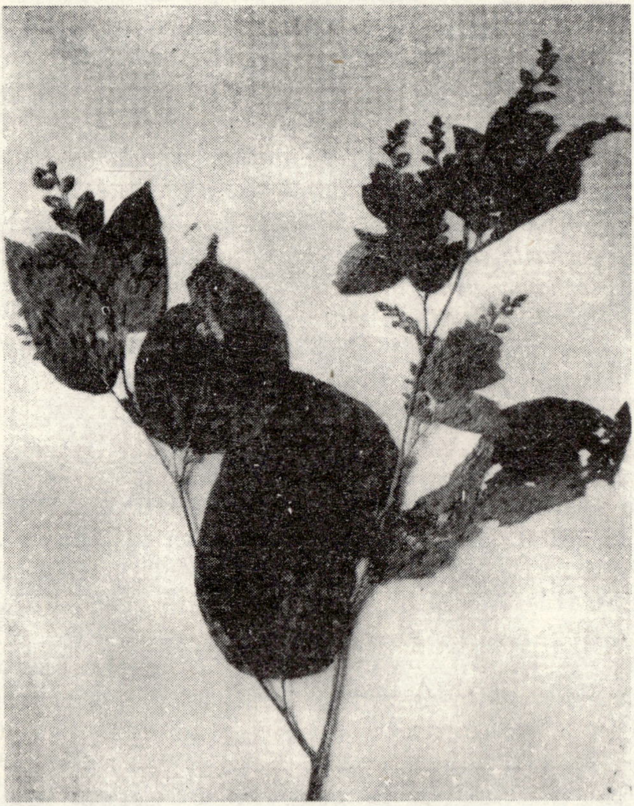

LEGUMINOSAE

FLEMINGIA STROBILIFERA R.BR.

HINDI- KUSRANT., **BOMBAY-** NUNDAR., **TEL.-** NALLABADDU., **MAL.-** KAMALU., **OUDH-** KASRANT.

A variable erect shrub 1-2-3 mm with simple leaves broadly lanceolate acute, silky haired beneath 5 - 13 cm. The infloresence is very conspicuous due to 2 ranks of large rounded pale green folded papery bracts. Braets are large ovate, folded enclosing small white fl ower clusters. Bracts 1.2 - 2.5 cm. long; flowers 2 or more in each braet, 9-10 mm calyx hairy, shorter than petals. pod small, swollen, 2 seeded, splitting into 2 valves; 9-10 mm, densely hairy, concealed by bracts.

It is found from Sind, Rajputana and Bengal to S. India and Andamans. It is reported from Tropics and Sub-tropics of Asia and America. To 2300 m sal forests shrubberies Sept October.

MEDICINAL USE : Roots used in epilepsy, and hysteria.

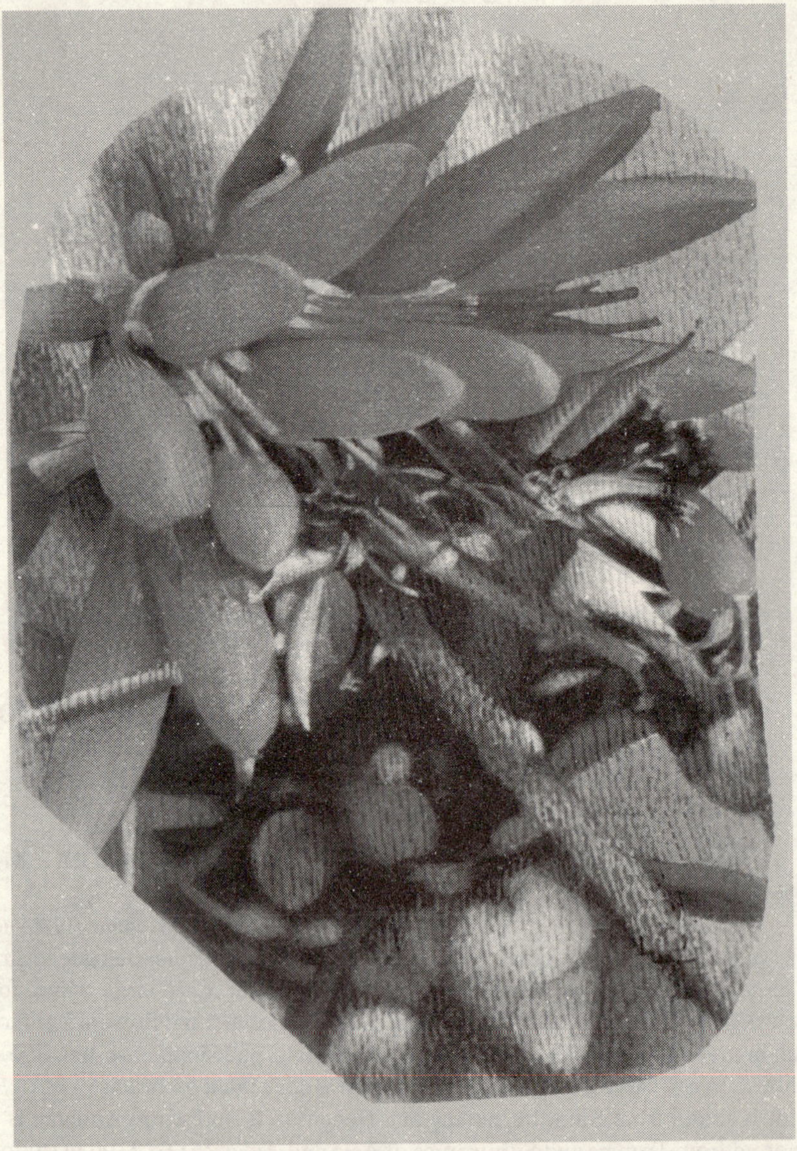

COMMELINACEAE

FLOSCOPA SCANDENS LOUR

LAKHIMPUR- KARAHIMLU., **TELGU-** KONDA - AMDIKAD., **TAMIL-** VAZPARLIPULLOO., **MALAYALI-** PRETIPULLOO., **ASSAM-** KANNA SHIMLOO.

It is found throughout tropical India, in Swamps from East Nepal, Sikkim and the Khasia Hills to Travancore. From Dehradun to Assam.

MEDICINAL USE : Juice of stem put in sore eyes in Lakshmipur Assam and in Malaya. This plant is used for repairing broken bones. Its stem is soft Leaves lanceolate and flower bunches are white or lilae in colour.

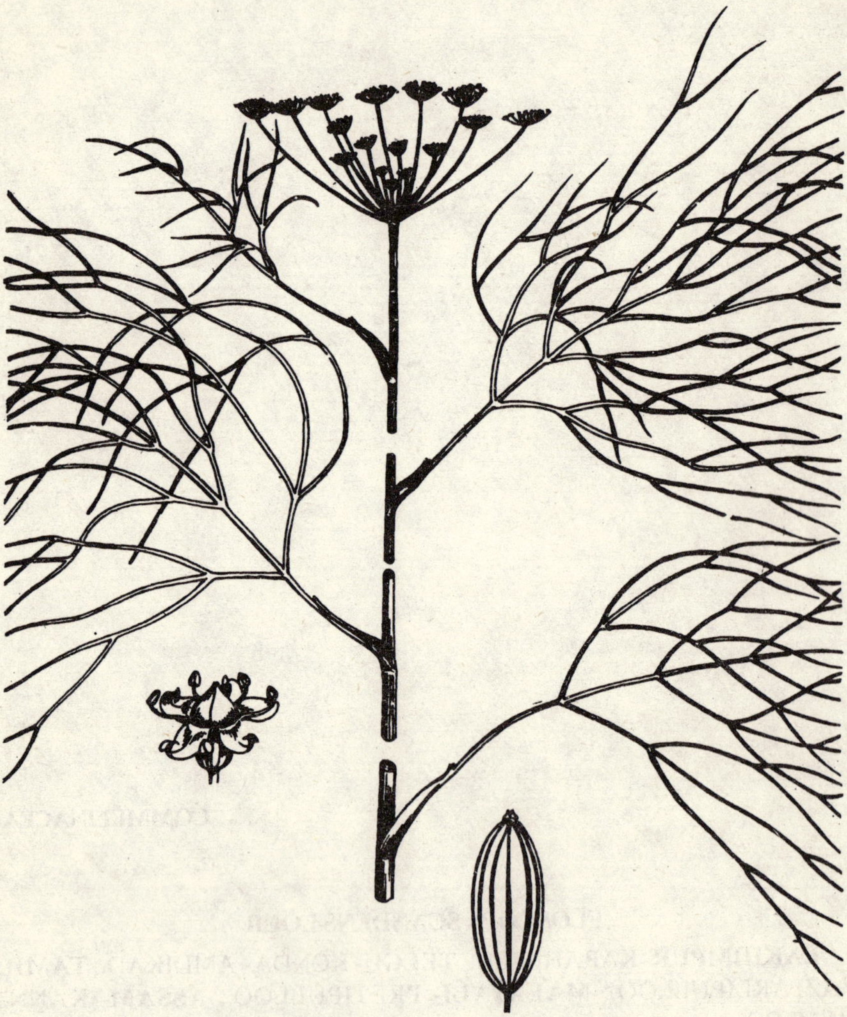

APIACEAE (UMBELLIFERAE)

FOENICULUM VULGARE MILL.

SANS.- MADHURIKA., **HINDI-** BARI SAUNF, SAUNF, SONP., **BENGALI-** PAN MUHIRI, MAURI., **BOMBAY-** BARI SHOPHA., **TAMIL-** SOHIKINAI SHOMBEI., **TELEGU-** PEDDUJILAKARAMU, SOPU., **ENGLISH-** FENNEL., **LOCAL NAME-** SONF., **GUJARATI-** WARRIALLI., **KAN.-** SOMPU

It is an erect stout glabrous aromatic perennial plant with leaves 2-4 pinnate, segments thread like flowers in yellow compound umbels; flower 1-2 mm in radius. Fruit is oblong or ellipsoid, ribbed 5-6 mm long, straight or curved. It is yellowish green or brown in colour. It emits a sweet aromatic aroma.

It is mainly a cultivated plant and is reported from all over India. It is also cultivated in USSR, Hungry, Germany, France, Italy, Argentina, Japan and U.S.A.

MEDICINAL USE : Fruits are stimulant, aromatic, stomachic, carminative and emmenagogue; leaves are diuretic and root is purgative. Oil from fruits used as a vermicide.

The seeds are considered a good digestive agent the extract of seeds is used for cough and bronchits.

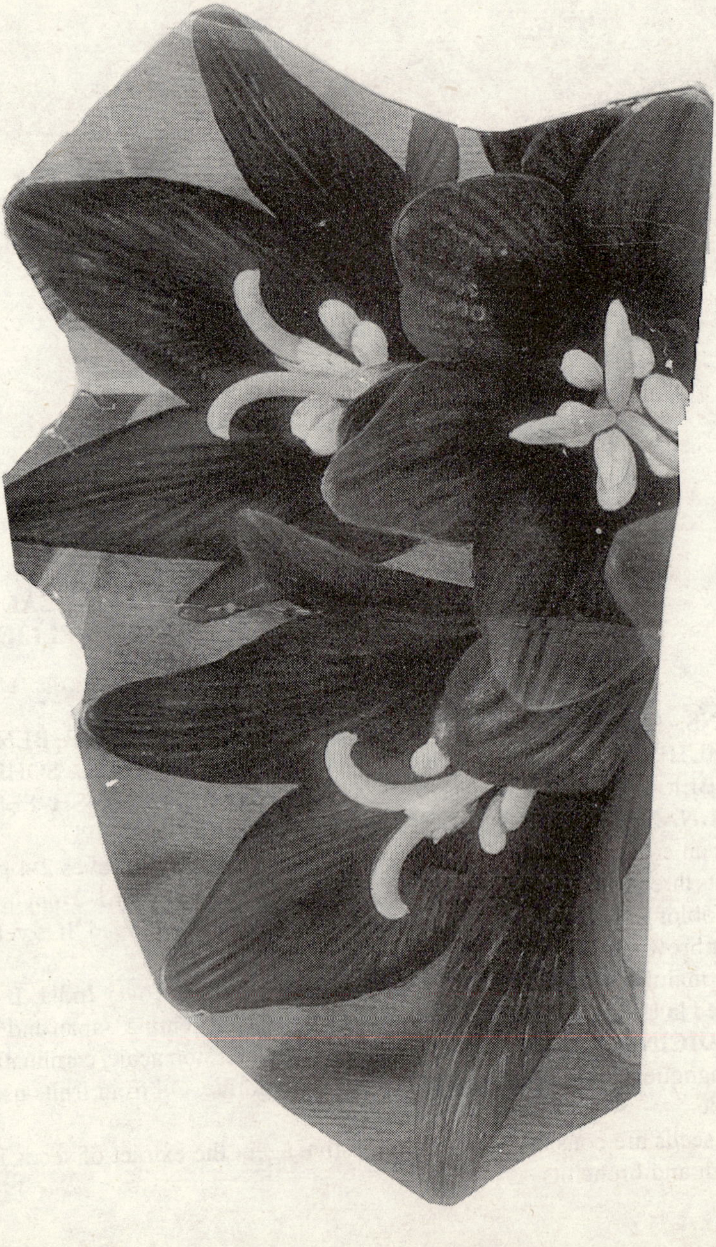

LILIACEAE

FRITTILLARIA CIRRHOSA D. DON.

It resembles F. ROYELI Hook in appearance. But it is more slender and often distinguishable by the coiled tips of the upper leaves. Flowers variable in colour, marroon yellow, green or purple, usually chequered, petals 3.5 - 5 cm narrow - elliptic blunt Blooming period May - June.

It is reported from Central and E. Himalayas and Sikkim, 11,000 - 16,000 ft.

MEDICINAL USE : Dried corms are used for asthma, bronchitis and tuberculosis. Its other speceis F. CAMCHALENSIS is widely used in indigenous medicine.

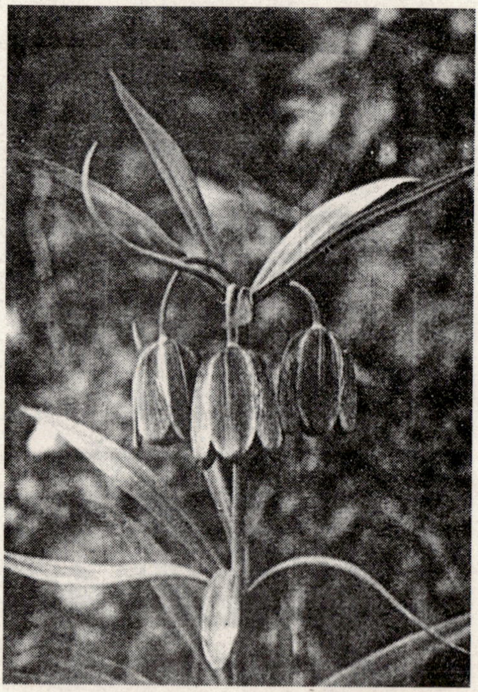

LILIACEAE

FRITILLARIA IMPERIALIS LINN

It is rather a robust leafy plant, with a terminal cluster of pendulaous yellow bell shaped flowers, topped by a crown of narrow leaf braets. Flowers 4-5 cm. not chquered. The stem robust 1-1.3 mm leaves lanceolate to 12 cm. the upper in whorls. The blooming season in April - May.

It is found in Kashmir at 1660 - 3000 m, abundant near Baramullah.

MEDICINAL USE : Bulbs are emolient resolvent and diuretic. Fresh plant is toxic.

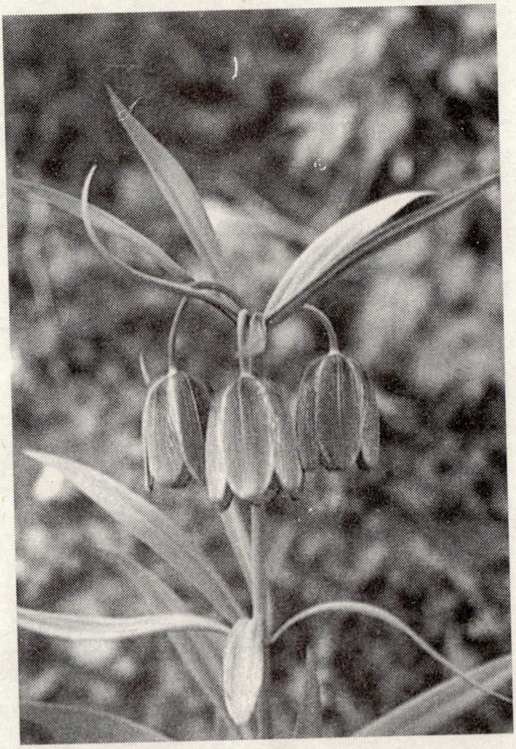

LILIACEAE

FRITILLARIA ROYLEI HOOK

It is bulbous herb, stem 15-60cm. Leaves linear lanceolate often long pointed, 5-10cm, Opposite 3-6 or in a whorl. Flowers yellowish-green to brownish purple usually chequered with dull purple, broadly bell shaped nodding; pendulous and usually solitary but sometimes 2-4.Petals narrow-ovate 4-5 cms. long, with a conspicuous neetary at base. The capsule is six (6) angled. The blooming period is June- July.

It is reported from pakistan to uttar pradesh. 2700-4000 m Alpine slopes, shrubberies, w, temperate, Himalayas 8000-13000 ft. from kashmir to kumaon.

MEDICINAL USE : The bulbs powdered and boiled with orange skin used for tuberculosis and asthma.

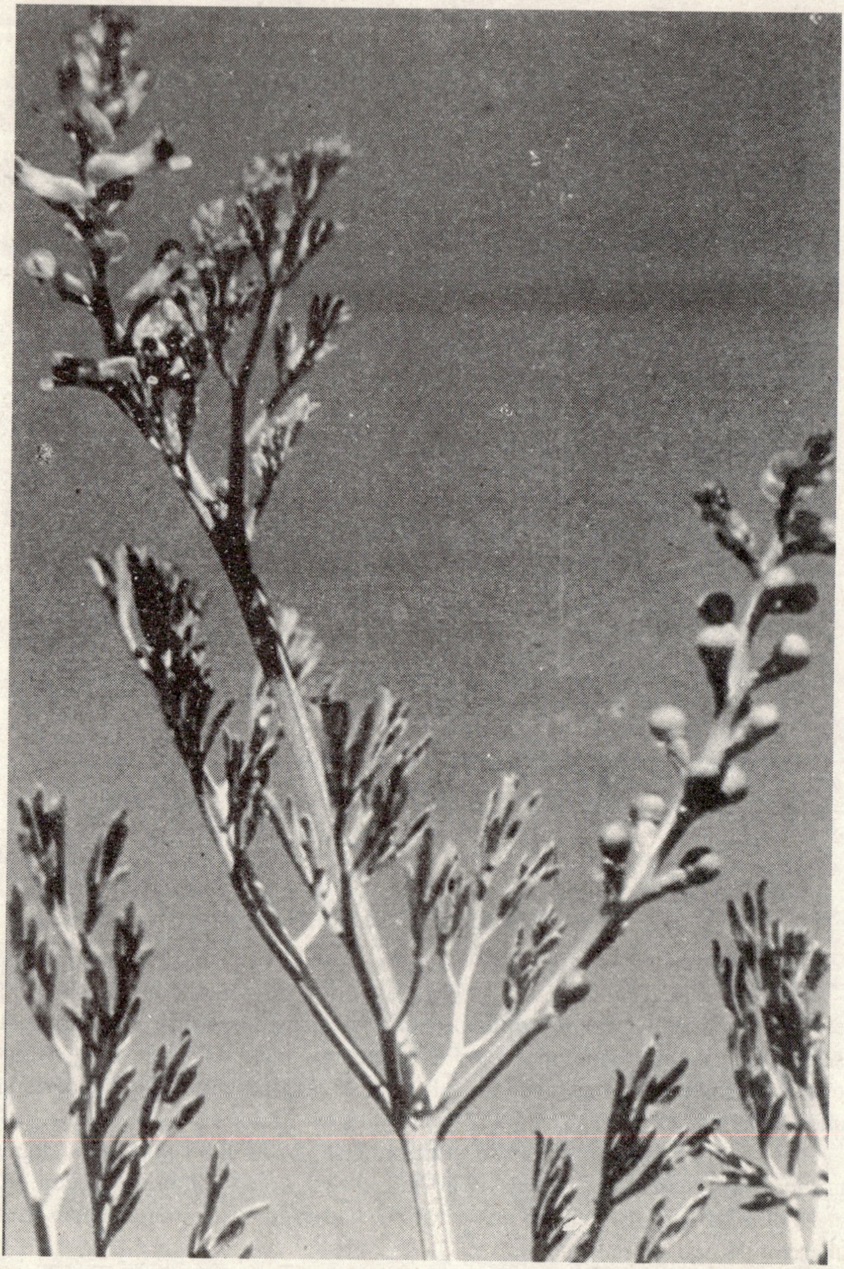

FUMARIACEAE

FUMARIA INDICA (HAUSSK) PUGSLEY
(SYN. F. PARVIFLORA LAM.

BENGALI- SHOTARA, PITAPAPRA SANSULPHA., **GUJ.-** PITTAPAPDO., **ENG.-** COMMON FUMITORY., **KANNADA-** PARAPATAKA., **HINDI & MARATHI-** PITAPAPRA., **KASHMIRI-** SHAHTEROH., **LOCAL NAME-** PAPRA, KILANO, PITPAPADA., **TAMIL-** TURU, THUSHA., **TELUGU-** CHATA - RASHI., **SANSKRIT-** PARPATAKA.

A delicate much branched, gloucous, leafy annual 5-30 cm. Latex watery. Leaves 2-3 times the bracts cut into narrow pointed segments C.1 mm wide. Flowers in clusters of tiny, pale pinkish, rosy - purplish or whitish each 5-6 mm long flowers stalks erect, equalling or slightly shorter than the lanceolate bracts. Sepals minute; upper petal with a short somewhat down - curved sae like spur; Fruit globular C.2 mm, are seeded, non spilitting. Flowers and fruits November - February.

It is found commonly as a winter season weed in cultivated fields and gardens beds or moist sandy soil. It is imported into the country from persia. Now it is found common throughout the Himalaya (April - May) and from Gangetic plain and Nepal down to Nilgiri mountains.

MEDICINAL USE : The plant is diuretic, diaphoretic, aperent, laxative and anthelmintic. It is used in low fever to purify blood and also in skin disorders. It is also considered as an efficient liver tonic and recommended for hepatic ailments, from simple biliousness to chronic malfunctioning of liver.

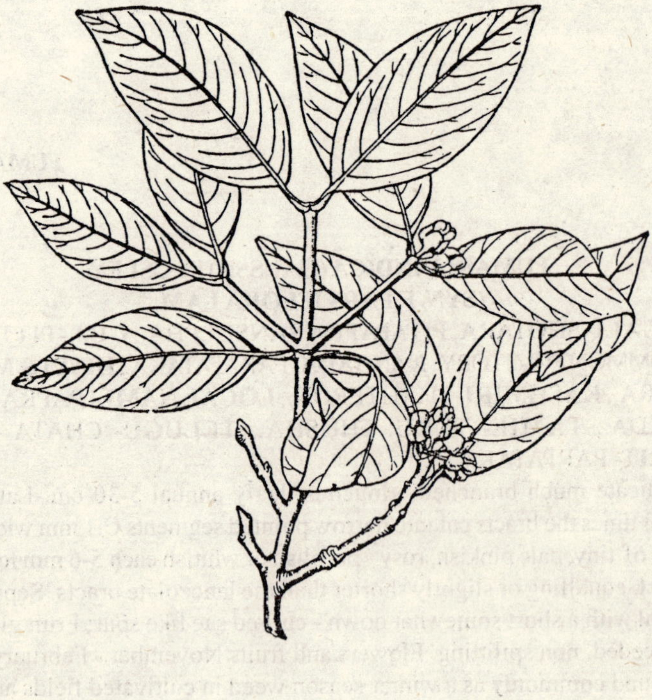

GUTTIFERAE.

GARCINIA CAMBOGIA DESR.

BOMBAY- VILATI - OMLI., **MARATHI-** ARADAL, DRAMBAE., **TAMIL-** SINCHINTH., **TELGU-** KODAKPULI., **KAN.-** UPPEMERA, SEEMAE HUNSAE., **MAL.-** KADUUMPULI, KODAPULI.

It is a small or medium sized tree, the branches spread in such a way that it gives a roundish or circular appearance to the tree. The leaves are paired and arranged in an opposite manner at the nodes. Ovate to accuminate 5 - 12.5 cm. long and 2.5 - 7.5 cm. broad. They are deep green in colour and shining. The flowers are in single bunch, axillary and terminal, sessile shining, blooming in summer. The fruit is oval to circular upto 5 cm. diameter and they ripe in rainy season. When ripe they become red or yellow ribbed in 6-8 stripes. The seeds are 6-8 and each one is enclosed in juicy pulp.

It is reported from mountains of the western Penninsula, from konkan to Travancore.

MEDICINAL USE : The decoction of fruit rind is given in dysentry and many diseases of the intestine.

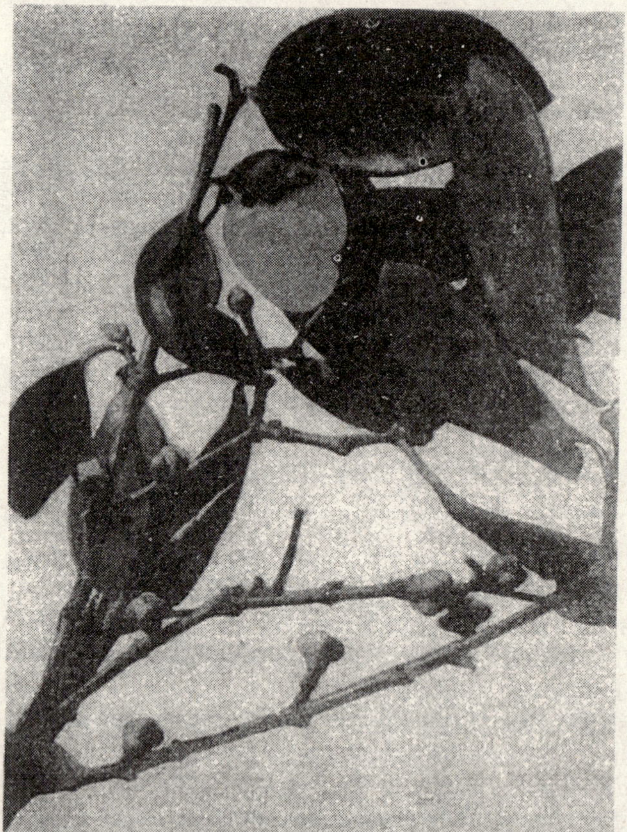

GUTTIFERAE

GARCINIA INDICA CHOIS (DUPETIT - THOUARSI) (SYN. G. PURPUREA ROXB.)

It is popularly known as kokam butter tree, Magosteen oil tree and bridonia talo tree.

HINDI & BOMBAY- KOKAM VISHAMBIL., **TAMIL**- MURGAL., **MAL.**- PUNAMPULI., **GUJ.**- KOKAN., **MARATHI**- AMMSOLE, BHIRAND, KATAMBI., **TAMIL**- MURGAL., **KANN.**- MURGALA., **MAL.**- POONUMPULLI KOKAM, RATAMBA.

It is delicate evergreen tall tree. The branches spread and are topmost. The leaves are oval to accuminate lanceolate 6.25 - 8.75 cm. long and 2.5 - 3.75 cm. broad. They are deep green dorsally and yellow coloured vertrally. Fruits are rounded in shape 2.5 - 3.5 cm diameter. When ripe theybecome deep blue or mouve. Each fruit contains 5-8 seeds. It blooms from November - February and the fruits ripe in April to May.

It occurs in evergreen forests of Western Ghats from Kokan Southwards and in Goa. Also cultivated in Southern Districts of Maharashtra and is reported to do well on lower slopes of Nilgiris. Kookan, N. Kanara, Western Ghats of Bombay, S. Kanara, Coorg, where it is often cultivated.

MEDICINAL USE : The fruits are vermifuge, heart tonic and is a remedy for piles, dysentry boils and internal wounds, and is found useful in reducing pain and heart diseases. The fruit juice is astringent and used to reduce acidity. The roots are bitter in taste.

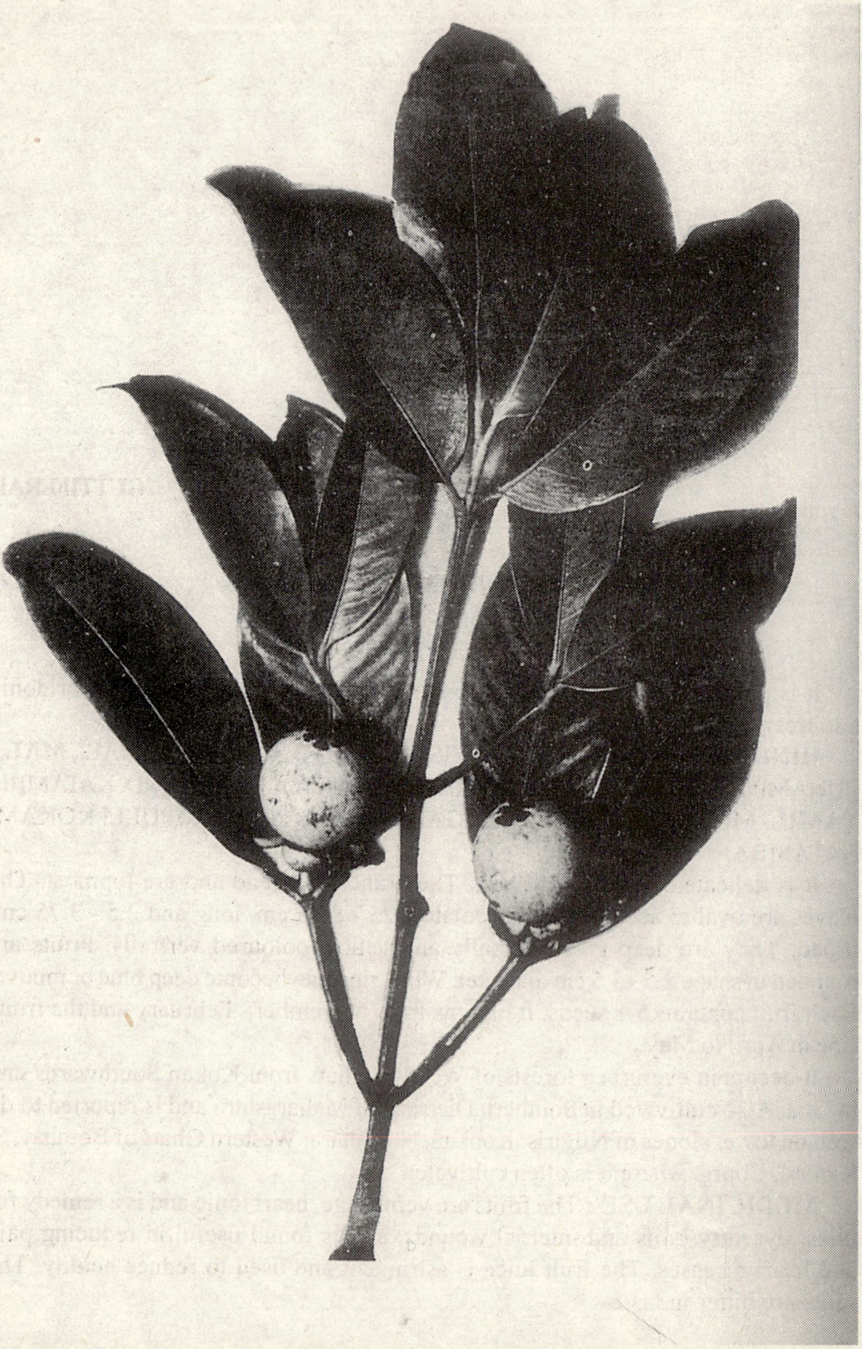

GUTTIFERAE

GARCINIA MANGOSTANA LINN

HINDI, BENGALI & BOMBAY- MANGUSTAN., **MAL.-** MANGGUSTO, MONGUSTA., **GUJARAT & MARATHI-** MONGASTIN., **TAMIL-** SULAMBULI, MANGUSHTANPAZAM., **ENGLISH-** MANGOSTEEN., **KAN.-** PANNERALE., **KON.-** TAVIR.

It is an evergreen small or medium sized slow growing tree reaching a height of 6 - 13.5 meters. The leaves are slender, paired elliptic to oblong pointed deep green, 15-25 cm long, leathery and glabrous on both sides . The flowers are solitary found at the ends of small branches. Each flower is 2.5 - 5 cm. in diameter pinkish with pulpy petals. The fruits are found exserted towards outer side of small branches on both sides. They are squarish to rectnagular, being 5-6.25 cm radius. The outer skin of the fruit is smooth, red or mouve. Seeds are found in nos. of 5-8 flattend and enclosed in white thick aromatic jelly like substance. The fruiting season is August to September and fruit is considered as propicalous. It is considered as a native of Malaysia and Singapore, East Indies and Philippines, cultivated as a garden escape in Burma, Malaya and Madras and lower slopes of Nilgiris. It is also recorded from Tamil Nadu, Java and West Indies.

MEDICINAL USE : Rind of the fruit is astringent used in chronic diarrohea and dysentry and bark and young leaves are used as gargle for sore mouth. Fruit is regarded as a remedy for leucorrohea, gonorrhea and gleet. It is considered as antifever and its decoction is given in respiratory problems. The outer portion of the fruit is used in making an ointment which is chiefly used for eczema, itching and like skin diseases.

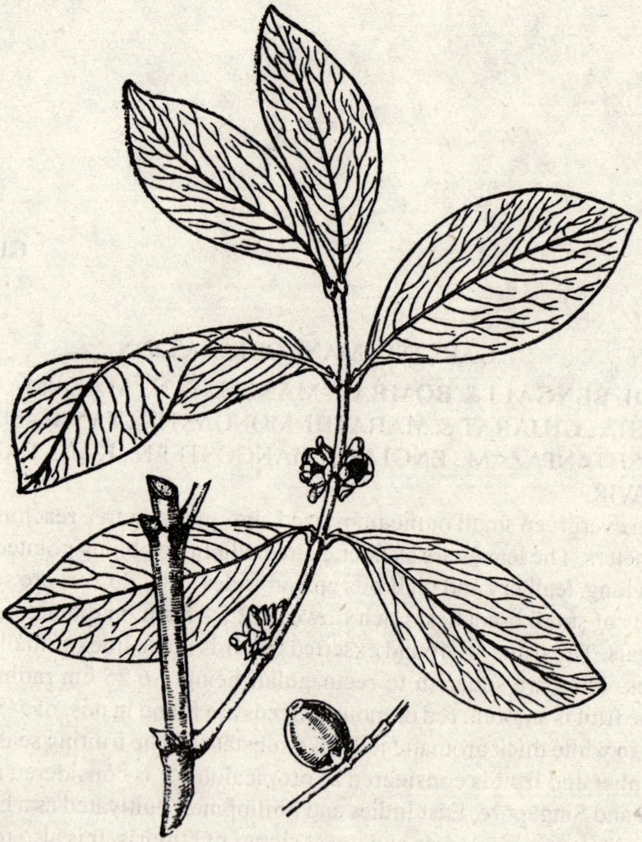

GUTTIFERAE

GARCINIA MORELLA DESR
(SYN. G. GUTTA WIGHT.
HENEOSTANA MORELLA

It is popularly known as Indian Gamboge tree.

ENGLISH- INDIAN GAMBOGE, CEYLON GAMBOGE., **MAR.-** KOKUM., **HINDI-** INDIAN GAMBOGE, CEYLON GAMBOGE., **MAR.-** KOKUM., **HINDI-** GOTAPHANBA, KOKAM., **TAMIL-** KORATAPULI - PUSPUVAR RAVEL, CHINNI., **KAN.-** KANGUSHTA, HARDALA, JARINOE, DEVEN BULII., **TEL.-** RIVAL - CHIRIPAL, MAKKI, SOLAIPUNLI., **BENGALI-** TAMAL., **MARATHI-** TAMAL., **MAL.-** CHIGGRI, DINUONBA, KURUKAMPULI, PINNARPULI.

It is an evergreen small or medium sized tree reaching a height of 9-15 meters, leaves are leathery 10-15 cm. long oral - accuminate, the marginal edges of leaves are thikened. Male and female flowers are seprate, the female flowers are larger than the male flowers. The fruits are small, almost the size of a plum. Each seed is 4 - valved, 4 chambered and 4 seeded. The seeds are flattened, rounded or pointed, dark brown in colour.

It is found in East Bengal, Khasia Hills, evergreen forests of N. Kanara, Western Ghats from S. Kanara and Mysore to travancore upto, 3000 ft.

MEDICINAL USE : Gum resin is used in dropsical affections. It is considerd as purgative, anthalmitic, amenor; obstinate constipation and as vermifuge.

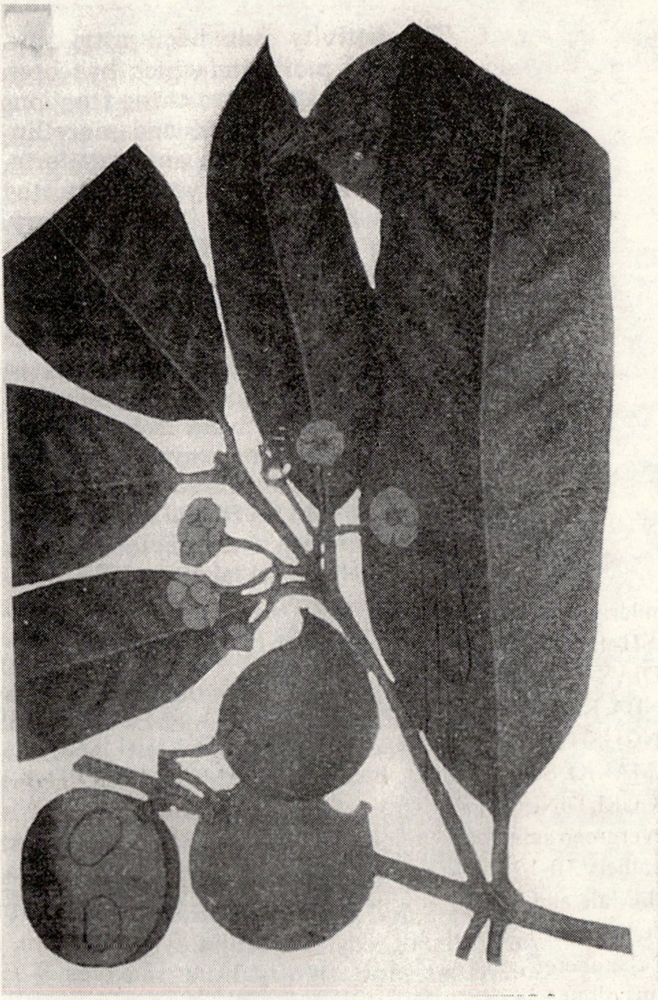

GUTTIFERAE

GARCINIA XANTHOCHYMUS - HOOK. F.
(SYN. G. TINCTOREA DON)

HINDI- DAMPEL, TAMEL., **BENGALI-** TAMAL, CHALAT., **MARATHI-HHARAMBI-** OTTA., **BOMBAY-** DAMPEL., **SANSKRIT-** TAMALA, TAPINJHA., **TAM.-** KULAVI, MALLAPACHHE, MUKKI, TAMALAM., **TELGU-** SITERHAN RAKU EVERUMUDDI., **GUJARATI-** KARMALA, OTTA., **KANNADA-** DEVGRIGAE, TAMLAMU., **MAL.-** ANNVAYA., **ORIYA-** CHEORO, SITAMBU.

It is a medium sized evergreen branched tree. The stem is straight the branches are angular. The leaves are leathery and glabrous 25 - 37.5 cm long and 3.75 - 10 broad arranged oppositely; margin entire; flowers axillary in bunches of three-many. Fruits when ripe are yellow; round and glacous 5 - 8.75 cm. diameter with a distinct beak seeds 1-4.

It is reported from East Bengal and E. Himalayas, N. Circars, Ganjam, W. pennisula on the ghats from Bombay to N. Kanara, Mysore, Coorg, Nilgiris, N. Travancore upto 3500 ft. and the Andamans.

MEDICINAL USE : Used for the same purpose as that of G. INDICA.

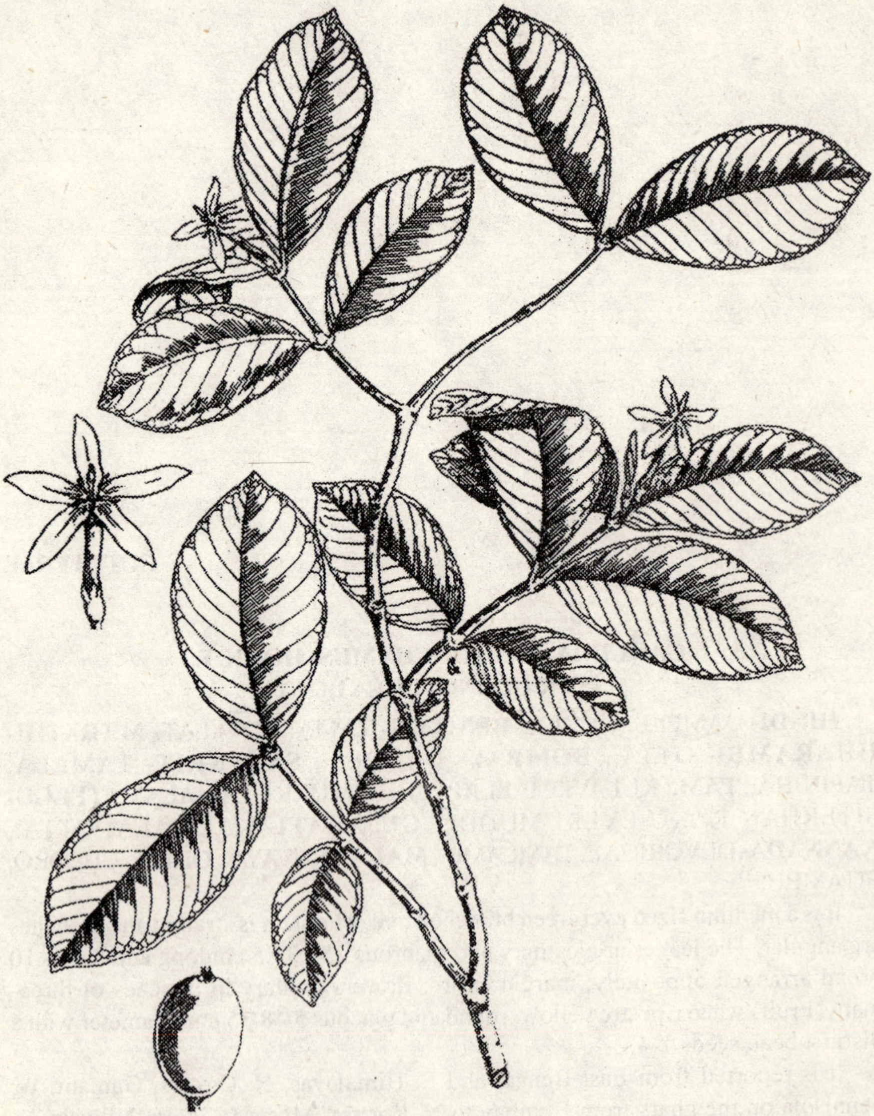

RUBIACEAE

GARDENIA GUMMIFERA LINN F.

BOM.- DIKAMALI, C.P.KARMARRI., **MARATHI, BENGALI & HINDI**- DIKAMALI., **TAMIL**- TIKKAMASLI, KANBALI PICHU., **TELEGU**- KARINGUBA, TELMANGA MUNCHIBIKKI CHITAMATA., **ENG.**- GUMMY CAPE JASMINE., **SANSKRITI**- PINDOV, NADI, HINGU., **GUJ.**- CAMARI, DIKAMLI., **KANAD**- SITTBIKKA KAMBINEANENA, DKAMLII, ORIYA GURUDU, VIRIDHICOLI.

It is a shrub with stout branches. The stem is not straight (bent) and 1.5 - 1.8 meter tall and 30cms. in girth. Branches are stout and curved. The bark is brown; the leaves are opposite or ternate, obovate to elliptic, corraceous. Flowers creamy-white, fragrant large solitary or paired. The fruits are pulpy with ovarian chamber.

It is cultivated in garden and hedges around bunglows. It is also reported from S. Mahrata country. N. Kanora, N. Circars Deccan and carnatic to the foot of the N. Ghats of Madras State and Malabar Coast. It occurs commonly in West. Pennisula.

MEDICINAL USE : Its gum resin is used medicinally as carminative stimulant and in dyspepsia. It is also supposed to be antiseptic and is used in veterinary medicine to keep off flies from sores. It is also well known in indigenous medicine as an antiseptic. Its other species such as G. JASMINOIDES ELLUS (Syn. G. FLORIDA LINN and G. LUCIDA ROXB.) are also used as medicinal plants more or less for the same above mentioned purposes.

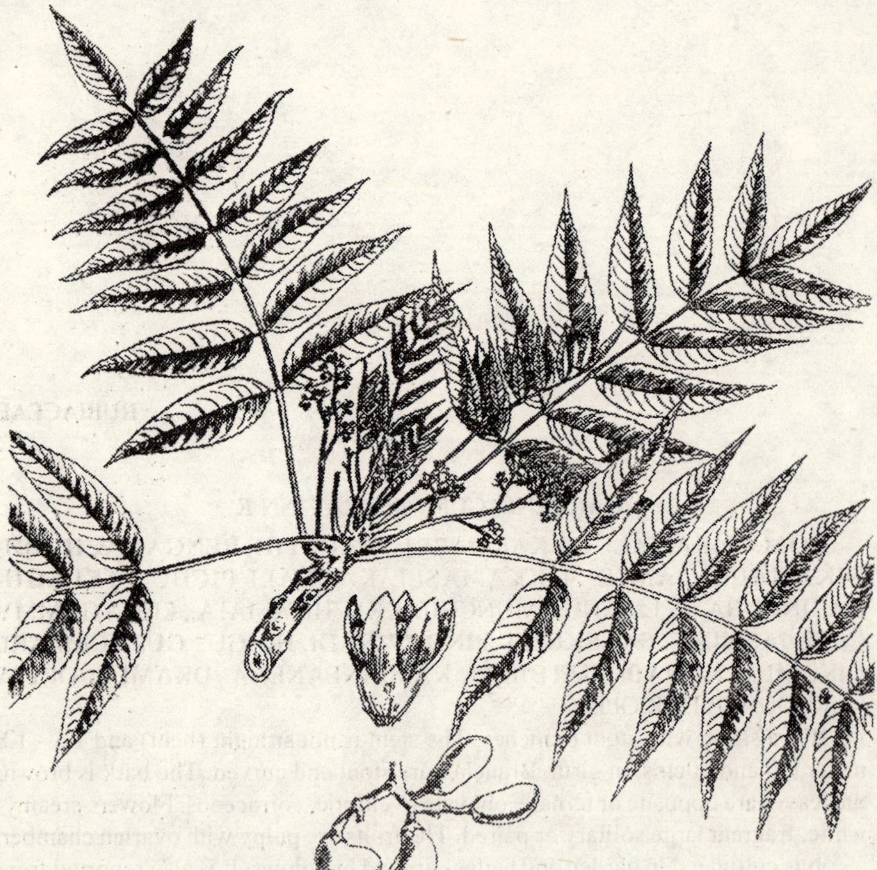

BURSERACEAE

GARUGA PINNATA ROXB.

HINDI- KAKAR, GHOGAN, TOMM, KERPATH., **BENGALI-** JUM, DUBDABAE, TOOM, KERPATT, NEEL, BHADI., **BOMBAY-** KURAK., **ASSAM-** GUDILIPOMA., **GUJ.-** KHUSIMB., **TAMIL-** KARUVEMBEI., **TEL.-** GARUGA, MARATHI GARUGO., **THOTMOLA -** ROHIMAL, POMMA, DEANG KHEANAG, GAINDLY, KAKAR, KUDAK, KURAK, KARAEVAMBU ARUNEELI., **KAN.-** HALABLUGGI, ARNELLI, GODDA., **MAL. -** KASARAMBA, KATHUKALINGAN, **ORIYA-** MOHI, SOMPAHI, ARMU., **BIHAR & ORISSA-** KANDAV, KARUR, ARMUDARU, KAKER., **NEPAL-** AANLAE, DUBDABAEAS.

It is a medium sized tree and reaches a height of 15 metres. The stem is crrect and straight and 6 - 7.5 m. tall and 1.8 m. in girth. The bark is dusty brown shelling down in flakes, irregularly. The leaves are pinnatifid with red glands, flowers yellow or greenish white hermaphrodite. Fruits differ in colour from black to yellowish green globular 8 mm in diameter with stones and pulp. The no. of stones varies from 3-4. It is reported from all over India.

MEDICINAL USE : Its fruits are considred as cooling refreshing and digestive. the juice of of the stem is used for eye trouble and good eye sight. The juice of the leaves mixed with honey is given for asthma. The deecoction of the root is used for lung troubles.

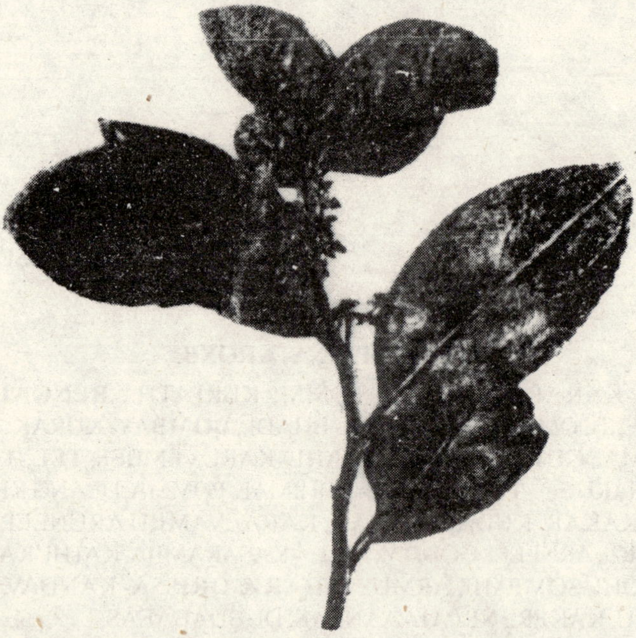

ERICACEAE

GAULTHERIA FRAGRANTISSIMA WALL

BENG & HINDI- GANDHPURA., **ENGLISH-** INDIAN WINTERGREEN, FRANGRANT WISNTERGREEN., **NEP.-** MACHINO, LEPCHA - KALOMBA., **KHASI HILLS-** JEERHUP, SHOLING - THREAT.

It is a robust branched aromatic shrub from 1-3. 6 m. tall. The leaves are ovate to lanceolate or acute, evergreen 5-10 cm. long smooth above, dotted with a bristles beneath, margins bristly - toothed. Flowers small fragrant white or pink globular found in numerous axillary spike like clusters. Flower clusters 2.5 - 8 cm. long, shorter than the leaves, flowers short stalked; corolla 4 mm by 3 mm broad. Fruit C.6 mm with dark voilet blue fleshy pointed - calxy lobes. Blooming period is April - May.

It is found in Uttar Pradesh to S.E. Tibet, Burma 1500 - 2700 in Forests, shrubberies very common in Nepal. It is also reported from Bhutan, Khasi Hills. W. Ghats, the Nilgiris and Tranancore Assam, pulneys and Travancore, above 5000 ft.

MEDICINAL USE : Volatile oil from the leaves is arommatic used in medicines as stimulant, carminative and in treatment of rhenumatism and neuralgia. Essential oil is an ingredient of several insecticidal preparations and hence knowns as antispetic.

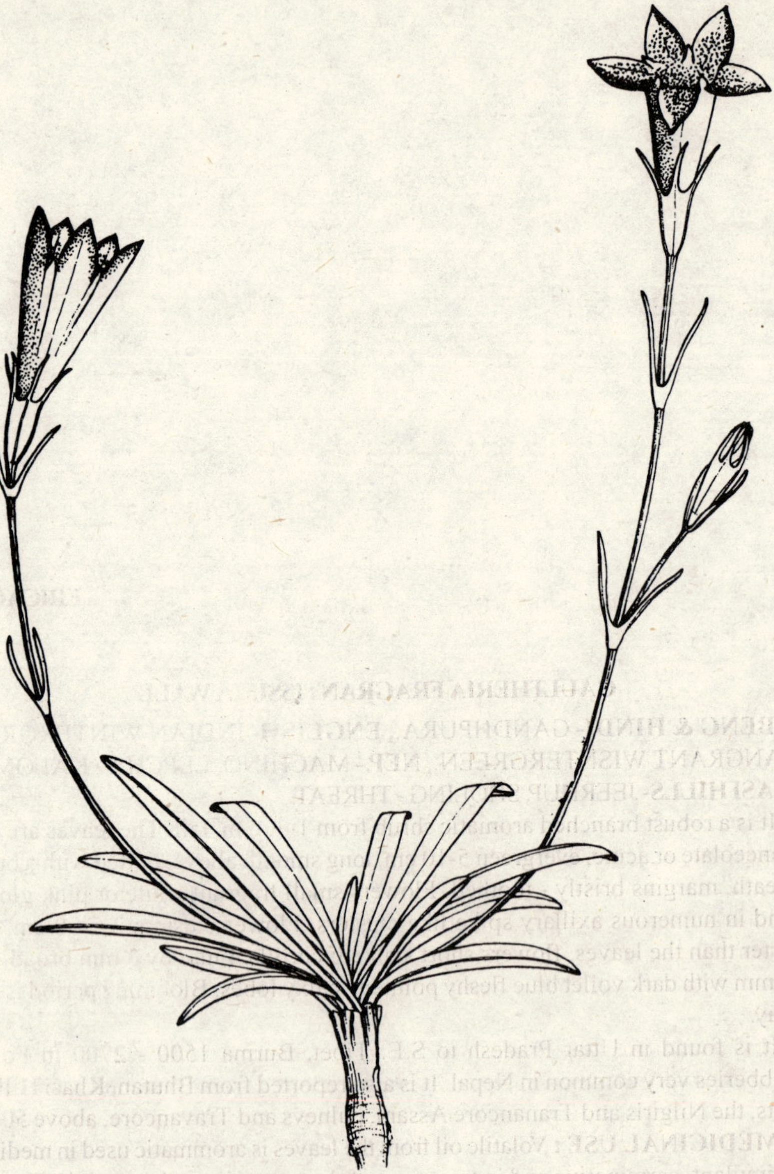

GENTIANACEAE

GENTIANA KUROO ROYLE
(SYN. G. CHINAVITA ROXB.)

ENGLISH- HIMALAYAN or INDIAN GENTIAN, CHIRETTA., **GUJ.-** KUDU CHIRAYAT., **HINDI & BENGALI-** KARU, KUTKI, CHIRETTA., **KANNADA-** NELABEBU., **KASH**.- KIRAITA., **KON.-** JARATE - KADDI., **MAL.-** KIRIYAT., **MARATHI-** KIRAYET., **PUNJABI-** NILKANT., **TAMIL-** NILAVEMBU., **TEL.-** NELAVEMU.

It is a herbaeous plant. Stem 5-30 cm, several unbranched branches arising from the stout root stock. Stem leaves 2-3 pairs, narrow linear to 2 cms. Basal leaves lanceolate. usually 10-12 cm. Flowers deep blue in colour, paler in the throat and spotted with green and white, usually 2 or more on each stem but sometimes solitary Corolla narrow funnel shaped to 5 cm with ovate acute spreading lobes and small triangular lobules; Calyx tubular, with narrow linear lobes 8-12 mm one half to two thirds as long as the calyx tube. The blooming season is August - October.

It is reported from Kashmir, Simla extending to N.W. Himalayas, 5000-11000 ft. Also from Pakistan to Uttar Pradesh 1800 - 2700 on Grassy slopes.

MEDICINAL USE : Root tonic, stomachic, febge, for urinary infections.

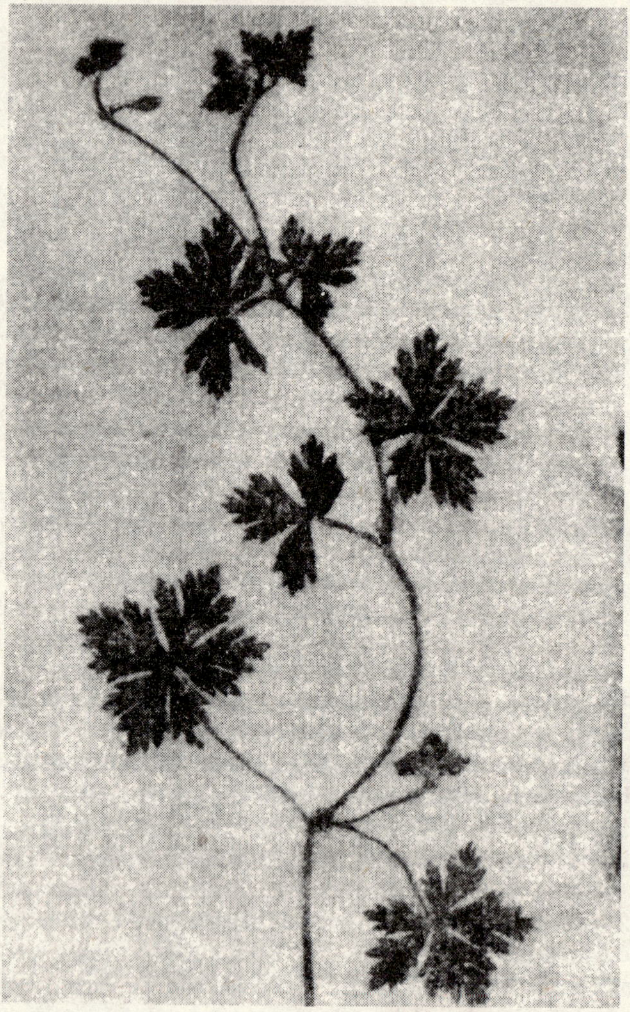

GERANIACEAE

GERANIUM NEPALENSE SWEET
(SYN. G. PRATENSE L. MEADOW CRANESBILL)

H. & P.- BAND, BHANDA., **ENGLISH-** NEPAL GERANIUM, NEPALESE CRANESBILL., **KASHMIR-** ROYAL.

It is perennial herbaceous plant. The stem is erect 15 to 45 cm. long and with spreading hairy. Leaves are lobed with stipules. Leaf blade 3-5 cm across, divided allmost to base into 5 to 7 ovate lobes which are further deeply cut into oblong acute toothed segments, flowers are in pairs, 2.5 - 4 cm across, usually bluish purple, with darker veins, but colour varying from almost red to blue, to white. Sepals 10-12 mm, individual flower stalks, beeoming reflxed after flowering, erect in fruit. Fruit C. 3.5 cm including beak. Blooming period June - August.

It is occuring in the temperate Himalayas, Kashmir, Khasi Hills and the Nilgiris, It is also recorded from Kuram Valley, Garhwal, Nepal, Sikkim, Manipur and pulney Hills. It is also found in Pakistan, temperate Eurasia, 3000-4500 cm. Shrubberies, open slopes, gregarious along irrigation channels in drier areas.

MEDICINAL USE : :Plant astin. used in certain renal diseases. Roots are used for colouring medicinal oils. These species are widely used in indigenous medicine.

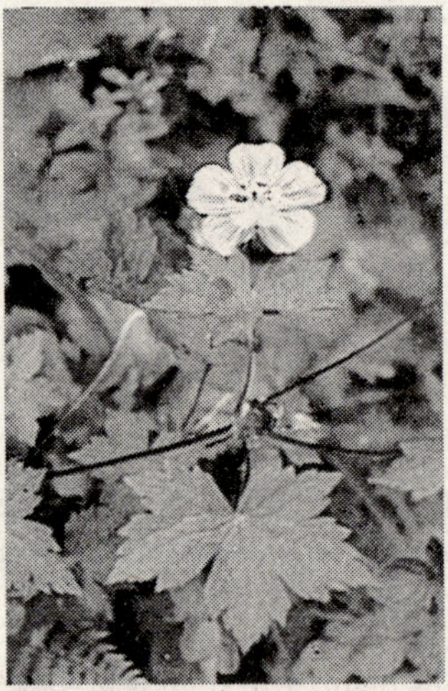

GERANIACEAE

GERANIUM WALLICHIANUM. D. DON EX. SWEET

H.- LAIJAHRI., **KASHMIR-** KAOOSHUD.

It is an annual or perennial herbaceious plant stems much branched 30 - 120 cm plant readily dstinguished by its large ovate often coloured stipules. Leaves mostly 4-8 cm across, 3-5 lobed, the lobes broad - rhombic often with a fine point and further lobed and toothed, flowers paired, rose to red purple with a pale centre, 2.5 - 4 cm across. Sepals bristly - haired on veins; stamen and filaments 5 - 7 mm. Flower stalks with two flowers. Blooming period is June to September.

It is reported from Kuram Valley, Kashmir, Simla and Kumaon. It is also found from Afghanistan to Bhutan. 2400-3600 m forests, shrubberies, open slopes,

MEDICINAL USE : Herb astringent, used as a cure for toothache, applied externally to eyes.

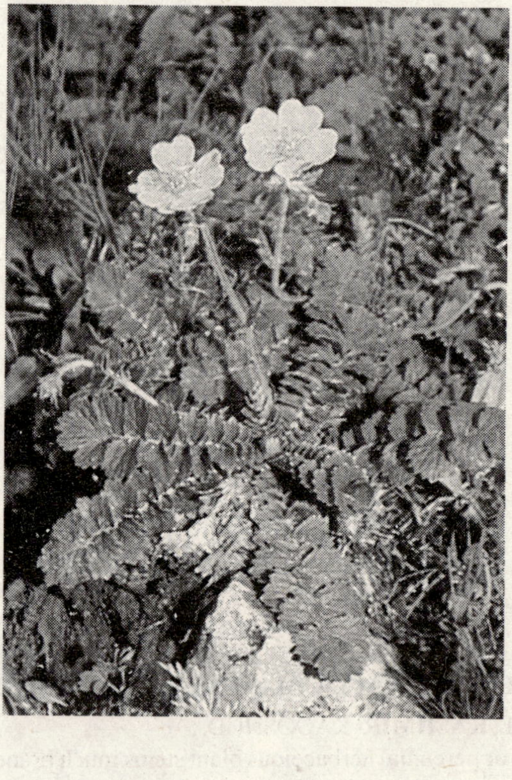

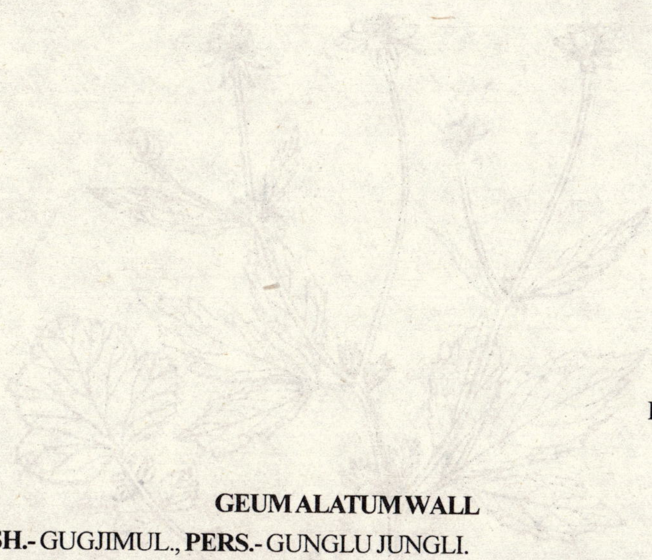

ROSACEAE

GEUM ALATUM WALL

KASH.- GUGJIMUL., **PERS.-** GUNGLU JUNGLI.

It is a perennial with pinnately - lobed basal leaves and with a few large yellow or rarely red flowers borne on sparsely leafy erect stem. Basal leaves are 5-30 cm, many pinnately cut into larger paired rounded and toothed broad - based stems 10 - 30 cm. alternating with much smaller lobes. Flowers 2.5 - 4 cm. across, erect or nodding petals 5, broadly obovate, much longer than the triangular calyx - lobes, epicalyx - lobes tiny. Fruit a globular head of usually hairy carpels with long nearly straight styles. Blooming June - August.

It is reported from Pakistan to S.E. Tibet 2700 - 4300 m. Shrubberies, open slopes. It is also recorded from subalpine and alpine Himalayas, from Kashmir 9,000 - 12000 ft. to Sikkim 12,000 - 15000 ft.

MEDICINAL USE : Herb astrin, styptie, tonic, febge, stomach used in dysen. diarr, sore throat and leueor. Roots considered astrin and antiseptic in Europe.

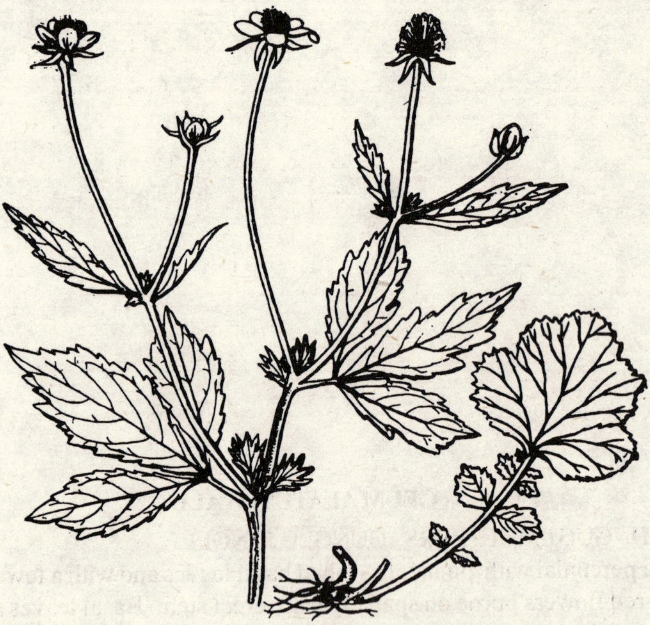

ROSACEAE

GEUM URBANUM LINN:
(IT IS VERY MUCH SIMILAR TO G. ROYLEI BOLLE)

ENGLISH- HERB BENNET

It is also known as wood avens of Europe

It is a herb with yellow flowers like the above plant but smaller in size 1.5 - 2 cm across and styles jointed in the middle. Upper leaves large 3 lobes, with leafy stipules, Basal leaves smaller unequally pinnate. lobed. Achenes bristly haired blooming period is June - August.

It is distributed in the temperate W. Himalayas, Afghanistan to C. Nepal 1800-3600 mtr. forests, shrubberies. From Kashmir to Kumaon.

MEDICINAL USE : uses similar to G. ALATUM.

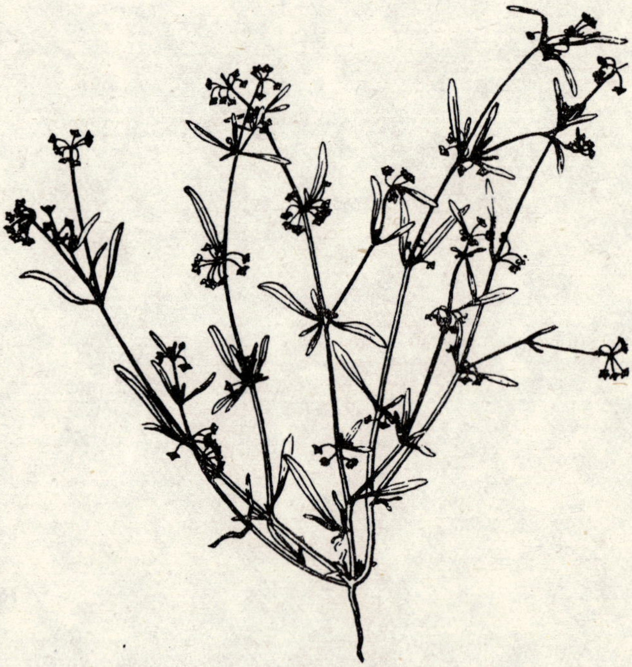

MOLLUGINACEAE
(AIZOACEAE)
(FICOIDACEAE)

GISEKIA PHARNACEOIDES LINN

HINDI- BALUKA SAG., **MARATHI-** BALUCHI BAJII., **SANSK & BENGALI** VALUKA., **BO.-** VALUCHI - BHAJI., **TAMIL-** MANALIKKIRAI., **M.-** PANEKIRAI., **TEL.-** ISIKEDANTIKURA, ISKADSARIKURA., **RAJASTHAN-** MORANG, SARAI.

It is an erect asending herb upto 20 cm. tall, branches subflexuouse. The leaves are 1.2 - 3x0.4 - 0.8 cm. linear lanceolate and subfleshy. Flowers small yellowish in lax, terminal and axillary cymes. Sessile. Fruit is a achene with five chambers, and seeds are black in colour. The flowering and fruiting season is July - September.

It is found as a weed mostly on dumat soil locally. It is also recorded from Punjab, Baluchistan, Rajputana desert, Sind, Gujarat, Kokan, S. Mahrata country, Deccan and Carnatic of Madras State.

MEDICINAL USE : This is an aromatic plant, astringent and vermufuge. The fresh plants paste mixed with water is given in the treatment of Taenia sp.

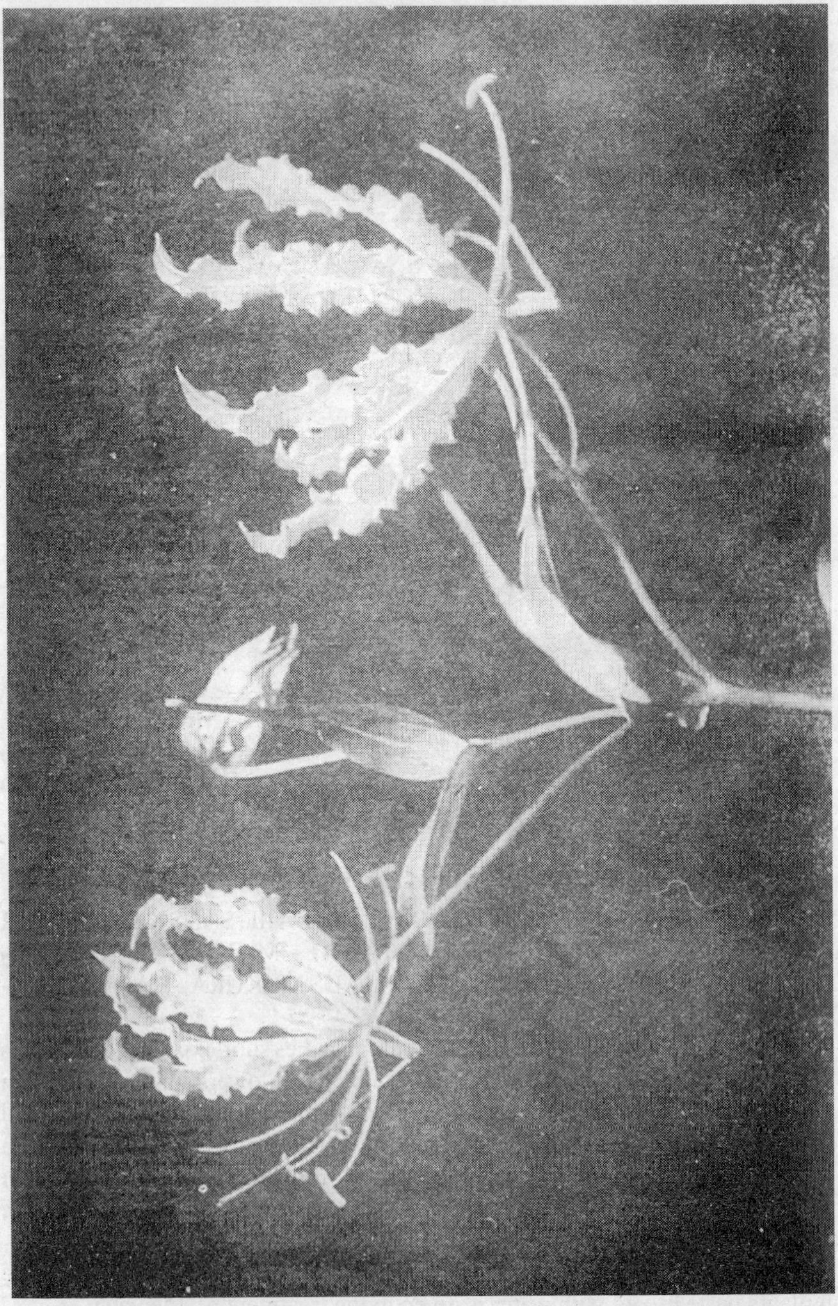

LILIACEAE

GLORIOSA SUPERBA LINN
GLORY LILIES
OR
CLIMBING LILIES
G. SUPERBA LINN

SANS.- LANGLAS, KALIKARI, AILNI, AGNISIKHA, GARBHAGHATINI, AGNIMUKHI., **HINDI**- KARIHARI, LANGULI., **BENG.**- BISHALANGULI, ULCHANDAL., **MARA.**- INDIA KARIAANNAG, NAGKARIA, KALLAVY. **GUJ.**- DUDHIOVAEHNAG, VARHVARDI., **TELUGU**- ADAVI-NABHI, KALAPPAGADDA, GANJERI., **TAM.**- KALIPPAIK-KISHANGA, AKKINICHILL., **KAN.**- AGNISIKHE, AKKATANGOBALLI, KARADIKANNI-NAGADDE., **MAL.**- MEDONI, MALATTAMARA, METTONNI., **ORIYA**- OGNISIKHA, GARBHOGHHAFONO, PANJANGALIA MAHERIAPHALO., **BOMBAY**- BACHNAG, KHADYANAG, KARIANAG., **PUNJAB**- KARIAR, MULIM, SANTAL-SIRIESAMANO.

It is small genus of ornamental climbing herbs native of tropical Asia and Africa, commonly known as GLORYLILIES OR CLIMIBING LILIES. One species occurs in India, G. SUPERBA LINN OR MALABAR GLORY LILY. It is an annual slender herbaeous climber common in low jungles almost throughout India up to an altitude of 6,000 ft. and in Andaman Islands. Root stock a chain of arched tubers, budding from the convexity above. The tuber is a fleshy perennial rhizome. The rhizome is cylindrical, bifurcated, usually V. shaped with the two limbs equal or unequal in length, pointed at the ends upto 12' long and 1.5' in diameter. Stem is 10-20 ft. terete, herabaceous, climbing and leafy. Leaves 6-8 sessile or shortly petioled, variable in breadth, many nerved alternate opposite or whorled, sessile or nearly so ovate-lanceolate with acuminate tips spirally twisted to serve as tendrils.

G. SUPERBA flowers in great profusion during the rainy season and is commonly cultivated in gardens. It is propogated by divisions of rhizomes planted before the rains in light rich soil with good drainge (Gopala Swamienger 490), Flowers pendulous with spreading stamens and styles, sharply deflexed at the extreme base through more than a right angle, so as to project from the flower horizontally showy large, solitory or corymbose with perianth 3-4 in diameter segments linear-lanceolate which have wavy margins, green-below it as are the margins and midrib. Filaments stout, golden yellow conective green, capsules 2 long. containing many rounded seeds.

It is distributed throughout tropical India; from the N.W. Himalaya's to Assam, Burma, Malacca and Ceylon, ascending to 5000 ft. also Trop, Africa, Malacca, Cochin & China.

MEDICINAL USE : The tubers are regarded as tonic, stomachic and anthelminitic when taken in doses of 5-10 grains. They are also used in leprosy, parastitical infections of Skin, Piles, Colic, in Snakebite and scorpion sting. It is an active ingredient of commercial Rumalaya cream.

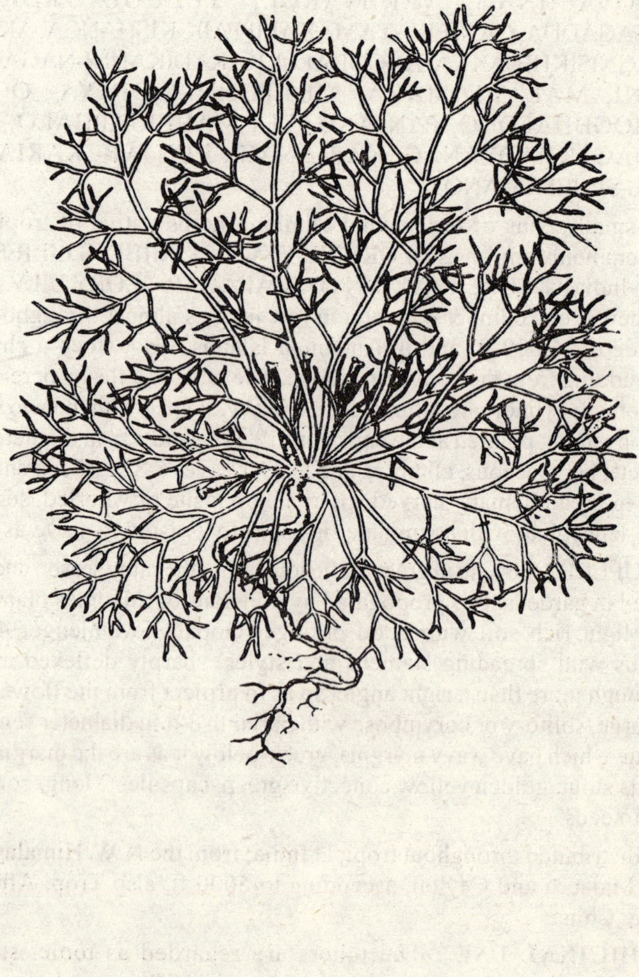

COMPOSITEAE

GLOSSOCARDIA BOSVALLIA LINN F. D.C.
(SYN. 1. VERBESINA BOSVALLIA, LINN F.
2. GLOSSOCARDIA LINEARFOBIA CASS.)

It is a small, prostrate or diffuse, tufted annual. The stem is 7.5 - 25 cms long and tunnelled. Leaves bipinnatisect. segments normally linear, heads small, yellow, heterogamous, about 8x8 mm Athenes densely bearded, especially along the edges. Awns spreadings blooming period is from July to Sept.

It occurs in sandy and rocky traets near Okhala and Faridabad. It is recorded from upper Gangetic plain, Madhya Bharat, Konkan, Deccan, S. Maharat country, N. Kanara and all plain districts of Madras State.

MEDICINAL USE : Plant is emmen. used in female complaints.

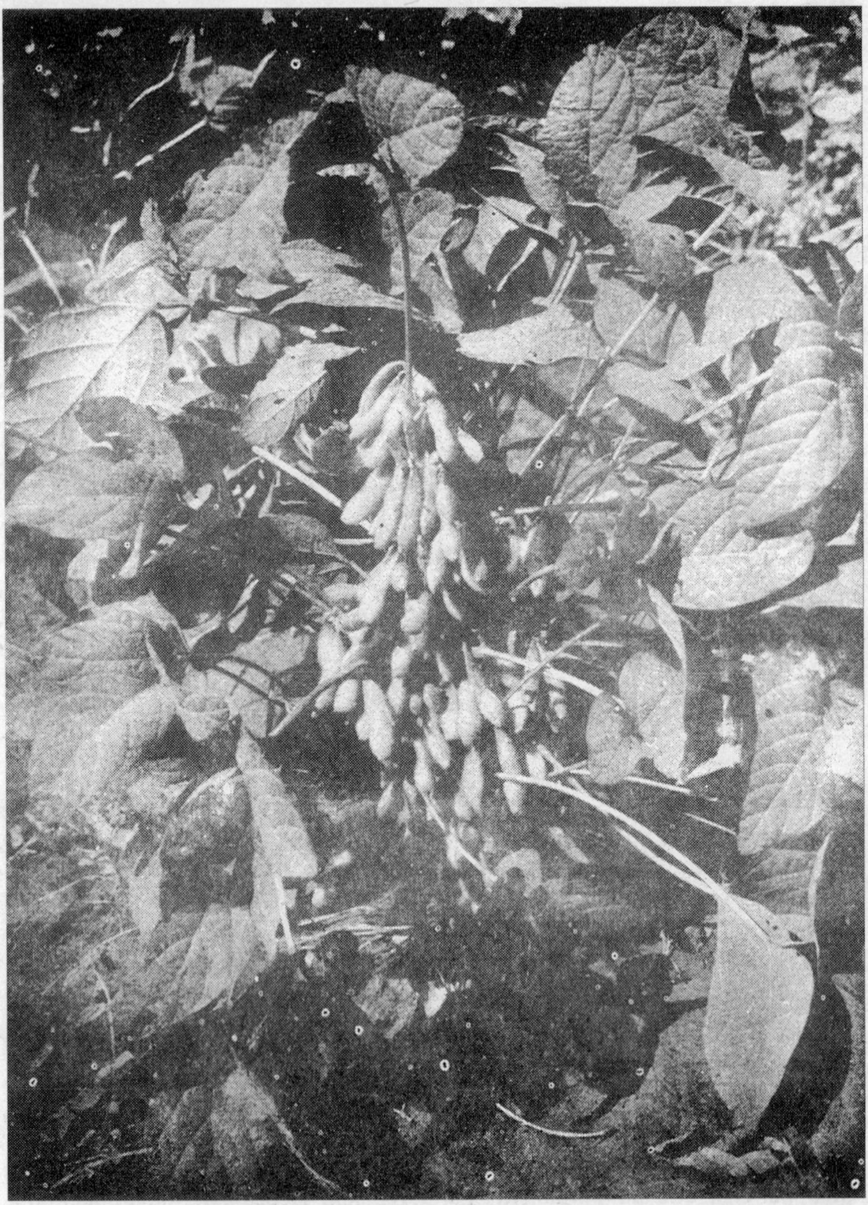

**FABACEAE
(PAPILIONACEAE)**

GLYCINE SOJA SIEB AND ZUCC
SYN. G. MAX MERA
"G. HISPIDA (MOENCH) MAXIM
"SOJA MAX (LI) PIPER

BENGALI- GARI-KULAY., **HINDI**-BHAT, BHATWAN, RAMKUNTHI., **PUNJABI**- BHAT., **ENGLISH**- SOYABEAN., **ASSAM**- PATNIJOKRA., **KASSHI**-RIMBAIKUTHULEGU.

It is an annual, erect or creeping or turning herb and densely hairy and reaching a height of 0.45-1.8 Mtrs. Stems appressed-denely hairy. Leaves oval to long-lanceolate long stalked, leaflets 3 (three) sub eoriaceous, pubescent beneath. Flowers white, mouve or reddish mouve, self pollinated small in axillary racemes. Pods 3.75-5 cm. long linear, oppressed-hairy, the remains of the style bent at right angles to the axis of the pod, each pod contains 2-4 seeds, The seeds are yellow, marron or black in colour.

It is considered as a native to S.E. asia and is now cultivate as pulse crop mainly in Punjab, Haryana, U.P., H.P., Maharashtra, Gujarat, Naga Hills, Manipur and Kashmir. This plant is unknown in the wild state.

MEDICINAL USE : Since it is rich in proteins, it is always mixed with food items which are required as protein rich items which are good for health people and as well as patients. Germinated soyabean is considered as a very good source of vitamin C. Decoction of the bark is astringent. It flour is considered ideal for dibetic patient. Its milk is substituted for cows milk for allergic children as it is easily digested. Soyabean oil is considered very valuable for eating purposes as it contains small guantities of fats and cholestrol and is kbown as Vital Oil commercially.

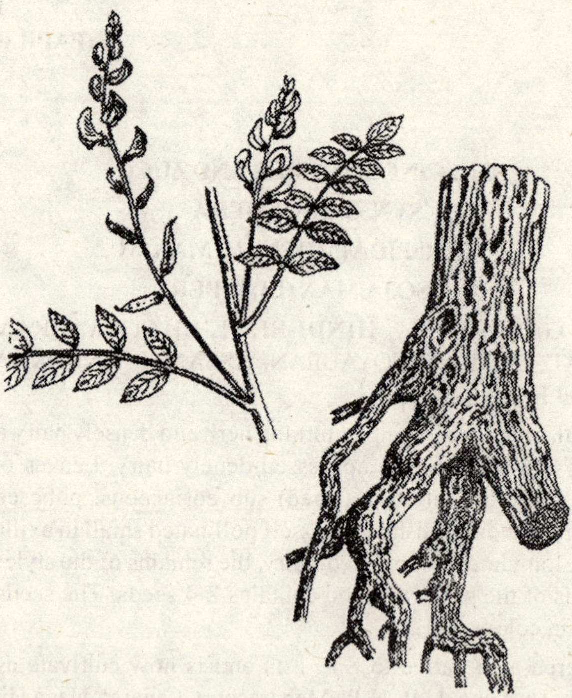

FABACEAE

GLYCYRRHIZA GLABRA LINN

SANSKRIT, BENGALI & BOMBAY- YASHTO - MADHU., **HINDI-** JATHIMADH, MALHAT TICE., **JASHTI-** MODH, MITHILAKDI., **PUNJABI-** MULETI., **TAMIL-** ATIMADURAM., **GUJARATI & MARATHI-** JASHTI KIDH., **KAN.-** JYESTHAMADHU, ATIMADHURA., **TEL.-** YASHTI - MADHUKUM - **ENGLISH-** LICORICE, LIQUARICE.

It is a perennial herb or under shrub, tall and erect. Reaching about a height of 1.5 metres, leaves compound, leaflets 4-7 pairs. Flowers are lilae or light voilet, small in slender axillary spikes which are equal to or slightly longer than the leaves. Fruit 1-3 cm long, flat densely covered all over with small spinous outgrowths. The root stock throws numerous additional roots, or in some forms there are several branched stems near the root stock remaining underground.

The plant is being cultivated in India, Kashmir, Punjab, Himachal Pradesh, Uttar Pradesh, Jammu and South India have been suggested as suitable areas for cultivation. It is also cultivated in Sub Himalayan tracts from Chenab east words, Sind and Peshawar valley. Burma and Andeman Islands. It also grows in Arabia, Persian Gulf, Afghanistan, Turkestin, Asia Minor, and Siberia.

MEDICINAL USE : The dried roots and the rhizone (stem) of this plant constitute the drug. It is useful in cough, sore throat, plant constitute the drug. It is useful in cough, sore throat, bronchitis, adbominal pains, consumption and epilepsy. For cough and sore throat raw liquorice is also chewed or sucked. It promotes urination and its diuretic activity as also antibiotic and antibacterial activity. Due to its sweet taste. It is used for making medicinal syrups and for masking bitter taste of medicines in mixtures and pills. It is useful in gastric and duodenal ulcers. Its powder mixed with butter and honey is applied on cuts and wounds. The leaves of the plant, if applied as a poultice are believed to be useful in scalds of the head.

It is a main constitutent of Glycodine Terpvasaka and cough pills. Used commercially. Glycyrrhizin a glycoside in root, is considered to be fifty times as sweet as sugar.

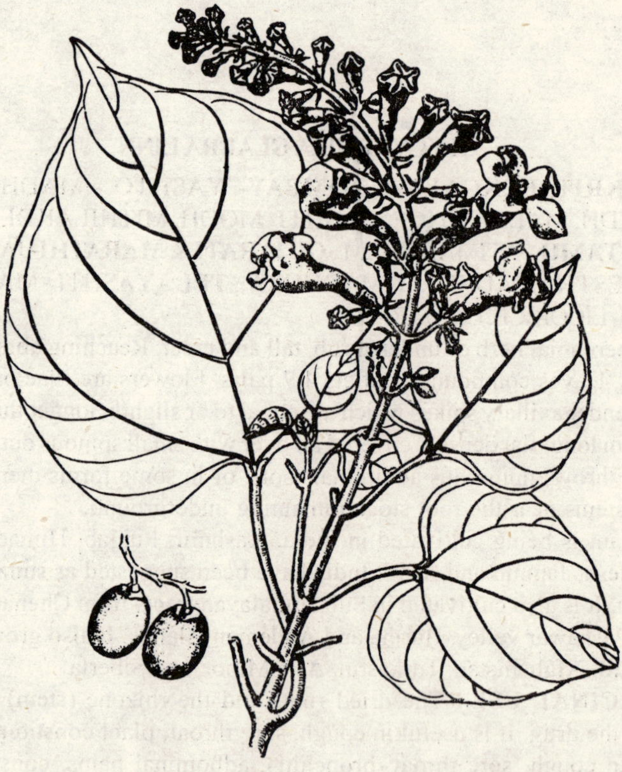

VERBENACEAE

GMELINA ARBOREA (LINN) ROXB.
(SYN. PREMNA ARBOREA ROTH).

SNAS.- GUMBHARI., **HINDI-** GAMARI, KHAMBHARI JUGANI - CHUKUR, GAMBHARA, SEWAN, SHEWAN., **BENGALI-** GUMBAR, KUNTAR., **MARATHI-** SHIVARASAL., **GUJARATI-** SHEWAN., **MAL.-** KUMBULA., **TAMIL-** KOTTAMAM, GUMADI, CUMMI., **TEL.-** GUMARTEK, GRIMMADI, GUMAR-TEK - PEDDAGAMROG, GUMUADUTEKU, TAGUMULA, GAMMADU., **KAN.-** SHIVANI, KULI., **MARATHI-** SHEVAN.

A small unarmed deciduous tree. Young parts clothed with pale yellow tomentum. Leaves broad, ovate accumnate; base cuneate; Flowers brownish yellow in paniculate cymes. Dupes pyriform or obovoid smooth; endocarpbony. Fruiting seasons is March to May. Planted in the lawn of garden. Most of the flowers fall off and only few develop fruits. It is distributed throughout India; lower Himalayas, the Nilgiris and the East and West Coast of India.

MEDICINAL USE : Juice of the leaves demule., used in gonor. cough and to inprove foetid discharges and worms from ulcers, Plant used in snake bite and scorpion - sting. G. HYSTRIX and like other species form an active ingredient of dashomoola in Abana, lukol and Rumalaya.

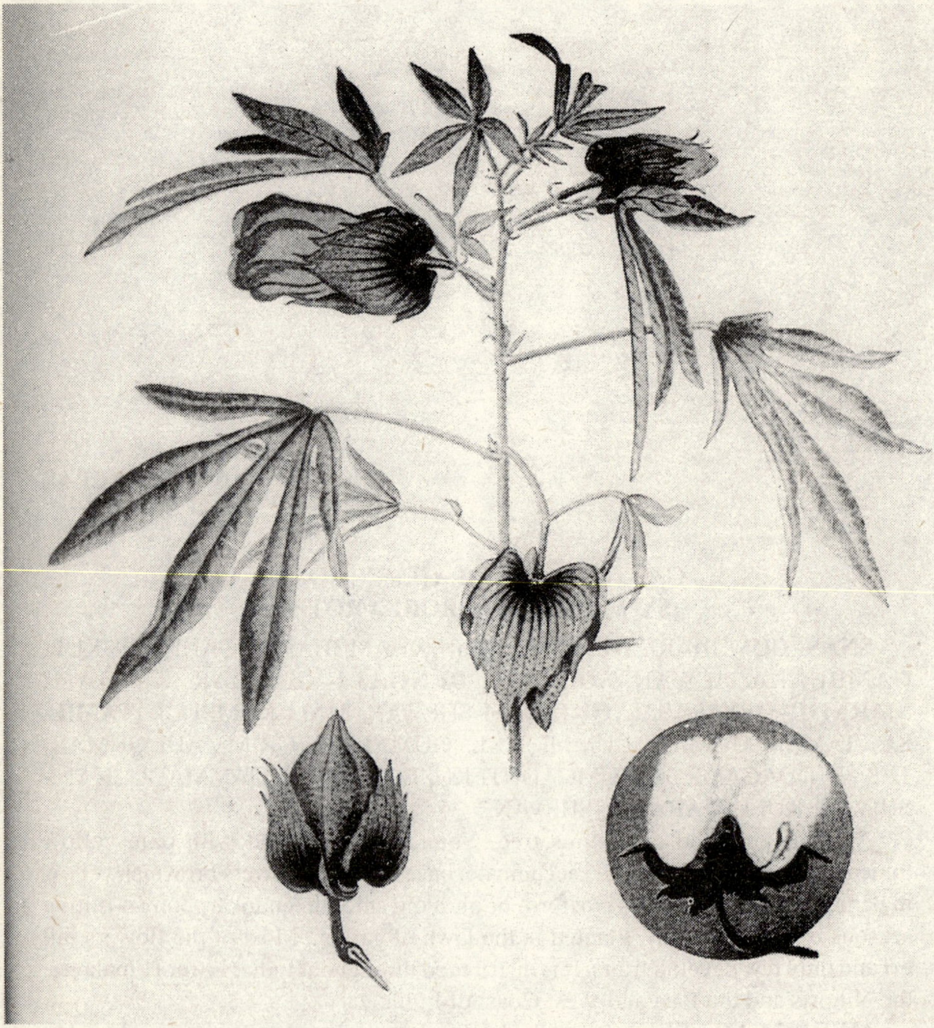

MALVACEAE

GOSSYPIUM ARBOREUM LINN
(SYN. G. NANKING MEYEN)
"G. INDICUM TOD
"G. NEGLECTUM TOD

HINDI- KAPAS, RUI, NURMA., **ENGLISH**- TREE COTTON., **PUNJABI**- KAPAS, BOMBAY DEOKAPAS., **MAL.**- CHEMPARUTTI, PANGI., **SANSKRIT**- KARPASAMN., **TAMIL**- SEMBARUTTI, PUNGI., **TEL.**- PATTI., **MARATHI**- DEOKAPAS-KANN, HALTI, ARALE TEY, PATTI, KARPSAMU., **GUJARATI**- KAPAS, TOOL., **ORIYA**- KARPASO, KOPA.

This is an annual or perenial plant. It reaches height of 60 cm to 3 meter. Commonly known as shruby pilose plant with thin woody mouve coloured branches. Leaves hairy, palmately 5-7 lobed more shining dorsally. Each lobe is oval, linear-lanceolate cordate at base. Stipules falcate. Flowers of the purple, yellow, red or white with a crimson center. Bractoles three in number united, 3-4 toothed. Capsules are oblong and pointed. Seeds are small hairy in two layers. Blooming period is monsoon. Flowers and fruits-October.

It is a cultivated plant and is grown all over India as a fiber plant.

MEDICINAL USE : Roots are used in fever. Seeds are use in gonnorrhea, Gleet, chronic cystitis and caterrh.

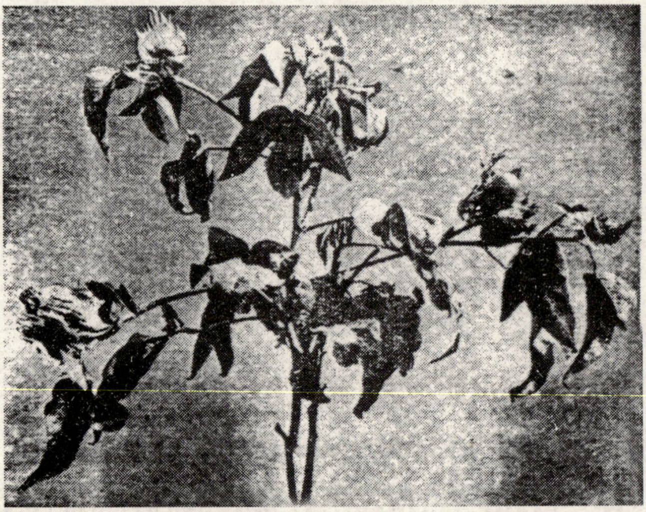

MALVACEAE

GOSSYPIUM BARBADENSE LINN
(SYN. G. ARBORIUM L.
VAR. NADAM (WATT) PROKH)

SANSKRIT- MAGHANI., **MARATHI-** PARUTTI., **MAL.-** CHEMPARUTTI., **TAMIL-** AVATTAM., **TEL.-** PAIDIPUTTI., **ENGLISH-** SEA ILAND COTTON, MISTRI COTTON, BRAZILANAN COTTON, PERU COTTON KIDNEY COTTON.

It is either annual plant reaching a height of 0.9 - 2 meter or perennials reaching a height of upto 4.5 metres. The stem is stout and spreading. Branches and new leaves are hairless to slightly hairy. The leaves are large with 3-5 lobules, lobules becoming narrower towards the base. Bracteoles 10 - 15 toothed, oral. Flowers large and contain oil glands. The seeds are kidney shaped, 3-4 in one chamber and covered with fibres.

It is native to tropical America and is grown mainly in Malabar and South Kanara.

MEDICINAL USE : Seeds in the form of an emulsion given in dysen. supposed to be pcectoral. Oil from seeds used to clear spots and freakles from the skin.

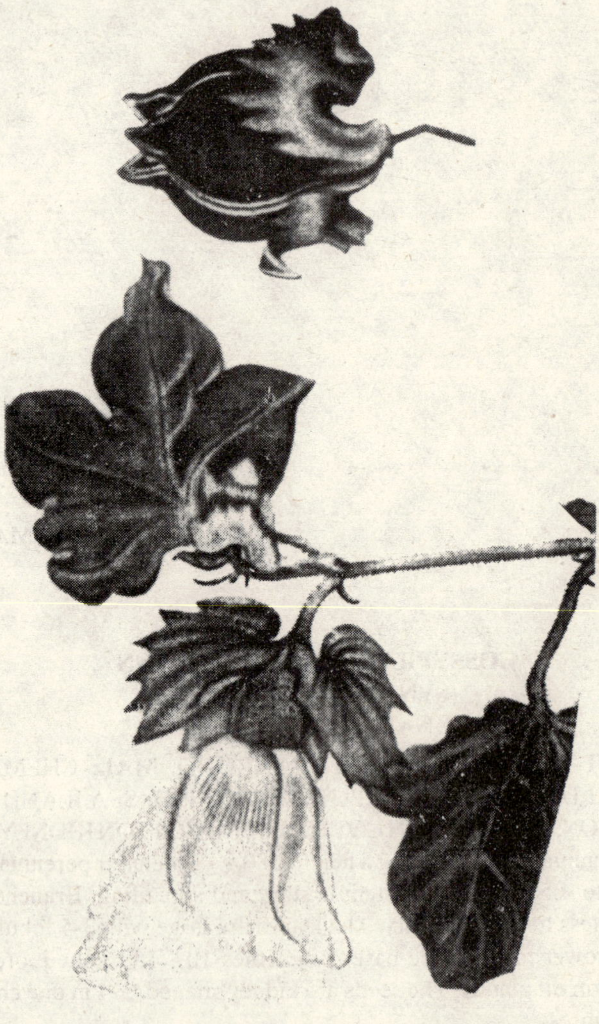

MALVACEAE

GOSSYPIUM HERBACEUM LINN
(SYN. G. WIGHTIANUM TOD
"G. OBTUSIFOLIA ROXB. P.P.)

ENGLISH- ASIATIC COTTON, LEVANT COTTON., **HINDI-** KAPAS., **SANSKRIT-** KARPASI., **BENGALI & BOMBAY-** KAPAS., **TAMIL-** PARUTTI., **TEL.-** KARPASAMU., **MAL.-** KARPPASI., **LOCAL NAME-** BARI.

An erect, shrubby hairy plant. It reaches a height of 60 - 2 metres. Stems woody. the leaves are broad, 3-7 lobed chordate at base; Each lobe is oval round, narrowed at the joint. The stipules are falcate. The bracteole. 3 in no. large entire or 6 - 8 toothed. Flowers large, yellow with purple centre, calyx beset with black glandular dots. Capsule ovate pointed. Flowering and fruiting season is September - October. The blooming period is monsoon period.

It is a cultivated plant. It is mainly cultivated in Maharashtra, Tamil Nadu, Andhra Pradesh and Karnataka. It is also reported from N.W. Frontier Province and Baluchistan.

MEDICINAL USE : Seeds demule, laxt, expect. galact, aphrodis, employed to procure abortion, considered nervine tonic, given in head ache, root and bark - emmen, galact. Juice of leaves used in Scorpion sting and snake bite.

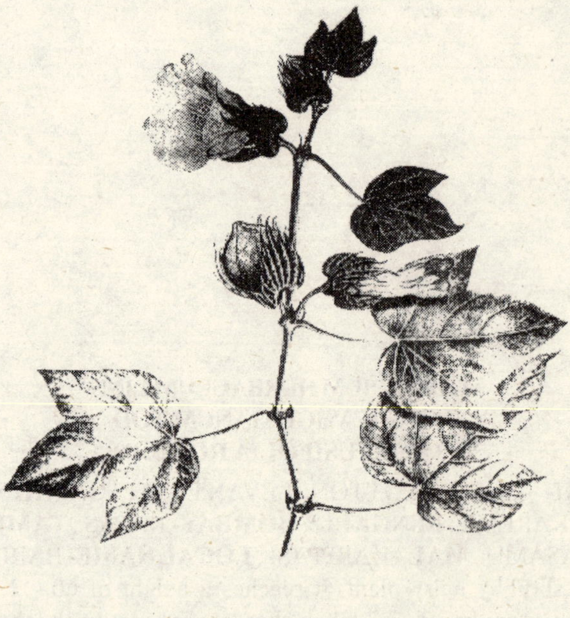

MALVACEAE

GOSSYPIUM - HIRSUTUM LINN (SYN. G. MEXICANUM TOD; " G. RELIGIOSUM L.)

HINDI- KAPAS., **ENGLISH-** UPLAND COTTON., **LOCAL NAME-** BARI.

It is an annual or perennial course, much branched bush clothed with woolly hairs. The stem is green brown or raddish brown. Leaves simple to five lobed, thick, lobes short, triangular, base chordate. Flowers yellow turning to pink, purple without a dark centre. Bracteoles long quite free with 7-12 teeth. Capules spherical. Seeds with a greyish, rusty or green tuzz; flowers and fruits September - October.

It is cultivated during rainy season and is grown chiefly in Punjab, U.P., Rajasthan, M.P., Tamil Nadu and Maharashtra.

MEDICINAL USE : In Guinea leaves and seeds are considered emole and roots emmen. Leaves and flowers (deprived of petals) contain glued. Gucrcimeritrin petals contain quercimeritrin and isoquercitin.

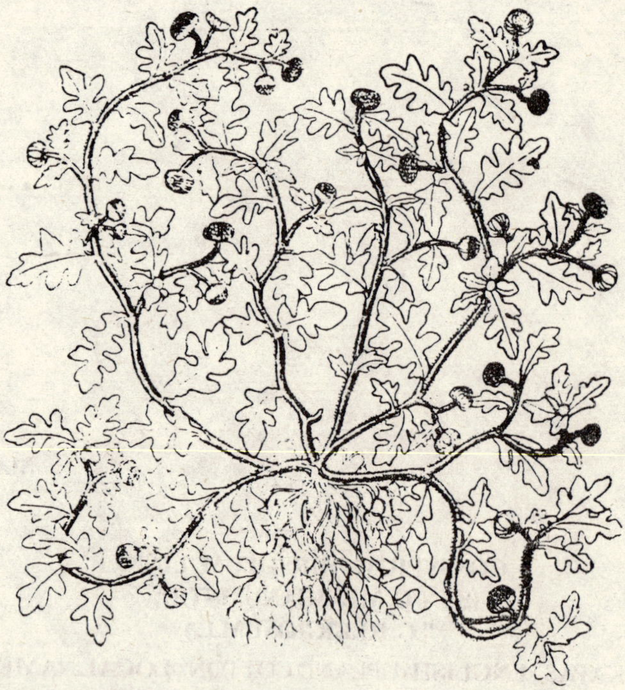

COMPOSITAE

GRANGEA MADERASPATANA (LINN) POIR
SYN. ARTOMISIA MADERASPATANA LINN).

HINDI- MUSTARU, MUKHTARI., **BENGALI-** NAMUTI., **MARATHI, MASHIPATRI GUJR-** TINKIMUNDI, NAHANIGORAKHMUNDI., **TELGU-** SAAVAE, MUSTAR, MEDRIPATIR., **TAMIL-** MASSIPATRI., **KAN.-** DAVAN., **MAL.-** NEELAMPALA., **BIHAR-** BHARIYACHEEM, BICHIBA.

It is an annual prostrate, tufted, leafly herb, forming circular patches. Leaves sinuately pinnatifid, thick, Heads yellow, disciform, heterogamous, about 6x9 mm. Pappus capsular. It keeps on blooming for the major parts of the year. Flowers and fruit through out the year.

It is found on dry, sandy, clayey soil and along Jamuna Banks on moist, silty soil. Commonly it is reported from all over India and Buluchistan.

MEDICINAL USE : Leaves stomach, antisept. deobstruent; prescribed in infusion and electuary in cases of obstructed menses and hysteria, and used in preparing antisep. and anodyne fermentations. Juice of leaves employed as a cure for ear ache.

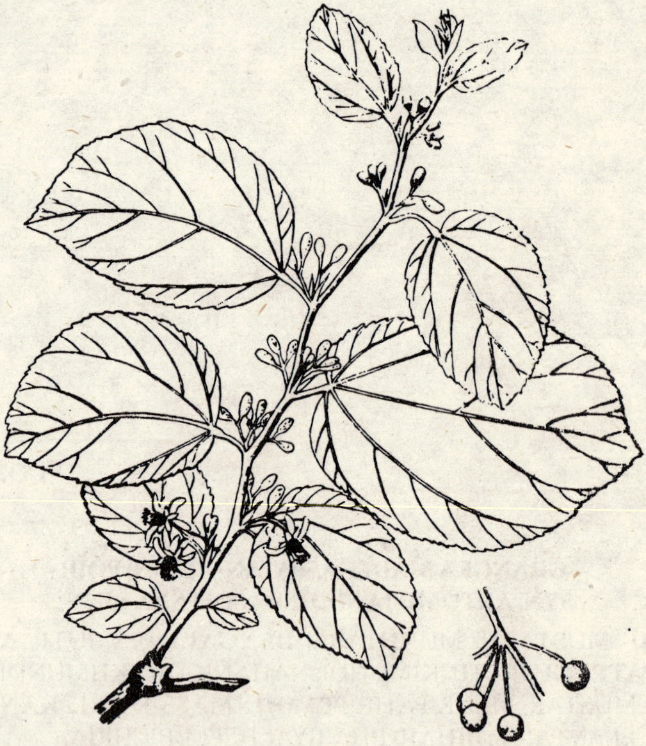

TILIACEAE

GREWIA SUB INAEQUALIS DL
(SYN. GREWIA ASIATICA MASTERS (NON. L)

ENGLISH- PHALSA., **MARATHI-** PHALSE., **TELGU-** JANA, NALLAJANA, PHOTIKI., **HINDI-** PHALSA, DAMIN, PERUSHA, SHUKARI., **LOCAL NAME-** PHALAS., **BENGALI-** PHALSA, SHUKRI., **GUJARATI-** PHALSA., **TAMIL-** PALISA, TADACHI., **KANNADA-** BUTTIYUDIPPE, TADASALA., **ORIYA-** PHARA SAKO.

It is a medium sized crooked tree with a spreading crown. Bark is rough and greyish white to brown. The leaves are variable the size ranging from 8-20 x 8x12 cm. Leaves acquire different shapes, such as conical, oral and obovate with irregular serrate margins. Peduncles in fasicles of 2-8 usually 3 flowered. The flowers are yellow axillary in position surrounded by a pair of subulate stipules. The fruits are roundish nearly the size of a pea containing stony pib. Hence it is known as drupe. They are green when unripe, red when semi ripe and dark purple when fully ripe, more or less globose pilose, nuts 1-2. The flowering and fruiting season is June - July.

It is found and cultivated extensively throughout India. It is unknown in the wild State.

MEDICINAL USE : Fruit astringent; Colling, stomach. Infusion of bark - demule . Root bark - in rheumatism. leaves are used as application for pustular eruptions.

This fruit is considered as digestive and hence eaten after meals. The juice of the fruit makes a drink which is very cooling and refreshing in extremes of heat.

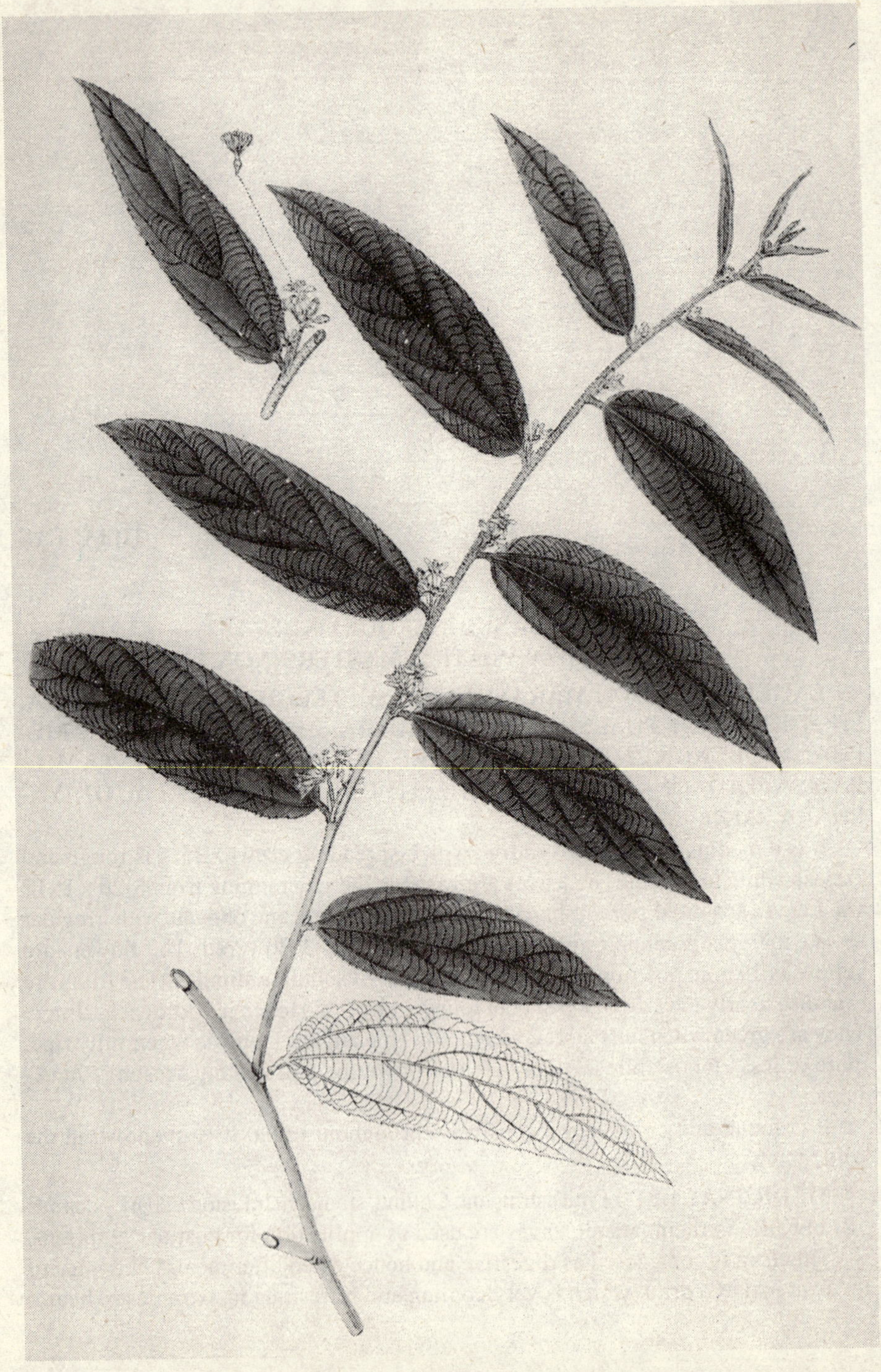

TILIACEAE

GREWIA HIRSUTA VAHL.
VAR. HELICTERIFOLIA
(SYN. G. POLY GAMA MAST
G. POLOSA ROXB.

HINDI- KUKURBICHA., **TEL.-** JIBILIKE., **MARATHI-** GOVIL.

It occurs in sub - Himalayan tracts upto 1500 m from Indus eastward; Bihar and Orissa.

MEDICINAL USE : Fruit and root are used in diarrohea and dysentry. Root is pounded in water applied externally to hasten suppuration and as a dressing for wounds.

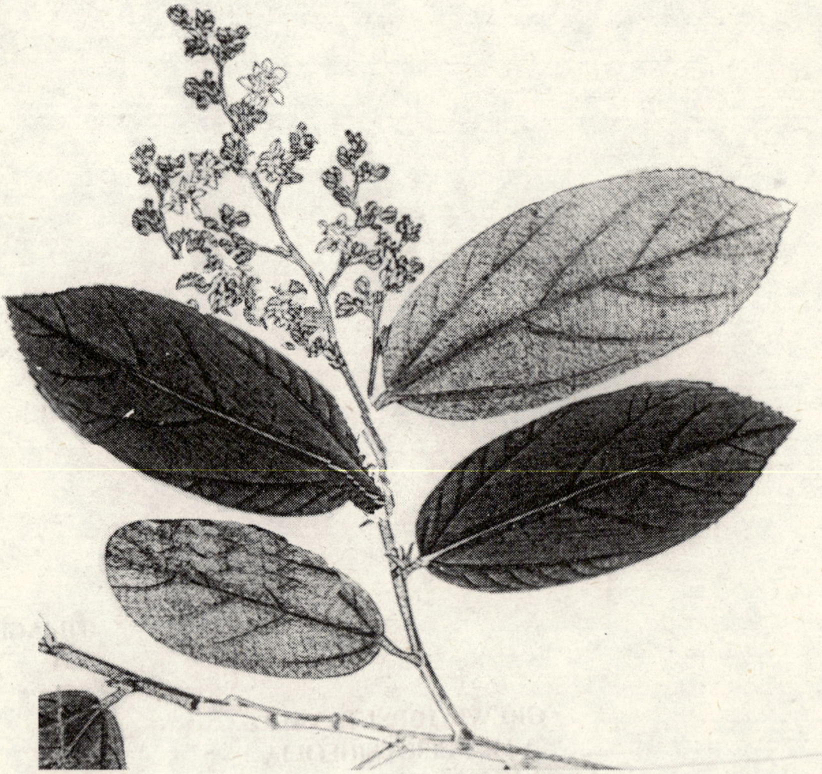

TILIACEAE

GREWIA MICROCOS LINN

BENG.- ASAR., **BOMBAY-** ANSALE, SHEERUL, ASOLIN., **MAL.** - KOTAKA, KOTTA., **KAM.-** ABRAINGU, BINNIAFRUNGU., **ASSAM-** THANGFRANKAE - ORONG., **TAM.-** KADAMBU,

It is a bush or tree which attains a height of atleast 15 mtrs. 1.5 m. thick. The bark is dark brown or black. The leaves are oral to orbicular and hairy. The flower branches are terminal and are of fading yellow colour. The fruits are round stony and of mouve colour (peasize). It is reported from East Bengal, Assam, Western Pennisula, Mysore and Anademan Island.

MEDICINAL USE : Plant in indign. typhoid fever, dysen. and syphilitic ulcerartion of the mouth and in small pox, exzem and itches.

The two other species known as G. SELENOPHYLLA ROXB. and G. VILLOSA willd are also used as medicinal plants in the treatment of cough and the diseases of the intestine and bladder.

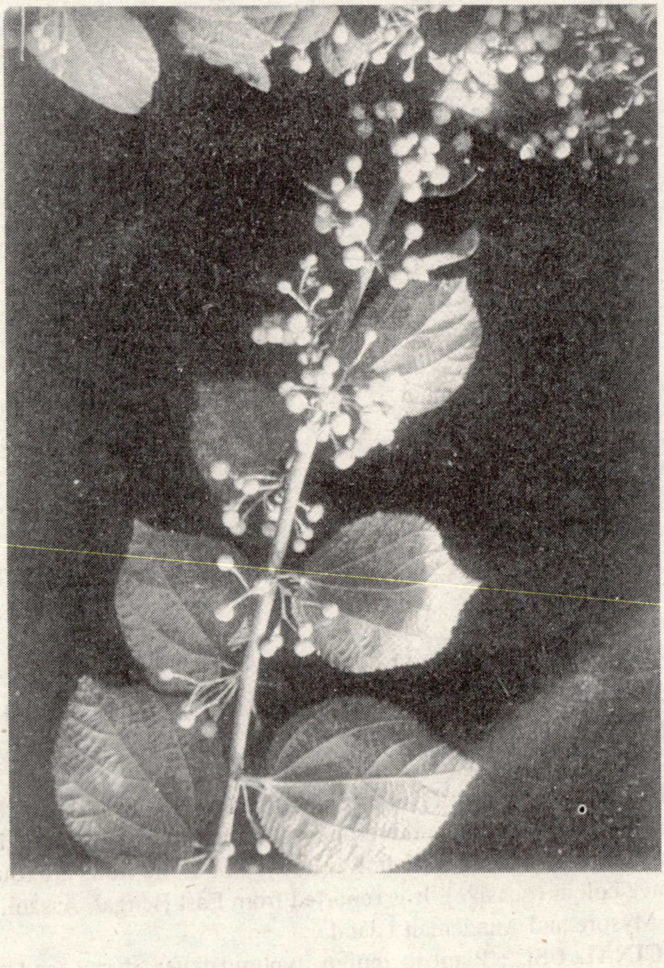

TILIACEAE

GREWIA POPULIFOLIA VAHL.
(SYN. G. TENAX (FOR S.K.) ASCHERS AND SCHWT.
"G. BETULAEFOLIA JUSS

PUNJ.- GANGER., **TEL.**- KALADI., **LOCAL NAME**- CHABENI, RAMCHANA, KHATOLA, GONDNI.

A much branched shrub upto 3 m. tall. Stems and branches whitish grey to grey. Leaves irregular in shape, subcoracious, Flowers about 2 cm long. buds oblong. Drupes 2 to 4 - lobbed, orange - red. Flowers July - August, Fruits - October.

It is reported from Punjab, Sind, Rajaputana and Western India down to the Nilgiris hills.

MEDICINAL USE : Mucilage of bark is used by women of west tropical Africa to clean the hair of vermun. It has pesticidal properties and the plant is also used in hilly areas of northern India in the treatment of tuberculosis.

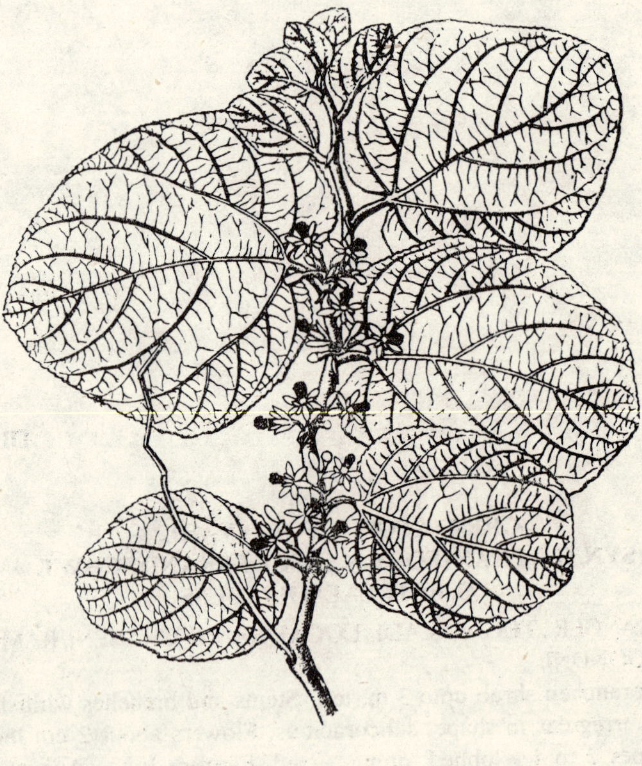

TILIACEAE

GREWIA TILIAEFOLIA VAHL

HINDI- DHAMANI, PHASA., **SANSKRITI**- DHARMANA, DHAMNI., **ENGALI**- DHAMIN, DHANUVIVISK., **BOMBAY**- DAMANU., **MARATHI**-)AMAN, DEMINI., **GUJARATI**- DALMON, DAMOA., **TAMIL**- CHARACHI, TTATARA, TARRA., **TEL.**- CHARACHI, JANE, SADACHI., **MAL.**- SATACHI, HADICHA, UNNU., **KAN.**- TARSAL, BUTALAE., **ORIYA**- DHAMAN, HAMARO., **COMMERCIAL NAME**- DHAMAN.

It ranges from medium to very tall tree. Its stem is 9 meters long and 2.1 m in irth. The bark is buff or dark brown. The leaves are stalked. Ovate to orbicular ith serrate margin. The flowers are small and thick on the main axis. The fruits are the size of a pea or gram, with stony pib, 2-4 chambered.

It is distributed in the upper Gangetic plain, Bihar, Bengal, Central and peninsular dia. It is also reported from Sub Himalayan region from the Jamna to Nepal upto 000 ft. Madhya Bharat, all districts of Madras State, Bihar and Orrisa.

MEDICINAL USE : The bark of the tree is used in dysen. employed externally remove the irritation from cow-itch. wood in powder form emetic, antid to opium isoning.

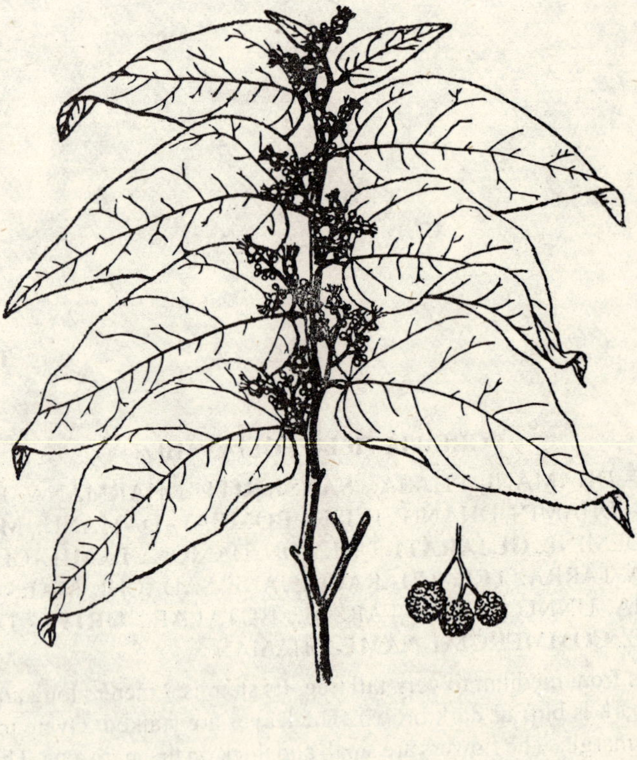

STERCULIACEAE

GUAZUMA TOMENTOSA KUNTH (SYN. GUAZUMA ULMIFOLIA LAMK)

BENGALI- NIPALTUNTH., **MARATHI-** TENMARAM., **TAMIL-** TENBACHI, TUBAKII, THANNARUM, RUDRALISHAK., **TEL.-** RUDRAKSHA, UDELREEK PUTT., **THANE-** CHETTOO., **MAL.-** RUDRAKSHAM, UTTARASHAM, UTTARASHAM., **KANN.-** RUDRAKSHEE BACHNAA., **ORIYA-** DEBODARU.

It is small or medium sized tree. Its bark is brown, rough and with spreading branches. It is condsidered as a shade plant. Leaves are elliptie to lanceolate to oval and hairy only. the flowers are yellow or blue in big clusters and papery. the fruits are woody elongated (almost 2.5 cm) and oval. Each fruit contains numerous oval brown seeds.

In some places it is cultivated while in others this is a wild plant. It is found near cities and villages. It is considered as a native of America. The above mentioned speices is grown in India.

MEDICINAL USE : Bark suddorific, tonic, demulc. Useful in skin dieeases and elephantiasis.

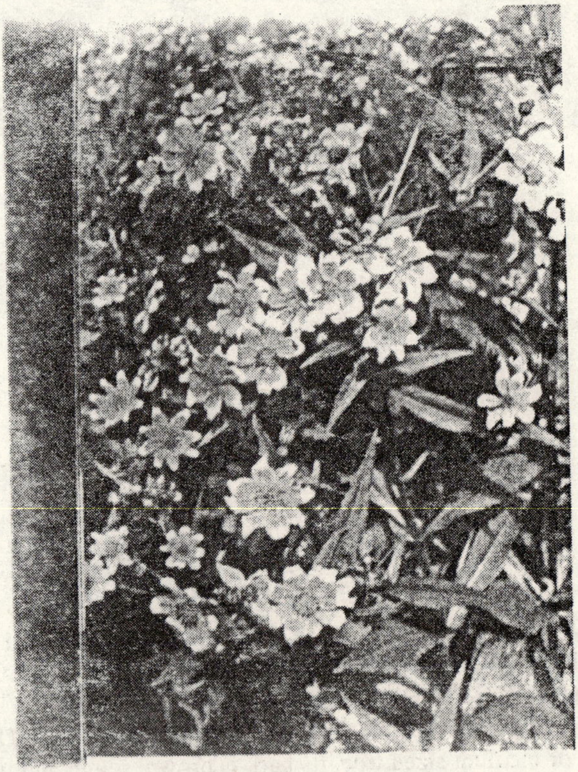

COMPOSITAE

GUIZOTIA ABYSSYNICA (LF.) CASS

BENGALI- RAMTIL, SIRGUJA., **BOMBAY**- RAMTILA., **HINDI**- KALATIL RAMTIL, SURGUJA., **TET.**- VALESULU., **ENGLISH**- NIGER SEED, RAMTIL, MARATHI KUHRASANI, KERALAE., **GUJARATI**- KALA., **TEL.**- RAM TEL., **TELGU**- BERYMUNUVAALU., **TAMIL**- PYALU, YUCHELU., **KAN.**- GURARDU, DU, HOOCHADUU, KARADDUU, BHOPAL RAMELI.

It is shout well built leafy annual reaching a height of 2 meters, stem is strong about 1.5 cm in diameter branched above. Leaves opposite, 7.5 - 12.5 cm toothed with a fine apical point clasping lanceolate to oblong. Flowers present in yellow heads in a lax branched terminal cluster. Flower heads 3-4 cm across, with ray florets few, broadly oblong, with 3 toothed apex, disk florets tubular, anthers longer, protruding, outer involucral bracts broadly ovate, blunt, green, receptacle with papery scales, seeds black, flatened. Blooming period is autumn.

It is considered as a native of tropical Africa, cultivated in various parts of India such as Madhya Pradesh, Orissa, Maharashtra and Mysore. Bihar, Andhra Pradesh, Tamil Nadu mainly.

MEDICINAL USE : It is mainly cultivated for the oil which is extracted from seeds. This oil is very useful and is used medicinally for several purposes such as rheumatism and its massage in children as well as grown up people is used for preventing cold in winter. It is used in many ointments which are made for skin diseases.

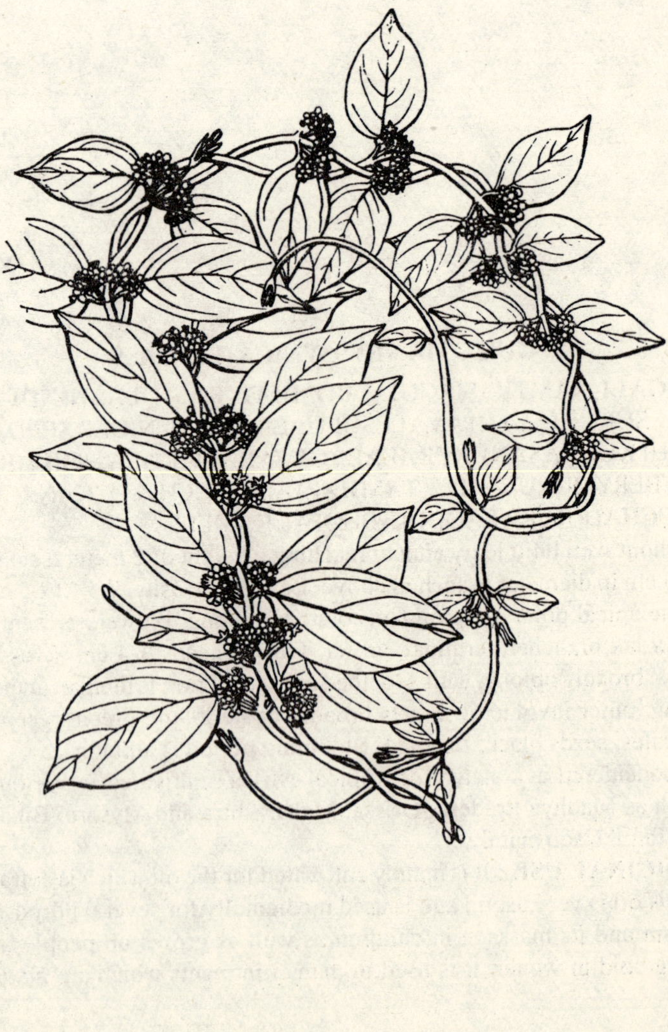

ASCLEPIADACEAE

GYMNEMA SYLVESTRE R.B.R.
(SYN. ASCLEPIAS GEMINATEA ROXB)

GUJARAT & MARATHI- KAVALI, KALI, KUNDORI, VAKUNCLI., **SANS.-** MESHASINGI HIDA MASHNI., **BOMBAY-** KAVALI., **HINDI & BENGALI-** CHHOTA, DUDDHILATA, GURMAR, MERA SINGI., **TAMIL-** ADIDUM, SHIRUKURANJA., **TELEGU-** BODAPANTA, BODAPATRI., **GUJARAT-** CHERUKURINJA, DULATI, MARDASINGI., **KANNADA-** SUNNGERA SAHAHEMBOO.

It is a woody elimber twining large, hairy densely or semi densely. Leaves are ovate lanceolate arranged in an opposite manner at nodes of the stem. Both surfaces of the leaf are pubsecent. They are non-glandular, profusely present all over the surface. The leaf is 3.1 - 5 cm x 1.25 - 3.1 cm. The flowers are small, yellow in colour, found in bunches in axil of leaf, sessile or a ray small pedicel is present. Folicles are lanceolate being approximately 7.5 cms.

It is reported from Banda, Karkan, S. Mahrata country, W. Ghats, N. Konera, N. Circars, Carnatic and Deccen.

MEDICINAL USE : The plant as a whole increase apetite, useful in cough, acidity, and sore-eyes. The roots are astringent, stomachic, tonic and refrigerant. The leaves cause hypoglycaemia in experimental animals but has got no such effect on human beings. It stimulate heart and circularory system, increase urine secretion and activate the uterus. The leaves have a peculiar property of neutralising temporarily the taste sensation for sugars and hence the name Gurmar is given to it.

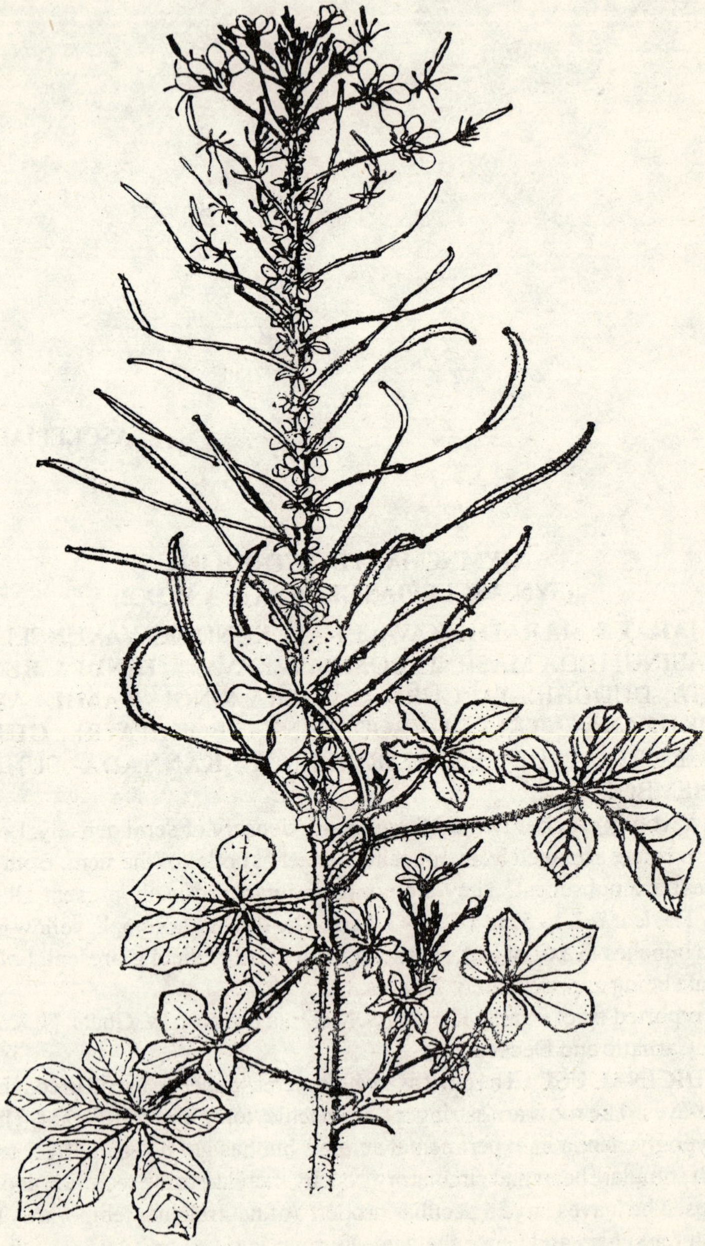

CAPPARIDACEAE

GYNANDROPSIS GYNANDRA (LINN) BRIQ (SYN. G. PENTO PHYLLA D. C) SYN. CLEOME GYNAMDRA LINN)

SANS.- SURJAVARTA, ARKAPUSHPIKA., **HINDI**- HULHUL, CHUROTA, GANDHULI., **BENG**.- SADA HURHURI, ANSARISAHA., **MAR.**- KANPHODI, MOTITILAVAN, PANDHARITILAVAN., **GUJ.**- ADIKYAKHARAN, SATITALVANI., **TEL.**- VAMINTA, VAINTA, VELAKURA., **TAM.**- KATTKADUGU, VELAI, TAIWELA., **KAN.**- NARUM BYALE SOPPU., **MAL.**- KARAVELA, TAIVELA., **BIHAR**- SETA KATA ARAK, CHAMANI, MARANG (HARMANI)., **PUNJAB**- KATHAL, PARHAR., **RAJASTHAN**- BAGRA., **LOCAL NAME :** HULHUL.

An erect or ascending glandular- pubesent annual upto 60 cm. tall, branching from the base. Leaves long stalked, digitately 3-5 foliate: leaf -lets unequal, subsessile obovate or elliptic-oblong : flowers white or purple bisexual to polygamous, in corymbose recemes. Capsules 2-4 mm. long striated, containg reniform, rugose brown or black seeds. Flowers fruiting - June to September.

It is met commonly in waste lands or caltivated ground throughout the warmer parts of India.

MEDICINAL USE : The leaves & seeds are used in indigenous medicine. Bruised leaves are rubifacient & vesicant & used as a cure for headache, neuralgia, rheumatisum & other local pains. The leaves are also used as cure for pus formation, leaf juice + oil is used for ear ache. The leaves are taken internally for billious disorders. The root is a mild febrefuge. Seeds are anthelmintic, rubefacient & a cure for expulsion of worms. An infusion of the seeds in given for cough.

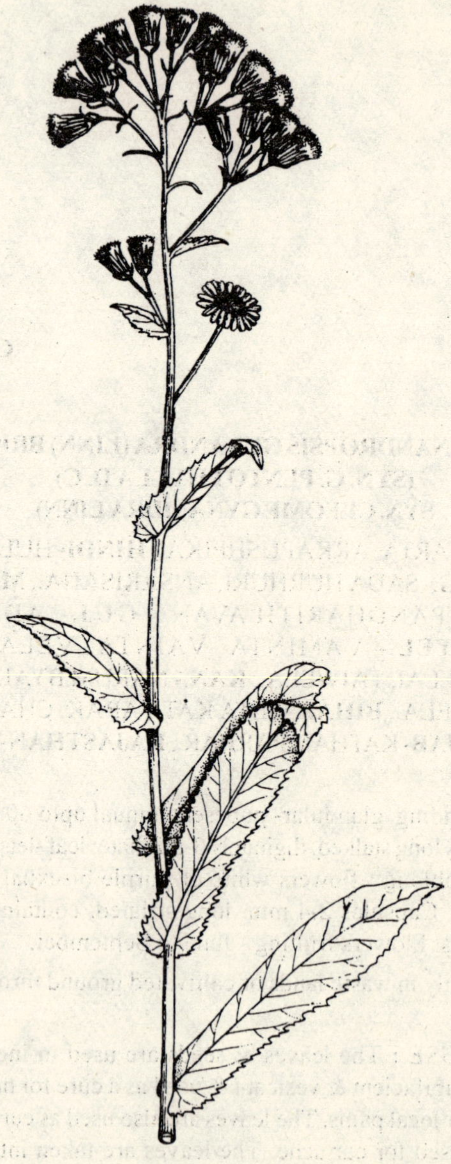

COMPOSITAE

GYNURA PSEUDO CHINA DC

It is a stout hairless perennial 1-2 m, with large obovate to oblong - long pointed leaves 15-30 cm or more, stalkless irregularly toothed, the upper narrower, clasping, flowers orange to orange yellow in large clusters placed terminally. Infloreceace widely branched; flower heads 1.6 - 2 cm. long, long stalked, several or many, involucre cylinderical, braets 10-12 equal, in one row, hairless and with papery margins, and with smaller linear, outer braets.

It is reported from Uttar Pradesh to South West China 1200-2400 m. Rocks open slopes. Flowering most of the year round. It is also reported from South India and Sikkim Himalayas at 2,000 - 4000 ft..

MEDICINAL USE : Plant, emol. resolv., used in poultice in erysipelas and for tumours on breast. Juice of leaves is used as gargles in inflation of throat.

Index

(B)

(C)

(D)

(E)

(F)